Praise for *The Compassionate Equestrian*

"Dr. Allen Schoen is an innovative, compassionate, and thoughtful veterinarian whose book emphasizes the responsibilities that attend the human-equine relationship. *The Compassionate Equestrian* provides practical information derived from a lifetime of caring for sport and pleasure horses. Dr. Schoen has a keen eye for animal and human behavior, and his book has value for the novice and the experienced equestrian alike."

Michael Kotlikoff, VMD, PhD, Austin O. Hooey Dean, College of Veterinary Medicine, Cornell University

"Dr. Schoen is an innovator in combining conventional medicine with holistic therapies. In *The Compassionate Equestrian*, he charts the rise of a unique field of veterinary medicine whose foundation rests on a profound respect for all life, and specifically for horses. This is compassion in its purest form, and it's revolutionary. Meticulously researched, *The Compassionate Equestrian* enlightens any reader on the benefits of applying sympathy and empathy to the core of all equine training and care. Practicing compassion is the essence of the bond between rider and horse, and of course between any two people."

Arriana Boardman, Member, ASPCA Board

"The horse just happens to be the perfect animal to help us understand ourselves better. He's far more physically powerful than us, but also more perceptive in many ways. Horses can see right through us, and they reflect our deeper selves back to us in a way that is undeniable. This much-needed book asks us to not only try to become better observers of our horses, but to think about that which we notice in a new and deeper way. Most importantly, it asks us to watch ourselves as we are interacting with our horses. The authors give us a path to follow, challenging us to use the powerful tools of self-awareness or mindfulness, and meditation (QFI in the book) to change our own behaviors and become better stewards of the horse, and then extend that to our interaction with other beings. Learning these tools takes work, but with effort it can become an integral part of our behavior. I know this because I have been on a similar journey myself, and the rewards gained in all aspects of my life—from my relationship with horses and people, to my ability to function in my businesses—are profound."

Doug Thal, DVM, DABVP, Creator of The Horse Side Vet Guide

"Dr. Schoen has always led by example, and lives a lifetime of connected joy with the horses that he treats and their owners. We will continue to benefit from his kindness and guidance through his new book, *The Compassionate Equestrian*. From backyard ponies to trail horses to show jumpers, it's 'all about the horse.'"

Paula Kennedy, LVT, Dean's Advisory Board, Cornell College of Veterinary Medicine

"Dr. Allen Schoen and Susan Gordon provide a thoughtful, provocative reminder that horses feed off our personal health and well-being. The rush of our daily lives, work schedules, and pressures to succeed can weigh heavily on veterinarians, trainers, and riders, and can influence our approach to the horse. The horse can sense this tension or stress. The book reminds us that personal mental/emotional well-being is important to ourselves and those (both horses and people) we interact with daily."

Ryland B. Edwards, III, DVM, PhD, DACVS, Fairfield Equine Practice, Newtown, Connecticut

Also authored and/or edited by Dr. Allen Schoen:

Kindred Spirits: How the Remarkable Bond between Humans and Animals Can Change the Way We Live

Love, Miracles, and Animal Healing

Complementary and Alternative Medicine: Principles & Practice with Dr. Susan Wynn

Veterinary Acupuncture: Ancient Art to Modern Medicine

The COMPASSIONATE EQUESTRIAN

25 Principles to Live By When Caring for and Working with Horses

Allen Schoen, DVM, MS, PhD (Hon)
and Susan Gordon

Forewords by
Hilary Clayton, BVMS, PhD, Dipl. ACVSMR, MRCVS
and Mary Ann Simonds

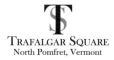

TRAFALGAR SQUARE
North Pomfret, Vermont

First published in 2015 by
Trafalgar Square Books
North Pomfret, Vermont 05053

Disclaimer of Liability

The authors and publisher shall have neither liability nor responsibility to any person or entity with respect to any loss or damage caused or alleged to be caused directly or indirectly by the information contained in this book. While the book is as accurate as the authors can make it, there may be errors, omissions, and inaccuracies.

This book is not intended to replace treatment by a veterinarian, licensed therapist, or other medical professional.

Library of Congress Cataloging-in-Publication Data

Schoen, Allen M
The compassionate equestrian : 25 principles to live by when caring for and working with horses / Dr. Allen Schoen, DVM, MS, Ph.D. (Hon), Susan Gordon.
     pages cm
 Includes bibliographical references.
  ISBN 978-1-57076-715-9
 1. Horsemanship--Moral and ethical aspects. 2. Horses--Training--Moral and ethical aspects. 3. Horses--Psychology. 4. Human-animal relationships. 5. Compassion. I. Gordon, Susan, 1960- II. Title.
  SF309.S37 2015
  636.1'0835--dc23
                    2015000721

Illustration of "Willie" by Susan Gordon
Front cover photo by Maurizio Migliorato (Copyright: www.123rf.com/profile_maury75)
Back cover photo by Doug Wahlsten
Book design by DOQ
Cover design by RM Didier
Typefaces: Caflisch Script Pro, Scala Sans Pro

Printed in United States of America

10 9 8 7 6 5 4 3 2 1

I would like to explain the meaning of compassion which is often misunderstood:

Genuine compassion is based not on our own projections and expectations, but rather on the rights of the other: irrespective of whether another person is a close friend or an enemy, as long as that person wishes for peace and happiness and wishes to overcome suffering, then on that basis we develop a genuine concern for his or her problems. This is genuine compassion.

Tenzin Gyatso, the 14th Dalai Lama

Contents

Foreword

by Dr. Hilary Clayton

I've been part of the equestrian world for over half a century, and during this time the world has changed in ways we could never have imagined. Technological innovations have allowed us to cram more and more "stuff" into our days, leaving less time to focus on the things that are truly important. We live our lives at warp speed with no time to think, no time to relax, and not nearly enough time to fully enjoy our lives and our horses.

In *The Compassionate Equestrian* readers are invited to slow down and smell the roses—or in this case, smell and feel and bond with horses. We are encouraged to step back from the modern-day equestrian world and allow our hearts and minds to experience the pure joy that comes from interacting with horses and other animals. Weaving together their perspectives—that of holistic veterinarian and that of a horse trainer—the authors take us on a journey that explores the multi-faceted relationship that can exist between a compassionate human being and a horse.

The 25 Principles of Compassionate Equitation that form the basis of this book (see p. 16) guide us toward a mutually rewarding human-equine partnership. The Principles emphasize treating every horse with the kindness and respect that we owe to all sentient beings (those able to feel pain/pleasure). After reading the Principles, I reflected upon how veterinary advances have affected our understanding of equine behavior in a way that has brought greater compassion to my own interpretation of the horse's responses during training. When I was young we were taught that some horses were "rogues"—they were innately evil, vicious, or dangerous. Many years later, after training several horses and looking at necropsies of many more, I realize that almost every horse that shows bad behavior does so due to pain, especially back or neck pain. Many horses do their best to accommodate our requests in spite of their own discomfort, but sometimes the pain becomes intolerable and the horse, physically unable to comply with the rider's demands, rebels against the request. On this basis, I believe that horses showing resistances should be given the benefit of the doubt and evaluated first for the presence of a physical problem, instead of forging ahead with increasing training demands.

This is a book for those who seek a mutually satisfying relationship with their horses. The Principles of Compassionate Equitation provide a road map for achieving such a relationship; we should read them carefully and often.

Hilary Clayton, BVMS, PhD, Dipl. ACVSMR, MRCVS

Professor and McPhail Dressage Chair Emerita
President, Sport Horse Science, LLC

Foreword

by Mary Ann Simonds

Two outstanding people have come together in *The Compassionate Equestrian*, bringing readers stories and science on how humans and horses should be interacting from both a horse trainer's and a veterinarian's perspective. Having lectured on equine behavior in veterinary schools and been involved professionally in the horse industry for over 40 years, I share many of the authors' experiences and sentiments.

It is an honor to support Susan Gordon and Dr. Allen Schoen in their efforts to raise awareness about our connection to all life, and in particular, about our special relationship with the horse. I share their love and passion for horses and for education, and I am delighted they took the time to write this guidebook of Principles *all* humans should embrace. The world would truly be a kinder and more compassionate world if everyone read their words.

Don't let the title fool you into thinking this is just about horses and riding, because it is not. While the target is to shift the paradigm of how we view, train, and treat horses, the message of the book extends far deeper. Readers should pause and contemplate the 25 Principles outlined on p. 16, listening to their hearts and minds, as the Principles will apply as easily to *all* forms of life as they do to horses. "Being reflective, treating others as we wish to be treated, helping to relieve pain and suffering" ...these are universal spiritual truths, as well as just a few of the 25 Principles for Compassionate Equitation.

If you love horses, you may feel you already subscribe to the Principles, and so this book will validate your beliefs. If you are of the many who have fallen into training "cults," then you may feel horrified upon the realization you have perhaps let go of your deep love and respect for horses. But don't worry, you are not alone. At almost every clinic I teach I ask people, "How many of you have done something a trainer told you to do, but you felt it was unfair to your horse?" Most everyone raises their hands and many start to cry. They admit they did what they thought they were supposed to do, not what their hearts were telling them to do.

The Compassionate Equestrian offers support to "do the right thing" for your horse. Listen to your inner voice and take action on behalf of what is good for horses. Learn to shift your view of the world from *human-centric* to *horse-centric*. This book challenges us to "slow down" and take a deep breath, examine our relationship with ourselves and with our horses. Using storytelling and personal experiences, combined with scientific research and a good dose of spirituality, these pages offer something for all readers. Whether you are a seasoned horseperson or someone who just loves horses and wants to share in the journey, the book promises discovery for all.

Mary Ann Simonds

Author, Lecturer, Founder and Director of the
Whole Horse and Equestrian Science Institute
www.maryannsimonds.com

Preface

Susan Gordon:

Dr. Allen Schoen and I have been involved in the equine industry collectively for more than 60 years. Once we began talking, we realized we were seeing the same issues in horses from our unique viewpoints as a veterinarian and a trainer. In the horse world there are so many personal belief systems and opinions that it becomes a challenge to bring the equine community together for the good of the "Global Herd" and welfare of all horses everywhere, including horses that become "homeless," unrideable, or neglected. It appears everyone is searching for ways to resolve the most pressing issues facing the equine industry, as well as finding answers to the sometimes-contentious atmosphere permeating equestrian activities due to the many different perspectives and opinions on training, breeding, and management. It is the purpose of this book to invite everyone involved with horses, all ages and levels, to embark on a program of self-discovery, reflection, and practice of compassion.

Compassion is defined by the desire to alleviate the suffering of another. Too often horses suffer due to a lack of mindfulness as to what may or may not cause them pain and distress. Many people are so busy in this modern "multi-tasking" world that they miss the very subtle clues horses use to convey their discomfort. With practice, the mind can be taught to become quiet, become more aware, and see all living beings—including ourselves—from a different view and with an open heart. Dr. Schoen and I have experienced the benefits of such practice in our own lives and are looking forward to sharing the stories of and reasons for our journey with our readers. We encourage each and every one of you to determine how you may develop an even deeper level of compassion in your life. Perhaps this will include changing how you go about your interactions with your horse and how you respond to the people you encounter at your barns, at events, and in other parts of your life.

After many years working with outstanding instructors and trainers up through the upper levels in the hunter-jumper, dressage, and eventing disciplines, and then a decade of teaching solo, I felt the need to retire and begin writing about the changes I have noticed in the equestrian industry. I did not ever aspire to be a "big name" trainer, just a very good one with a focus on creating happy, competitive horses and confident riders who could think for themselves. Over time I began to see more lame and distressed horses trained in a manner that did not develop the correct musculature for carrying a rider. I was frustrated and often heartbroken at seeing the same problems cropping up over and over again. There were too many sore, unhappy horses whose discomfort, behavioral problem, or outright lameness may have been the result of how they had been ridden and trained. The fundamental questions became, "How can these horses be helped, and how can people be made more aware of their effect on their horses, especially when mounted?" I often wished I had a veterinarian by my side to confirm what I was seeing and feeling in the horses, especially a veterinarian with the background and integrative approaches pioneered by Dr. Schoen.

Our book will take you through our 25 Principles of Compassionate Equitation (see p. 16). Each Principle describes a part of the process for developing compassion toward horses, yourself, and all sentient beings. We have used the term equitation in preference to horsemanship due to the prevalence of misunderstandings around the definitions of horsemanship. Today there is a style, perhaps more of a trendy "label," placed on horsemanship that is occasionally demonstrated without a foremost concern for safety, standards of welfare, and basic riding skills that translate appropriately from good ground work to the saddle. Equitation, we feel, refers to standards of riding that are best for the horse. This traditionally means a balanced seat, good hands, and correct application of the aids. Equitation is also inclusive of proper ground training, handling, and management.

There have been many new research studies released in recent years that support what long-time horsepeople already know about the emotions and intelligence displayed by horses. We have included links to these resources and studies in neuroscience, mind-body medicine, and equitation science. We acknowledge the practice of compassion alters biochemistry and neurophysiology, and look forward to future scientific research that will better identify the link between a compassionate brain and heart and the correlating physiological responses in our equine companions.

A long time ago I was just another little girl in love with horses, like many of you. I can think back on all the major events in my life and relate to them according to which horse I had at the time and where I was riding. I found my niche as a trainer and leapt at every opportunity to ride whenever, wherever, and whatever kind of horse that came my way. From ponies in the park, to rented trail horses, and finally the magnificent show jumpers I schooled for clients, they all contributed to aspects of my development as a human being, as well as a rider. Through a combination of being in the right place at the right time, determination, and a lot of studying, I developed a sensitivity and method for identifying the root issues in "problem horses." Eventually I acquired enough skill to be successful in helping them find their way to a more satisfying and comfortable life, and often a second career.

One horse of particular influence was an old Hanoverian gelding that showed up as I was on hiatus from riding as a professional. You will meet "Willie" throughout this book, and you will follow his stories as we support you on your journey as a Compassionate Equestrian. It was as though my meeting Willie was destiny. Our paths crossed at a time when I wasn't really looking for a horse, and nobody was looking for a horse like Willie. Through a challenging reschooling process, I developed a deeper level of empathy and compassion for older horses, especially those that had been pushed over the edge of tolerance and had nowhere else to go.

My goal is to be of service to horses and humanity. Along with Dr. Schoen's mutual vision, invaluable veterinary experience, insightful thoughts, and co-creativity, I wish to inspire people to become more mindful of how we interact with horses and other horse people. By becoming more aware of how our thoughts and actions affect others, we can open our hearts in recognition of how similar we all are, rather than how different we all are. Everyone has this ability for becoming more "open" and "aware."

In the process of writing this book I've had to let go of the last remnants of my old trainer's mindset that I felt necessary to keep things in control at the barn and in my personal life. I now see that in many ways over the years, I likely provoked some of the very circumstances I would love to see change between other horsepeople and in how they interact. The practice of compassion is not an easy path, but it is one that creates an extraordinary lightness, joy, and palpable difference in the areas of our lives that most need improvement.

Consider this is an invitation to join Dr. Allen Schoen and me on an interactive journey to becoming a Compassionate Equestrian. There are many options as to how you can read and peruse this book, explained further in "Before You Begin Your Journey" (see p. 6). Please consider becoming part of our ongoing dialogue and let us know how the step-by-step process of deepening and practicing compassion works for you, your horse, and all others who benefit from your loving-kindness.

Dr. Allen Schoen:

Welcome to *The Compassionate Equestrian* safari trip! You are cordially invited to join Susan Gordon and me on a *different* type of trail ride. This ride is both an "inner" and "outer" ride: it begins in our hearts and minds, meanders through our horses' hearts and minds, and joins all others involved in the care of our horses, including their grooms, riders, trainers, veterinarians, farriers, and kindred spirits. This ride offers a unique perspective on our interactions with horses and their care-givers at barns, shows, and backyards throughout the globe. *The Compassionate Equestrian* offers a traveler's guide to a new, yet ancient perspective on **how** we interact with another species—the horse.

The 25 Principles of Compassionate Equitation that Susan Gordon and I developed (see p. 16) are based on an integration of the latest in neuroscience and quantum physics, along with practical equine experience and knowledge. They are written with Susan Gordon's 30-plus years of practical, in-the-saddle and on-the-ground, holistically-oriented horse-training experience, as well as my 35 years of clinical equine veterinary practice, developing my own unique integrative approach that combines the best of conventional equine medicine along with veterinary acu-puncture, chiropractic, musculoskeletal alignment, and other natural approaches to equine health care. Over my decades in equine veterinary practice, I have seen a full spectrum of health care offered by those involved in tending to our horses. I have been impressed with the empathy and compassion of many, as well as been exposed to those who, I'm sad to say, have either lost their kindness and tolerance somewhere along the way or simply have not ever been aware of how they treat their horses.

Through all these experiences, my own professional and personal spiritual journey has led me on an exploration, searching for new approaches to becoming a better veterinarian and help animals that cannot be helped any other way. I began this quest as an idealistic animal lover who simply wanted to *help*. My grandfather often joked that the first words out of my mouth were "animal doctor." As far back as I can remember there was an "inner knowing" that I would be a veterinarian. As a young child I once wrote my mother a note saying that I was one day going to be a veterinarian who helped animals that could not be helped in any known way. As I struggled through the challenges of a tumultuous public school, I inherently believed that I would one day go to the prestigious Cornell University College of Veterinary Medicine. Prior to receiving my veterinary degree from Cornell, I also followed my passion for understanding animal behavior and received a master's degree in Applied Animal Behavior and Neurophysiology from the University of Illinois. This combination allowed me to view animals from a medical perspective, as well as a behavioral perspective.

Following in the footsteps of the world-renowned veterinarian and author, James Herriott, I began my practice in New England, treating "all creatures great and small" as he did in his famous books. In a few years of practice, I found myself looking beyond the limitations of conventional medicine and surgery, and searching for new approaches to help animals that did not respond to what my veterinary training could offer.

My search began with an introduction to the scientific basis and clinical applications of veterinary acupuncture through my first teachers of this discipline, Dr. Sheldon Altman and Dr. Marvin Cain, in addition to others. Once my doors of perception opened to a new reality that there was *more* to healing than medications and surgery, my personal journey seemed to suddenly move at light speed. I studied and began integrating into my practice the scientific basis and practical applications of acupuncture, traditional Chinese botanical (herbal) medicine, chiropractic care, osteopathy, holistic nutrition and nutraceuticals, homeopathy, laser therapy, and physical therapy, as well as other complementary modalities. Dr. Ihor Basko was the first veterinarian to introduce me to the practical use of Chinese herbal medicine in animals. I was asked to teach my unique integrative approach throughout the world and became a Clinical Assistant Professor both at Colorado State University College of Veterinary Medicine in Fort Collins, Colorado, and Cummings School of Veterinary Medicine at Tufts University in North Grafton, Massachusetts.

During this time I was asked to edit *Veterinary Acupuncture: Ancient Art to Modern Medicine* (Mosby, 1992 and 2001) and co-edit the first textbook on complementary medicine: *Complementary and Alternative Veterinary Medicine* (Mosby, 1998). In addition, I was asked to share my personal journey in my books *Love, Miracles and Animal Healing* (Simon & Schuster, 1995) and *Kindred Spirits: How the Remarkable Bond Between Humans and Animals Can Change the Way We Live* (Broadway/Random House, 2001). In *Kindred Spirits* I shared my vision as it was in 2001. I realized then we—all creatures—are kindred spirits. I am elated to see now that much of what I wrote about then has unfolded. I discussed my visions of how we could create and benefit from equine-facilitated therapy, concepts that were quoted in Linda Kohanov's bestselling *Tao of Equus* (New World Library, 2007). It brings me great joy to see how so many of us benefit from and are friend-and-family to animals.

The Compassionate Equestrian is taking that vision and sharing it again, 14 years later, from a continually evolving perspective, and now focusing on the ideas I've developed through my equine practice as I asked myself, "What is Ultimate Healing?" I have explored many perspectives. Some were dead ends, some were detours, and some right on. I appreciated the accuracy of the title of one of my favorite books *The Path to Enlightenment Is not a Highway* by one of my teachers, Baba Hari Das (Sri Ram Foundation). It has been a long and winding road to this point of awareness. In my search for Ultimate Healing, my insight *at this moment* is that *compassion* may indeed be one of the key foundations for *all* our interactions.

This is what led me to create this book with someone who has come to a similar awareness through her own circuitous route. I have realized that innately, within all of us, we are *truly compassionate*. In some, it is continuously and actively present, in others, it seems to have been obscured by their past or by less than positive experiences with other humans and animals.

Writing this book has actually stimulated in me a reevaluation of where I am compassionate and where I can continue deepening my compassion for all beings, including that which I allow for myself. It reminded me of my own innate compassion and how that has impacted my veterinary journey, my interactions with all animals under my care, my staff, colleagues, and clients, friends, and family.

The great news that has come to the foreground recently is that based on the latest in neuroscience and quantum physics, we can heal old destructive "imprints" (the "wounds" or "emotional wounds" that make it difficult for some to feel compassion for others and for themselves). There are ways to create new neural and emotional pathways that can assist us in being happier, healthier, kinder, more tolerant, and of greater benefit to all other beings as we share space, time, and earth.

The purpose of this book is to be a guiding support for deepening our relationship with horses, all animals, all people, and nature through transforming a heart and mind through compassion. I invite all of you to take this safari ride with us. It may show you various lions, tigers, and bears from your past and how they may have impacted your relationships with horses and people. It may float you down a river of thoughts and introspective insights as to how you can integrate compassion into your horse life—and the rest of your life. You may have to climb a few hills or mountains, and struggle to look at various aspects of yourself that you might realize you would like to improve. You may find yourself getting lost in the clouds, in a place with too much "mind traffic." You may find yourself taking deep dives into old "wounds" as you make the choice to now let go of them so you can imprint new, healthier neural pathways. You may feel like you are being drowned by endless waves of fear and concern, only to suddenly realize *you are the peaceful ocean below the restless waves*. You may fall off your proverbial horse, realize you *can* get back in the saddle, and be ready to ride on, blossoming even more.

I feel like *The Compassionate Equestrian* is just the beginning of a new dialogue among horsepeople about how we can expand our love of horses and to be of greater benefit to the world. I envision the book to be the beginning of a co-creative journey between you the reader, all other horse lovers, and Susan Gordon and me. I look forward to the book being the foundation for a compassionate animal movement that can thereby help create a more compassionate society based on loving-kindness for all.

Introduction

The teachings of all the great mystical paths of
the world make it clear that there is within us an
enormous reservoir of power, the power of wisdom and
compassion. If we learn how to use it—and this is the
goal of the search for enlightenment—it can transform
not only ourselves but the world around us. Has there
ever been a time when the clear use of this sacred power
was more essential or more urgent? Has there ever
been a time when it was more vital to understand the
nature of this pure power and how to channel it and
how to use it for the sake of the world?

Sogyal Rinpoche
Glimpse After Glimpse: Daily Reflections on Living and Dying
(HarperOne, 1995)

Susan Gordon:

We are human, they are not. They don't look like us, and they do not speak our language. We can train ourselves to do all kinds of brilliant things during our time on this planet, creating a multitude of materials and objects of desire that fulfill every need we have or think we have. Humans make and exchange goods and property, and carry on making everything bigger, better, louder, faster. We whip ourselves into frenzies or fall into deep depressions, and indulge in many other states of being in between. This is how we keep the "wheel of existence" turning again and again.

Horses—and other animals—must look at us with great curiosity and wonder what we are up to much of the time. They happily allow us to house, feed, and care for them, and seem compliant with whatever environment in which we choose to keep them. Some become geniuses at things like untying knots or opening stall doors. They display feelings and emotions. Some exhibit a sense of humor. They have been observed mourning at the loss or death of a friend. Even though they do not look and think like us, there are enough similarities in our physiology and life processes that we must look at them with as much curiosity as they must feel when studying us.

They may not understand our words but they are quick to react to the moods we are in, the things we strap on them and prod them with, and the little boxes we coax them into for travel or living quarters. They are not human, but they certainly have served humanity in many ways for a long time. Their history deserves considerable respect.

Many of us say we love horses. Are they capable of loving us back? If we offer them compassion, can we expect compassion from them in return? In describing a great equine athlete we say, the horse "has heart." The heart is described as being the *center of compassion*—the loving point from which we develop empathy and the desire to relieve the suffering of others.

In other words, just how "human" are these non-humans?

When we observe a being that does not use elaborate spoken languages like humans do to communicate with others, it appears they still understand the concepts of friendship, fear, happiness, and sadness, among other emotions. Remarkably, they seem to understand *our* emotions in relationship to their own. They even exhibit signs of reading deeper into the human psyche than we are willing to admit. This seems especially true when we are under considerable stress. They have access to their *primordial psyches*—the old part of the brain that connects to ancestral knowledge—without the blocks that humans tend to place around their own. We create many reasons for not letting our true, loving selves radiate from our center. What are we afraid of that horses are not?

That which we lay before you in *The Compassionate Equestrian* is not designed to be an easy path to follow. The Principles of Compassionate Equitation which we introduce to you on p. 16 are a deep, personal set of commitments that may enhance your experience as a horseperson and as a person in general. Becoming a Compassionate Equestrian will allow you to take the peace, calm, and heart-centered techniques from this book and put them into practice with yourself, your horses, and everyone else you encounter. May you find this to be an enlightening experience, a validation of all the wonderful love and care you provide for your horses already, and of tremendous benefit to your heart and soul, and all other beings, in the days ahead.

Dr. Allen Schoen:

We are all interconnected via an integral web of interactions from everyone's mind and heart. You know, they joke and say there are actually over seven billion human "*youniverses*" on the planet—and each person is their own *youniverse* unto him- or herself. Each horseperson is seeing that same horse barn through a unique filter based on his or her own life's experiences. Every person in the barn brings perceptions and responses to it, and the horses bear the brunt of the good, the bad, and the ugly. Horses, too, bring their own experiences to the barn. Whatever number of horses there are on the planet, that's how many horse universes ("*equiverses?*") there are.

One of the things I have found with all animals that interact with people (as compared to those that *do not* have to interact with people) is that they have actually evolved to a different level of awareness in consciousness. I chuckle and say, "When a horse is in a herd, he is just 'horsing around.' He's just being a horse." When the horse interacts with people though, he becomes a great student of human behavior. He watches us from his predator-prey point of view—he feels like prey and interacts from a fearful and cautious mind. From there, he can evolve into the most compassionate, loving being or the most dangerous, frightening, 1,200 pounds on the earth. He can either love you or hurt you. Perhaps both companion animals and their people subconsciously evolve to a new level of interconnectedness, becoming more like each other, based on the foundations of my *Transpecies Field Theory*, which I introduce on p. 7.

What it boils down to is that it's not just our minds, but our hearts *and* minds, and the heart and mind of everyone in the barn or at the show, from the grooms, trainers, and riders to the horses, dogs, cats, and birds. To me, *Ultimate Healing* is bringing this awareness to all animal and horse lovers everywhere. There is an opportunity that has arisen as neuroscience has advanced and continues to develop, documenting ancient spiritual traditions that claim the benefits of loving-kindness and compassion. As these two areas converge into a new field, sometimes called *neurospirituality* or the *neuroscience of behavior*, we can better understand the positive or negative impact we have on the animals with which we interact.

The topic of *neurohealth* was discussed at the 2015 World Economic Forum in Davos, Switzerland. Dr. Philip Campbell, the editor-in-chief of *Nature* magazine, stated that, "If the twentieth century was the century that successfully tackled *infectious* disease, the twenty-first century will hopefully be known as the century that tackles *chronic* disease. And no chronic disease (heart, cancer, diabetes combined) takes as big a toll on society than brain disease and mental illness" (Tapscott, D., "Davos 2015 Wrap-up: Get Ready for Breakthroughs about the Brain," The Huffington Post Blog, February 2, 2015). It was also said that neuroscientists needed to look at *neural circuitry* as well as *neurochemistry*. This is what we are discussing in this book when we mention *neural networks* and *mindstreams* (see p. 49, for example). As I read Tapscott's wrap-up, I realized how relevant this book is in our current world situation. At Davos, the world's leaders, cutting edge thinkers, and wealthiest business people all converged and voiced their concerns about the state of the world, climate, violence, and the unpredictability of the current situations. I was impressed that amidst all of that, they acknowledged that the *neurohealth* of the population is an essential component of remedying these situations.

I feel that the essential foundations for the human-animal bond, evolutionary biologist E.O. Wilson's concept of Biophilia (an innate desire to be with all life, as outlined in his book *Biophilia,* Harvard University Press, 1986), and neurohealth are intimately interrelated. Understanding the Transpecies Field Theory (p. 7), therefore, is one of the keys to helping all of us out of the stress and depression that permeates this world. This is why we see many more households include pets as we become more urbanized. This is why so many people who have the ability to share their lives with horses feel that connection in their lives is *imperative*. Sharing our lives with animals in a compassionate way can improve neurohealth and make the world a better place.

This book offers two separate, yet converging views of how we can better treat our horses. Susan and I have chosen to collaborate on this book because we recognize that there are significant benefits to sharing our different perspectives and also appreciate the commonality of our insights. I am not a horse trainer and do not have the awareness or expertise in horse training that Susan has. There are aspects of certain training methods and approaches of which I am not fully cognizant. Susan shares her knowledge of these by describing her personal journey with her horse, Willie, in her own words. Alongside and around Susan's contributions, I bring perspectives based on over 35 years of pioneering and integrating innovative veterinary approaches to equine health care, as well as my passion for animal behavior, neuroscience, and consciousness studies. Together, I feel that our two unique, yet complementary perspectives can offer different benefits to each reader, depending on the kinds of insights you would like to take from this book. I often add this invitation after all that I share in speaking and in writing: "if you agree with my views, resonate with them, and if my perspectives are of benefit, integrate them in your life in whatever way feels right. If you do not agree with anything, just let it go." No one has all the answers. We are all on our own unique journey in the midst of the collective journey called life on earth.

I appreciate the value and benefits of conventional practice, yet, have also undertaken a personal, professional, and spiritual journey, realizing there are many additional options for healing animals and people. That healing is a full circle: The more we become aware of how we can benefit through developing loving-kindness and compassion in ourselves, the more we can help the animals in our lives, and subsequently, the animals become all they can be, and they will then support us in becoming all we can be. Full circle.

The more we understand neuroscience and comparative neurobiology, the more we realize we share similar brain patterns and brain programs with animals. We share more similarities than differences. In fact, one of the paramount paradigm shifts I would like to see is to change from having to prove *what is the same* to having to prove *what is different* in regards to the way our thoughts and moods function as compared to those of animals. Recognizing "sameness" as the foundation, rather than always separating "self" from "other" by looking at differences is a concept I call the "Commonality of Biophilia." This is an immensely powerful change of purview that has innumerable ramifications in how we see the world and how we treat all animals.

I would like this book to become a catalyst for recreating compassion and loving-kindness as the foundation for all our interactions with every living being we encounter... two-legged, four-legged, and winged! Thank you for choosing to become a Compassionate Equestrian.

Before You Begin Your Journey

Before you begin your journey as a Compassionate Equestrian, we would like to explain some basic understandings that comprise the foundation of Compassionate Equitation.

Building the Foundation

What follows is the Mission Statement of *The Compassionate Equestrian*:

> Compassion becomes the foundation for all decisions that an equestrian makes with regard to his or her horse and all people involved in the equine community, as well as the global community. Through choosing compassion as the common ground for all decisions, equestrians can together become a movement for creating a kinder, happier, healthier, more compassionate world.

With this Mission in mind, there are three components that form the triangular foundation of The Compassionate Equestrian Approach. These include the following (and see below for further exploration of each component):

1   The *Charter for Compassion*—understanding and joining this movement to embrace the core value of compassion.

2   The *Transpecies Field Theory* (TSFT)—understanding the interconnectedness of all beings through the interdisciplinary perspective of the Transpecies Field Theory.

3   Short periods of *Quiet Focused Intention* (QFI), including routinely asking, "What is the most compassionate choice for my horse, and for all beings, in this situation?"

The Charter for Compassion

The Charter for Compassion (charterforcompassion.org) is a vision and a document developed by prominent religious historian and bestselling author Karen Armstrong, which invites all people, communities, organizations, and religions of the world to embrace the core value of compassion. The Charter has been translated into 30 languages and has inspired a global movement. Armstrong won the TED Prize (awarded to an individual with a creative, bold vision to spark global change) in 2008 when she proposed the concept of the Charter and requested assistance in creating and spreading its message. The Compassionate Equestrian is doing its part in inviting the equine community to embrace Armstrong's Charter of Compassion. (Our page may be found on the charter's website here: charterforcompassion.org/node/6612.)

The Transpecies Field Theory (TSFT)

The second component of the foundation of the Compassionate Equestrian is the Transpecies Field Theory (TSFT), which proposes that there is a dynamic, behavioral, energetic field that affects all of us who interact together. This continuously interactive, energetic, behavioral field impacts all living beings. When every being in the field is behaving based on various "past programming" (their habitual behavior patterns), they will have certain effects on everyone involved. Dr. Schoen's TSFT theory is based on the combination of various other interdisciplinary theories in the fields of physics, new biology, psychology, and sociology, to name a few. It is a *transdisciplinary exploration* of the interconnectedness of all that is.

Once we recognize that the Transpecies Field exists, the next exciting step is realizing we can actually have a conscious impact on it by focusing our intention on a particular positive thought or emotion, such as compassion. This is the basis for the Compassionate Field Theory (CFT—see p. 10), as well as for the entire Compassionate Equestrian Approach. Wow! You can actually improve the all-around "energy" in your horse barn! You can have a positive impact on everyone, everywhere you interact with horses, other animals, and people. (Dr. Schoen discusses his theory in more depth beginning on p. 48.)

Quiet Focused Intention (QFI)

The third component of the triangular foundation for the Compassionate Equestrian is a commitment to take short periods of Quiet Focused Intention on compassion for all beings prior to interacting with your horse. This component is based on the latest neuroscience research unfolding from the University of Wisconsin Neuroscience Lab and the Center for Investigating Healthy Minds at the Waisman Center, University of Wisconsin-Madison. There, neuroscientist Dr. Richard Davidson and his associates have found that simply focusing intention and meditation on compassion for 10 minutes a day for two weeks can *actually change* our fMRIs (functional Magnetic Resonance Imaging, measuring brain activity), our brain function, and help us become happier people. After reviewing the research from these institutions, Dr. Schoen had an epiphany and thought, "What if we extrapolated these concepts to the equine community? What if every equestrian committed to taking 10 minutes to quietly focus on compassion for all beings *prior* to walking into the horse barn or driving to an event or riding into an arena?"

Our sense is that simply taking 10 minutes of QFI, feeling compassion for your horse and for all beings you interact with, could have a profound impact on you, everyone you see in the barn, and everyone you interact with in the horse community. Essentially, we are proposing that one possible solution to the twenty-first century challenge of *neurohealth*—as discussed at the 2015 World Economic Forum (see the Introduction, p. 4)—may be the integration of 10 minutes of intention on compassion whenever we are connecting with animals.

Integrating these three components into your equine life offers you the potential of becoming part of a more expansive paradigm shift, where conscious, intentional choices based on compassion can help all beings live a healthier and happier life.

The 25 Principles of Compassionate Equitation

Upon our foundation, we then can begin to build a *Compassionate Self*. This book begins by listing the 25 Principles of Compassionate Equitation, which are followed by 25 chapters that explore each principle and why it is important to the horse industry. The 25 Principles of Compassionate Equitation describe a process of learning, awareness, and practice on your path to becoming a Compassionate Equestrian. In regards to riding and horsemanship skills, developing good *equitation* is necessary to become a good *equestrian*. It is the means to an end, so to speak. So it is with The 25 Principles. They are a set of progressive teachings that help you become more aware of your compassionate nature and how it may be organized and applied to your relationship with your horse—and beyond.

Compassionate Equitation is the guiding set of principles for this teaching program. A *Compassionate Equestrian* defines the horseperson who emerges as a result of studying and applying the Principles.

The Layout of the Book

The Compassionate Equestrian is a progressive journey: You begin by understanding compassion and how it relates to the equine world. Then you examine how to apply compassion to your equestrian lifestyle. Finally, you'll consider a mind-body approach to compassionate action, and how to take it *beyond* horses. Compassion takes practice. It is an acquired skill, just like learning how to groom, tack up, post a trot, apply the correct aids to canter, maintain position without stirrups, and any number of other lessons accrued along the way to becoming a good rider. When riders become highly accomplished, they often apply their expertise to teaching others. This is one goal of this book: to nurture an understanding and practice of compassion that may be extended to include what we term the "Global Herd"—our worldwide family of horses and fellow equestrians. As we have already expressed, we feel Compassionate Equestrians will also have a positive influence on their non-horse-related friends, family, and businesses so as to become community and global leaders in creating a compassionate world for all. *Every one of you reading this book* has the opportunity to help make this world a better place. Our horses can help facilitate that journey.

KEYWORDS AND CONCEPTS

There a number of keywords and concepts used throughout this book that may be new to some of you. Some are terms that have been defined by and used in various fields of study, such as neuroscience. Others are words or phrases that we use creatively with some "poetic license" to describe certain concepts. Some of these terms and our use of them are briefly described here. They appear in alphabetical order, not in order of appearance or importance.

Breath: A slow deep inhalation with a brief stationary moment in our abdomen followed by a slow relaxed exhalation.

Calm: A sense of inner peace and quiet in our heart and mind.

Center/ing: A calm place in our hearts and minds. To "center" yourself, locate your "physical center of gravity" (usually visualized about 2 inches below your navel) and focus your mind on this part of your body to feel stable, calm, and in control. When our minds are cluttered, racing, or stressed, we can redirect the energy to our center, breathe, and find a place of calm.

Collective Intentionality: According to the Stanford Encyclopedia of Philosophy, this is the power of minds to be jointly directed at objects, matters of fact, states of affairs, goals, or values. Collective intentionality comes in a variety of modes, including shared intention, joint attention, shared belief, collective acceptance, and collective emotion (Schweikard, David P. and Schmid, Hans Bernhard, Summer 2013 Edition, Edward N. Zalta ed., http://plato.stanford.edu/archives/sum2013/entries/collective-intentionality/).

Compassionate Field Theory (CFT): A dynamic, interactive, energetic field exists between humans and animals and can be based on Quiet Focused Intention (QFI) of compassion for all beings, thus positively impacting the behavior of all involved in the Field, creating a collective intentionality of compassion.

Conscious Awareness: The "observation of one's own thoughts," which then provides the clarity and insights into our feelings and behaviors, some of which may stem from beliefs and parental imprinting.

Disruption: Disruptive thoughts; thoughts that interfere with our equanimity.

Ego: The sense of self, especially as contrasted with another self or the world.

Equitation Science: As defined by *International Society for Equitation Science* (www.equitationscience.com): Equitation science promotes an objective, evidence-based understanding of the welfare of horses during training and competition by applying valid, quantitative scientific methods that can identify what training techniques are ineffective or may result in equine suffering.

Imprints/Imprinting: Programmed responses in our brain based on previous experiences—worry, anxiety, fear, or compassion, for example.

Intention: A mental state that represents a commitment to carrying out an action or actions in the future and involves mental activities such as planning and forethought. A determination to act in a certain way.

Interpersonal Neurobiology: The use of this term in this book involves a new field of study investigating the interaction of neurobiologic activity between individuals, both humans and animals. Dr. Dan Siegel, executive director of the Mindsight Institute and author of *The Developing Mind* (Guilford Press, 2012) defines this field as one that seeks the similar patterns that arise from separate approaches to knowledge. It invites all branches of science and "other ways of knowing" to come together and find the common principles from within their often disparate approaches to understanding human experience (www.drdansiegel.com).

Manual Therapies: Therapies administered by hand from a person to a horse including chiropractic, osteopathy, and various methods of massage therapy, among others.

Metta: A strong wish for the welfare and happiness of others.

Mind Traffic: The busy thoughts that travel through our mind endlessly.

Mindstream: In Buddhist philosophy, this is the moment-to-moment continuum of awareness that provides a continuity from one life to another. In this book it is

Continued ➜

used more simply to just define the continuous moment-to-moment continuum of thoughts in this lifetime.

Mindfulness: A gentle, intentional, non-judgemental focus of attention on your emotions, thoughts, and sensations in the present moment.

Neural Imprints: Neural pathways imprinted (see above) into our brain based on repeated thoughts, emotions, and actions.

Neural Net: In neuroscience, a biological *neural network* (also sometimes called a *neural pathway*) is a series of interconnected neurons whose activation defines a recognizable linear pathway. In this book the term *neural net* is used more simplistically as a series of neural pathways that are programmed based on previous behaviors and experiences.

Neuroscience: The scientific study of the nervous system. Traditionally, neuroscience has been seen as a branch of biology. However, it is currently an interdisciplinary science that collaborates with other fields such as chemistry, computer science, engineering, linguistics, mathematics, medicine (including neurology), genetics, philosophy, physics, and psychology.

Neural Wiring: The interconnectedness of our neurons to create various pathways in our brains that manifest as particular repeated behavior patterns.

Neurohealth: The new awareness of the importance of the health of the brain and nervous system for overall well-being.

Neurospirituality: A new field of study investigating a neuroscience basis for spiritual experiences.

Patterning: Programming recurring thought processes in our brains.

Quantum Field: Merriam-Webster states that the interaction of two separate physical systems (as particles) is attributed to a "field" that extends from one to the other and is manifested in a particle exchange between the two systems. Everywhere atoms and molecules are constantly exchanging information—that is, there is a field of interconnectivity at a subatomic level.

Quantum Physics: A simplistic definition from Wikipedia states that quantum mechanics is the science of the very small. It is the body of scientific principles that explains the behavior of matter and its interactions with energy on the scale of atoms and subatomic particles. In this book, the term *quantum physics* is used to refer to the behavioral interactions between matter and energy.

Quiet: A deep sense of inner calm and equanimity.

Release: Letting go of all tension from body and mind.

Slow Down: Quieting your thoughts and your mind; creating a sense of inner and outer calmness and peace; easing the frenetic pace of modern-day life.

Transpecies Field Theory (TSFT): This hypothesis proposes that there is a dynamic, behavioral, energetic field that affects all of us who interact together. When every being in the field behaves based on all their various past programming (their habitual behavior patterns) they will have certain effects on all others involved. This theory is based on the combination of various interdisciplinary theories from the fields of physics, new biology, psychology, sociology, and interpersonal neurobiology, among others. It is an interdisciplinary exploration and explanation of the interconnectedness of all beings (see p. 7 for more on TSFT).

Transpersonal Psychology: Transpersonal psychology is a sub-field or "school" of psychology that integrates the spiritual and transcendent aspects of the human experience with the framework of modern psychology. It is also possible to define it as a "spiritual psychology." The transpersonal is defined as "experiences in which the sense of identity or self extends beyond (*trans*) the individual or personal to encompass wider aspects of humankind, life, psyche, or cosmos." It refers to development beyond conventional personal or individual levels.

Where It All Came From

The chapters ahead include the many resources we considered while forming our own ideas and intentions regarding horses, the equine community, and our place in the world. We share them in detail in the hopes that some of these resources will provide others the evidence they need to make a change, as well. We do not provide all the answers as much as we ask the questions and list the reasons we would all benefit from *seeking* those answers. This process is something we both have experienced in our own lives. This book, therefore, isn't so much a directive as, in fact, a journey in which "wandering and pondering" are part of the solution. The change needs to come from *within each of us*. We see this book as the catalyst, but we cannot tell any one person to change as much as each of us must find the reasons to on our own.

This book is for all levels of equestrians. There are tidbits of training and veterinary information that might be "old hat" to you, and you might just as often discover entirely new concepts. All are meant to be ideas that you can eventually explore further, should you desire, as there is a bevy of websites, online seminars, and great books already available on many of the topics we discuss. We provide extensive referencing throughout the text, should you choose to educate yourself further in areas that we feel are beyond the scope of this book.

Two Views, Two Voices

As we explain in our Introduction (see p. 5), this book offers two different perspectives on the possible next steps for the equine world to consider, as well as demonstrating their synergistic convergence. With that said, as you saw in the Introduction, throughout the pages ahead you will notice two different "voices" in the writing, one from "Susan Gordon, Horse Trainer," and the other from "Dr. Allen Schoen, Integrative Veterinarian." We chose to present the book in this way in order to accurately reflect the distinct personalities of each author.

The chapters begin with "the trainer's viewpoint" followed by that of "the veterinarian." In some chapters we have combined the dialogue in places as we have shared experience or do exactly the same thing in a given circumstance. Some ideas introduced in early chapters may be expanded on in later ones. These are marked with references forward. If you feel some information is repeated, know that this is intentional as there are important messages contained within.

Repeated information may be related to subject matter in more than one context, or expanded on later, well beyond its introduction in an earlier segment.

Why?

The Compassionate Equestrian is meant for horse people who love being with their horses but may have noticed—as we have—certain issues when dealing with other horsepeople; with situations at barns and horse shows; or with business related to the equine industry. For example, maybe you are frustrated by the number of horses you see in your riding group that are not staying sound. Maybe you work with a rescue organization that's overwhelmed by requests to take on even more "unwanted" horses. Perhaps you struggle to maintain peace amongst boarders at your barn. This book is a close-up look at what may be at the root of some of these issues, along with some insights to help resolve them via a path of personal awareness. We intend this to be a mutually beneficial journey: as we are sharing our experiences as a trainer and veterinarian, we are also looking to you, our readers, to assist in spreading the 25 Principles of Compassionate Equitation to your equestrian discipline, favorite breed, or particular field of interest within the industry.

For many of you, some of the concepts in this book will simply confirm how kind, tolerant, and forgiving you are at present. You may want to use this book as a vehicle for a more focused and organized approach to being a Compassionate Equestrian. By prioritizing the 25 Principles of Compassionate Equitation in everything you do with your horse, you might find a shift in your "mindstream" (see p. 11) and worldview. This book is for *all* of us to work together in harmony to help develop a more humane, considerate, and sympathetic horse world—and society at large. We can create a *collective intentionality* of compassion within each horse barn, event, or anywhere we are together with others (see p. 10).

Read and study with an open heart and mind and decide what *you* would like to add to the conversation. As you are reading, jot down your own ideas for expanding the concepts presented in this book. We have already noticed that just by making others more aware of the need for compassion, we are beginning to change the journey, and we thank you in advance for co-creating the future world of Compassionate Equestrians with us.

The 25 Principles of Compassionate Equitation

1

We recognize the sentience (ability to feel pain/pleasure) of horses, as well as all beings. We acknowledge that the horse is a willing, thinking, living being with most of the identical emotion-creating molecules found in human beings. We recognize that the horse has bones, muscle, nerves, and organs, as does a human, and that these structures are just as susceptible to injury, damage, and disease as those of people.

2

We treat animals as we wish to be treated ourselves, with respect and compassion, to the best of our abilities.

3

Compassionate Equitation is based on an underlying foundation of respect, compassion, and loving-kindness.

4

Compassionate Equitation is based on the latest in neuroscience and equitation science, and the benefits of a compassionate brain and heart for all interactions.

5

We make time for self-reflection and reevaluation of various areas of horsemanship. Do our choices meet basic humane standards of respect for all life?

6

We take a few moments of silence to become heart-centered, allowing for the release of any destructive emotions, prior to working with any horse in any way. This allows both the individual and the horse to interact from a place of inner calm, peace, awareness, and mindfulness, thereby allowing for the most positive, constructive outcome from all interactions between humans and horses.

7

Compassionate Equitation accelerates the evolution of joy, respect, and gratitude between humans and horses, and allows for a more expansive, conscious interaction between humans and equine companions.

8

We acknowledge that a peaceful, quiet environment is of benefit. Research suggests that classical and country music are conducive to a peaceful environment for animals.

9

We agree to act with patience, kindness, and consistency, avoiding any intentionally harmful, aggressive, violent behaviors, including actions out of anger or egoic self-interest.

10

We allow for the creation of new, more respectful, humane, and considerate approaches to horsemanship and all training methods.

11

We acknowledge that common sense is a component of compassion. We agree that our hearts be open to the bigger picture of how the horse industry has evolved, and how it will evolve into the future, as kindness, tolerance, and forgiveness are restored to all aspects of the equestrian world.

12

We are committed to educating everyone involved with horses in the understanding of how pain and discomfort are expressed by a horse.

13

We recognize that horses may exhibit subtle behavioral signs of discomfort and pain. These signs could indicate the early onset of potential lameness and lead to chronic, serious problems. We agree to increase our mindfulness, awareness, and understanding of such subtle signals conveyed to us by the horse's silent language.

14

We acknowledge that all beings deserve to live in a holistic, balanced, healthy environment. This is imperative to preventive health care, both physically and mentally, of humans and horses, and includes the creation of barns and environments free of toxic compounds.

15

We embrace a holistic, integrative approach to equine health care, merging the best of conventional and complementary approaches that help horses heal, and relieve their pain and suffering as quickly as possible.

16

We offer the most natural food sources and supplements available.

17

We acknowledge neurobiology and quantum physics as a foundation for interspecies communication, the Transpecies Field Theory, and the Compassionate Field Theory.

18

We acknowledge that compassion is the common foundation shared in the world of equestrian activities. Grounded in individual responsibility, respect, loving-kindness, and a true willingness to alleviate another's suffering; compassion is the unifying force that transcends all labels, beyond breeds, discipline, health care, and medications. The essential question is, "What is the most compassionate choice for our horses and all involved, in this moment?"

19

We embrace compassionate rehabilitative programs. A cradle-to-cradle equestrian model ensures a humane life from birth to death for all horses.

20

We choose to restore compassion to the center of all equine-based facilities, horse training techniques, and equestrian sports, and to clearly understand and acknowledge the difference between what constitutes kindness to horses and what does not. We cultivate responsible compassion toward all horses, including those deemed feral, unwanted, "homeless," aged, or unrideable for any reason.

21

We allow for an authentic bond based on compassionate care to form between horses and humans, leading us into a new paradigm of training and understanding that brings our worldwide community of horse lovers together with peace, awakened compassion, and loving-kindness for the good of all.

22

We recognize the importance of applying a life-cycle assessment and sustainability model to the equestrian industry.

23

We acknowledge the importance of healing "old wounds" as an integral foundation of heart-centered horsemanship. Healing old wounds allows us to be the absolute best human beings we can be. Removing these harmful "filters" allows us to see the world with clearer vision, unobscured by destructive patterns and emotions.

24

We acknowledge that by the acceptance and practice of the 25 Principles of Compassionate Equitation, we are on the path to becoming compassionate global citizens and extending the message of *The Compassionate Equestrian* to the entire world.

25

We acknowledge that forgiveness is a key to healing emotional and psychological wounds, and pain and suffering within ourselves. We recognize the importance of forgiving ourselves, as well as forgiving all others—horses and humans—as a foundation for improving health and happiness. We commit to working on forgiveness within ourselves for the benefit of all beings.

CHAPTER ONE

The Sentience of All Beings

We recognize the sentience (ability to feel pain/pleasure) of horses, as well as all beings. We confirm that the horse is a willing, thinking, living being with most of the identical emotion-creating molecules found in human beings. We recognize that the horse has bones, muscle, nerves, and organs, as does a human, and that these structures are just as susceptible to injury, damage, and disease as those of people.

Susan Gordon:

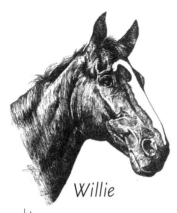

Willie

When I first saw Willie all I could think was, "Yep, that's a Warmblood all right...What the heck happened to him?"

He was 18 years old and very thin. He had been sold to an unknowledgeable owner as part of a package deal for trail horses and was kept on a small, dry desert lot north of Phoenix, Arizona. His deep chestnut coat was bleached by the sun and roughened due to a lack of grooming. On top of his poor condition, he seemed angry. Very angry.

The owner tried to make an excuse for his emaciated frame and warned me that the horse would "cow kick." A rare and obstinate form of definitive hostility...a hoof carefully aimed sideways and punched with authority at the object of the animal's disdain. As if on cue, Willie took aim at the hapless fellow and demonstrated his prowess with a well-executed stab of his right hind leg. Fortunately, the guy knew this horse's range and was smartly out of reach.

I hesitated with the long-bristled body brush for a moment, amazed at the horse's obvious dislike for his current owner. Many years of experience with all kinds of horses, including a stallion, had given me a "sixth sense" of sorts—an ability to quickly read and react to equine body language, as horses do with each other. I knew this was an animal that demanded respect and became difficult when he did not get it.

"What's his name?" I asked.

"Willie," said the slight blonde fellow. He looked like he belonged on a California beach brandishing a surfboard instead of the dirty bridle he held out in his hand, still keeping a distance from the big chestnut. "His papers say 'Wilhelm,' though. You can have a look at them."

"Papers, huh?" I thought. Willie did not sport a brand on his left hindquarter as is typical of most Warmbloods (a symbol of their breed registry). For horses born in Europe the brand denotes the region from which they come. I was beginning to wonder what I was doing even looking at this horse. If it hadn't been for the pretty little barnyard and three empty stalls I had back home, it would not be happening.

I finished grooming and threw my trusty old Crosby jumping saddle on Willie's back. This saddle and I had been through a lot in the 15 years I had owned it. The rich, smooth leather was soft and broken in where my leg could settle into a horse's sides like a hand into a perfectly fitting glove. It had helped me stay on horses' backs in many a difficult situation.

Willie seemed to have a permanent sneer etched on his face, which did not do much to add to his already pathetic look. As we headed to the nondescript riding area, surfer guy mentioned, "He likes to run when you point him toward home." At that point I knew we had a problem.

I climbed aboard and began to direct Willie around a slightly worn track in the hardened footing. I was concerned about the lack of fencing should he decide to bolt and head for the road. I gave the grumpy gelding a pat on the neck and attempted to prod him into a more active walk. His lack of feed undoubtedly contributed to his lack of wanting to go forward, and I found myself uncharacteristically pounding his sides, concerned about bruising his ribs if I kicked too hard. He was otherwise unresponsive to my leg.

Somehow I was able to convince him to try a lazy trot, and it told me that somewhere, way back in that unhappy subconscious of his, there was a well-trained horse that had just ended up in a desperate situation. Now I was even more curious. I asked for canter, and he tried very hard to comply, but he had absolutely no energy. His ears relaxed forward a bit, perhaps realizing I was not going to do anything nasty to him. I had given him a free rein as an invitation to move out as much as he wished. I tired as quickly as Willie did since my full-time riding days were in the past, and my legs did not have the strength to continue pushing this giant of a horse around the dusty desert track. Besides, it was one of Phoenix's famous oven-with-a-hair-dryer days—we both risked overheating after about 15 minutes of exertion.

When I'd seen the newspaper advertisement for a Hanoverian for $2,000, I thought a zero was missing. Even in their teens, Warmbloods tended to go in the five-figure range. As I hopped off Willie however, I had to think the asking price was too much and it wasn't worth the risk to bring him home. He had other issues: huge windpuffs (fluid-filled sacs, bulging around his hind fetlocks); two very unusual lumps of hard tissue in his throatlatch area at the base of his jaw; and one hock appeared to have thoroughpin, while the other hock was not clean either. But my curiosity stayed with me and I decided to humor the owner and have a look at the papers once Willie was untacked and returned to the yard. What I saw deepened the mystery of his current state even further.

He'd been imported from Belgium as a five-year-old and was sold to an equestrian center in Malibu, California. He was originally named Vasall, and the name had been changed to Wilhelm after he arrived in the United States. Soon after his arrival in California, Willie was brought to Arizona via an eventing trainer I was familiar with.

"Hmmm," I thought. "Those little indicators of good training were not false."

This horse was trained in Europe, and usually that meant a very good start in the classical system, which produces a horse that is straight, obedient, trainable, sound, and athletic, providing they continue to be ridden correctly. Along with Willie's import papers from Belgium, there was an old bill of sale, his AHSA identification (now known as the United States Equestrian Federation), and his United States Dressage Federation lifetime registry number. It looked like he'd had a full show career in several disciplines. Then there was his state-required hauling card. He'd changed hands so quickly in the past year of his life that the card had not been transferred to any of the previous three owners. Nobody had bothered to fill out the paperwork and send it in to the Department of Agriculture.

I told surfer guy I would think about taking him and went home to make a decision.

I wanted to see a horse in my empty barn, and the big German horses had long been my favorite breed, but after so many years in the horse business, I knew what I was getting into with such a difficult rehab project. I had to think it wasn't a smart choice for me.

After a day or two the phone rang, and it was the fellow who was selling Willie.

"You have to buy him," he said. "I'll even drop the price. Nobody else wants him, and he'll be going to the killers if nobody takes him."

Those were the magic words. Now this was a rescue case, even though I still had to pay $1,200 for the privilege. I promptly set about arranging payment details and a delivery date. My backyard was about to have a new occupant.

At the beginning of many great equine-human relationships is a little girl in love with horses. The majority of people in the horse business are women—about 80 percent of total horse owners, in fact. Whatever the magic between girls and ponies, horses have held our hearts captive since their usefulness for war and transportation waned. Somehow boys suddenly show up at the more advanced levels of jumpers, rodeo, and polo, and the girls who grew up spending their days at the barn wonder where all the boys came from! We tend to find something very exotic and wonderful about a man who handles horses and rides them with the same love and care we are so easily in touch with. Some display a natural skill with horses, perhaps embedded in their DNA, a shared lesson from the men throughout history who depended on horses for their safety and prowess on the battlefield. Both women and men learn early on that life's ride is an endless cycle of emotions, ranging from elation to hardship. Never mind that we as horsepeople are inviting non-human beings to come along on the ride with us!

We know from our interactions with other humans and those of our own and opposite gender that we harbor tremendous egos and feelings of pride, and those feelings can be hurt if we are betrayed or rejected. We experience love for another, and revel in the touch of one who loves us back. All of us recognize the proverbial ups and downs of living. We have inevitably experienced and responded to an endless list of mental and physical highs and lows throughout our lifetime, no matter how old we are, what we do, or where we are. The Principles of Compassionate Equitation help us recognize the benefits of identifying and gaining control over swinging emotions and mental distractions that can lead to difficulty when working with horses and with other people, both in and out of the equine environment. By becoming more heart-centered and understanding the feelings of others, including horses, the process becomes a daily habit and progresses to a continuous practice of truly possessing empathy for others at all times, and being of help when you can.

When did you fall in love with horses? Do you remember how it felt the first time you rode a horse?

I was one of those horse-obsessed little girls. From the age of 11, I wanted to be a horse trainer. Before my parents conceded to the purchase of my first horse, I trained our mixed-breed, black-and-white dog, PJ, to jump obstacles and pull a wagon. She also trained *me* to pull *her* in the wagon when she got tired. Such was my symbiotic relationship with animals from an early age. I found solace in them and had an easier time communicating with animals than I did other humans.

My entry into the world of horse ownership began at age 12 with an unruly ranch horse. She, like PJ, was also a mix of unknown origins, a stocky white mare named White Cloud. Nothing made me happier than being with that horse. As the years went by and I worked my way up to professional standards, it did not occur to me that something was still absent in my profound understanding of the equine world.

You do not get much closer to experiencing herd dynamics than when living in a barn yourself. You sleep when the horses sleep and are awake when they are. You learn each horse's personality, individual scent, his particular nickers and whinnies, and recognize his emotions. You notice subtle changes in his health. You even begin to feel like one of the herd members yourself and are reluctant to leave the others for even a short time.

Have you ever sat in a pasture just watching a group of horses? If not, try it sometime. If you have, go do it again. There is always something to be learned from herd dynamics.

For three decades I immersed myself in the horses' world. Although several times I left the business due to sheer physical burnout; I ultimately returned anew with recharged enthusiasm and additional wisdom as to how to keep everything in balance. With no family of my own to care for, my time and resources have always been devoted to the horses under my care and training.

After retiring from riding full-time at the age of 42, grateful for my many years of riding and competing with no serious injuries, I began teaching instead. I was also meditating regularly, a practice I started in my twenties. It wasn't until my mid-forties that the "missing element" began to materialize. After all those years of observing horses I began to see what I had not seen before. It was as though an angel had stood before me in human form, but I only recognized the person, and did not see an angelic presence. The "aha!" moments eventually emerged at a more conscious level: The horses—those beautiful animals with the deep liquid eyes—I *knew* when they felt happy and sad; when they were stressed, with legs tender from jumping; when they needed comfort on a cold day with warm bran mashes; when they were excited by the arrival of a new friend. I was spending more time watching each horse, and he watching me, now as I was on the ground teaching instead of on his back riding. It made sense. The horse cannot see you when you are on his back, nor can you see the expression in his eyes when mounted.

In decades past, I was as careful as could be with the tools at my disposal. There weren't therapeutic saddle pads on the market early in my career, so I made my own out of foam mattress camping pads. Custom saddle fitting was rare, but each saddle I used was checked according to wither clearance and shoulder angles. The horse and his environment were kept as spotlessly clean as possible so as to prevent problems from the hooves on upward. Yet still, how could I, after so many years of being so conscientious about my horses' comfort and immersed in their herd life, have failed to fully recognize *exactly* and *specifically* what I was sitting on?

Visualize what's beneath the surface of your horse's coat. From muscles to molecules, take a good, long look at what you're sitting on.

Look at these animals. I mean, *really* look at them and study them closely, even if you already consider yourself a competent horseperson. Be mindful of every detail, beginning with the outer form, and then visualize what's below the surface of that shining coat. Imagine yourself sitting on those living tissues and think of the horse as a whole being. You are sitting on the skin, bones, nerves, muscles, and organs of another living creature.[1]

Understanding and caring for the musculoskeletal system allows riders and caregivers to ride, train, and manage their horses efficiently and effectively. Keeping this system in optimum condition and appreciating how it functions leads to a supple, comfortable horse able to maximize his range of movement and perform at his best. Check out Gillian Higgens' Horses Inside Out *(www.horsesinsideout.com) and Susan Harris'* Anatomy in Motion *(www.anatomyinmotion.com).*

When I took up competitive running at age 48, six years after retiring from full-time horse training, it felt as though I was finally feeling in my own body what my horses had been experiencing as a result of all the intense training and exercise they were getting. The kind of workouts we put them through "in training" isn't so much what horses would do by themselves given the option. An athletic program is not part of their "genetic makeup." [2]

According to the University of California, Davis publication Suspensory Ligament Injuries in Horses *(Ferraro, Gregory L; Stover, Susan M; Whitcomb, Mary Beth), all horses are subject to tendon and ligament injuries, regardless of breed or whether they are performance horses or ridden for the occasional trail ride. Of course, athletic horses by their occupation are at greater risk. These injuries can occur in both the forelimbs and hind-limbs and can be serious enough to end an athletic career or lifestyle (www. vetmed.ucdavis.edu/ceh/docs/special/Pubs-SuspBrochure-bkm-sec.pdf).*

A deeper sense of empathy for horses ensued, and I began to register "discomfort" when a horse was thought to be exhibiting behavioral issues. This went beyond thinking, "He just doesn't want to do that," or "He doesn't like to jump." I felt as though I was seeing for the first time the *true* physicality of these beings, becoming more aware to what the horse might be feeling after stepping on a rock, stumbling after a fence, or slipping on a wet spot in the arena. It is one thing to have good communication with an animal, but still another when empathy and mercy are also a part of that dialogue, as well as the subsequent response.

WHAT MAKES MUSCLES "HURT"?

A good rider is a physically fit rider, and a fit rider also knows how to slowly condition his or her horse for peak performance. Our muscles respond to exercise similarly to horses. Here's how lactic-acid buildup affects both the human and equine athlete:

Working muscles require fuel. During *aerobic* activity (not too strenuous), fuel stored in muscle tissue is combined with oxygen from the blood to provide energy and movement. When exercise activity increases and you push your heart rate to an *anaerobic* intensity of beats-per-minute, or your horse's heart rate to that degree, the oxygen in your blood or your horse's is being depleted faster than it can be supplied. When this happens, muscle cells switch to an energy system that doesn't require oxygen. *Sport-specific heart-rate training* is an exceptionally useful tool to track cardiovascular fitness. Heart-rate monitors are available for horses, as they are for human athletes.

This *anaerobic* system requires more than 10 times the amount of fuel to produce the same amount of energy. This system also produces *lactic acid*, a metabolic waste product. If too much lactic acid accumulates in a muscle, it can result in extreme discomfort. The result of pain from overworked muscles can linger and cause you or your horse to be resistant and stiff in subsequent rides.

Have you ever run hard, or done an intense anaerobic workout of any kind, where you taxed your system and felt the results of lactic-acid build-up? It only takes a couple of minutes of fast, hard running to push your body into anaerobic mode. Symptoms of lactic-acid buildup (also known as *lactic acidosis*) include: a burning feeling in your muscles, rapid breathing, cramps, nausea, weakness, and a feeling of exhaustion. Keep in mind these symptoms are in the moment and are a sign to stop, or at least back down from the intensity of the activity. Unfortunately for the horse, he can't relay the information back to you if his muscles are reaching such a threshold. The purpose of Principle 1 is to confirm your horse as a sentient being, albeit one that can't verbally convey his feelings to you. Rather, he will explain his thoughts and emotions through his body language and behavior.

A good way to ensure your horse's comfort as he is reaching a new level of fitness is to limit the time spent in anaerobic activity, as is recommended for runners. Otherwise, you spend too much time dealing with extremely sore muscles and a lot of inflammation. When you ride your horse in this condition, you set him up for lameness and a sour attitude to work. Long, slow cool-downs for both human and equine athletes help the blood oxygen levels return to normal and remove waste material from muscle tissue.

My concerns were raised for every sore, tight spot in the horses' bodies. I imagined how cruel the jerk of a rider's hand felt, and how the muscle fiber was pulled and torn in an overstretched neck. My students became acutely aware that any activity causing pain or stress in a horse was unacceptable. They were taught the importance of correct hands and seat, to yield to the horse for optimal movement, and to recognize the precise timing necessary when applying the aids. When students rode unsupervised they were expected to remain mindful, ensuring that any emotions that surfaced or "corrections" they felt necessary to make were as kind and productive as those used during their lessons.[3]

As my awareness grew I also developed an understanding that deep breathing, proper rest and recovery, standard treatment protocols such as massage, and long, slow distance work apply to humans and horses alike, and have the same therapeutic benefits.[4]

In "Muscle Pain is a Form of Lameness that Limits Movement in Horses" from My Horse Daily, we are told that muscular aches, pains, and stiffness impact a horse's performance and his attitude. Caught early, they can be managed effectively. If undetected, muscle pain robs your horse of comfortable, free movement. Just think of how you feel if you've overdone it and have muscle pain or injury. It's not fun. See more at: http://myhorse. com/redirects muscle-pain-form-lameness-limits-movement-horses/

And in her video, Exercise Physiology: Are Horses like Humans & Other Species? *Dr. Erica McKenzie of Oregon State University, an Ironman triathlete, shares what exercise physiology research in humans and dogs can tell us about our horses (www.thehorse.com/videos/31915/exercise--physiology--are--horses--like--humans--other--species?utm_source=News-letter&utm_medium=welfare--industry&utm_campaign=06--27--2013).*

What are you working on when you ride? Do you make an exercise "plan"? Do you break your session down into cardio, strength, and flexibility? How about a suitable warm-up and cool-down? Do you include recovery periods?

It became my specialty to evaluate and plan a rehabilitative program for even the most difficult equine cases. I did so by deconstructing the circumstances that caused training and conditioning problems in the first place and using gentle, classical techniques based on the dressage *Pyramid of Training*, sometimes also referred to as the *Classical Training Scale*. This allowed for progress to occur over a period of time determined by the horse himself. No shortcuts or gimmicks have ever worked with horses, to my knowledge. If you cover up a problem, it will resurface, usually at the most inopportune time.

We will do a tremendous service to horses if all those who are in contact with them learn to see each horse for what he truly is. With that recognition, we are better equipped to acknowledge with care and attention the degree to which the physical and mental states of the horse are affected. We are asking this horse to pay full attention to us; therefore, it is in all fairness to the horse if we offer the same in return.

WHAT CAN BE PAINFUL FOR HORSES

- Rough, jerking hands
- An unbalanced seat
- Deliberately pulling a horse's head around or tying it down
- Tightening a girth too soon and/or too much
- Abusive application of artificial aids (spurs, whip)
- Overtightening the noseband
- A poorly fitted bit, or one that is adjusted too high or too low
- A poorly fitted saddle
- Hard, rocky footing
- Working the horse beyond his physical capabilities
- Gastric ulcers from stress

Dr. Allen Schoen:

As mentioned in my preface, in the beginning of my veterinary career I was an idealistic animal lover with the vision of being able to help animals in any way possible. I was fascinated by animal behavior and animal health care in general. My journey took me to studying animal behavior and pursuing a master's degree in animal behavior at the University of Illinois, and from there I followed my real desire to become a veterinarian and be able to relieve the pain and suffering of animals. At Cornell University's College of Veterinary Medicine I received one of the best trainings possible in conventional medicine and surgery. It was the foundation for my lifelong exploration of the question, "What is ultimate healing?"

My pursuit of an answer to this question began with a solid foundation in the anatomy, physiology, and pathology associated with conventional medicine and surgery. I appreciated the benefits of medications and surgery as well as their indications, limitations, contra-indications, their side effects and potential side effects. At that point I found my passion in veterinary medicine was looking for *other* options to help animals heal when they weren't responding to Western medicine and surgery, or where surgery was not an option, or where there were harmful side effects.

My journey then took me down other avenues: first into veterinary acupuncture. Once I opened my mind and my heart, recognizing options other than drugs and surgery exist and that acupuncture is based on neurophysiology, I thought, "There are so many other ways we can care for animals." Then acupuncture led me to Traditional Chinese Medicine for animals, including Chinese herbal medicine, Western botanical medicine, chiropractic and manual therapies, osteopathy, stretching, physical therapy, homeopathy, nutritional supplements, the human-animal bond, and mind-body medicine.

Certain behavioral health issues an animal was experiencing seemed to possibly relate to the choices the person in the animal's life was making, and to that person's thoughts and emotions.

What I started noticing over 35 years of veterinary practice with all animals, and in particular with horses, is that some issues the animal might be experiencing could possibly be related to the choices the person in the animal's life was making. The person's thoughts and emotions could also impact the care and well-being of the animal. I started to realize how integral that was, and it made me really begin to appreciate that one of the key issues in question was not just the human-animal "bond," but the compassion and the love that people actually have for their animals. People have animals because they want to share their lives with them.

As I spent time considering the incredible impact human thoughts and emotions have on horses and their well-being, I found myself initially being quite judgmental for a while. But over the years I realized people were just trying to do the best they could from where they were at a particular moment in time. Clearly, with this in mind, one of the most important elements involved in the ultimate healing of horses is training the minds and hearts of their human caretakers.

People have animals because they want to share their lives with them. They want to experience relationships with different species. There are more multi-species households in America now than not. In the Biophilia philosophy proposed by Dr. E.O Wilson of Harvard University, there is an innate desire to share our lives with nature and other beings (see p. 4). I believe that horse barns are an extension of that desire—to share our lives with other species.

Over decades of traveling from barn to barn in my veterinary practice I realized there was such a different feel, a different energy going from one facility to the other. If everyone was happy in the barn, the horses would be happy. If everyone was unhappy, the horses would be unhappy. Therefore, the key to making horses as healthy and happy as they can be, which is my primary duty as a veterinarian, involves improving the conscious awareness of *everyone* in the barn. This includes the owners of the barn, the trainers, the riders, the grooms, and anyone who visits. The secret to all of it is developing everyone's heart and mind to be active proponents of integrating wisdom and compassion into a person's daily interactions with animals.

I've been asked if I really practice this technique at all the barns I visit. I do it to the best of my abilities in a particular moment, depending on where I am inside my own heart and mind. And I do it in different ways. Sometimes I have a groom who may or may not speak English that well, holding a horse, and I can pick up on certain things just by the way he is holding the horse. Is he holding the horse too hard or being kind and tolerant? Does he love the horse he is caring for? In this scenario I might use very simple, *positive feedback training*, saying, "Thank you for holding this horse so gently. Thank you for being so compassionate with this horse." Then, the groom smiles. All of a sudden, he's brought into *conscious awareness*—he's not just generally aware of his surroundings and the horse he's holding because his senses tell him that it is so, he's *fully mentally* present, in the moment, and aware of *how* he is holding the horse. Perhaps now he does so much more gently, and then I can see that we are all working together in a more aware way.

With so much of what we do, improved care is simply bringing specific concepts into *conscious awareness*, and once that happens, everyone present is aware of and wants to be a part of a more harmonious resonance.

Sometimes all it takes is a gentle "thank you" to put a smile on someone's face.

I have noticed that as I treat a horse, the other horses in the barn often have their heads out of their stalls, watching, and they actually seem to *want* to walk out and be next in my hands, especially if I have treated them before. I have observed this over decades of practice and being with horses. The horses are talking, they are communicating, and they are interacting with us all the time. The only thing that blocks this communication is our perception, or lack of perception, of what is going on between us. It is so simple! It all comes back to our own minds.

"The root of all phenomena is your mind. If unexamined, it rushes after experiences, ingenious in the games of deception. If you look right into it, it is free of any ground or origin, in essence free of any coming, staying or going."

Sogyal Rinpoche, *Glimpse After Glimpse: Daily Reflections on Living and Dying* (HarperOne, 1995)

EXERCISE IN COMPASSION

Which YOU "Showed Up"?

1 Take five minutes right now and sit down with pen and paper, or your computer or tablet.

2 Imagine and briefly describe a particular situation with you and your horse—for example, grooming your horse and getting ready to go for a ride.

3 Explore which person "in you" showed up to be with your horse and how it manifests. If your ego is in charge and is being hysterical, garrulous, demanding, and calculating, how are you interacting with your horse and with everyone else at the barn? If you ride at a boarding or training facility, this includes the grooms, your trainer, and the other riders. If you ride at home, this may include family, friends, and other animals.

4 Read what you have written, and if the ego is in charge in your description, say, "Okay, let's switch over." That inner voice of wisdom—your *wise guide*—whom you've only rarely heard or tended to must be awakened. Once you become

What I found over years of hard lessons and challenges is that there is a difference when I try, to the best of my abilities, every morning, before I go off to treat animals and see patients, to do a minimum of 5 or 10 minutes (and ideally 20 minutes) of "quieting my mind" and bringing in the intention of being of benefit to all beings I meet that day. I call this Quiet Focused Intention (QFI—see p. 8). And remember, I want to be of benefit not just to the horses, but the grooms, the trainers, the riders, the owners, the barn cats and dogs, the birds in the hayloft—all the beings that share time and space with me.

If I begin my day and I am two hours late already, and I am feeling rushed as I think of the long list of horses and dogs and cats that I have to see that day, the first horse I approach is the greatest 1,200-pound biofeedback "instrument" you've ever seen. He gives me a look and seems to say, "Don't touch me. I have two words for you, and they are not 'Happy Birthday'!" I look at the horse, and he is giving me the "hairy eyeball," and his ears go back, and at that moment I simply say, "Thank you."

aware of it, you will be able to develop it more and more. How does that feel? What kind of differences do you feel within you?

5 Now imagine what your day with your horse will look like with the voice of your wise guide becoming clear. How will you act today? As you interact with your horse, what kind of responses might he have toward you?

6 Apply this same approach with your trainer, with other riders. How are you now going to treat *all beings* in your barn today?

As you write these steps down and examine them, the exercise becomes an interactive, co-creative project.

Practice it regularly and see if you hear your personal inner wise guide *more* and *more* each day. Consider how that shifts your perception and experience of each moment shared between you and your horse.

The beauty of that is, in an instant, I've just slowed my breath, changed my awareness, and shifted my thoughts from the worry over my list of future patients to the one that is standing before me in the present. I say, "Thank you, I am here for you, and how can I be of benefit?" I take in a slow deep breath, and oftentimes the horse will breathe deeply at that moment, too. His eye will change. He'll lower his head and seem to say, "Okay, *now* we can work together."

Horses are the greatest biofeedback "instruments" ever created.

I have similar experiences with dogs and cats. Each animal we are with is a beautiful biofeedback mechanism if we are *open* to that awareness and even more so if we have been exposed to the benefits of *mindfulness* and *mindfulness-based stress reduction (MBSR)* as developed by Dr. Jon Kabat-Zinn at the University of Massachusetts Medical Center. There are many terms used to describe elements of these techniques now. One variation on these approaches is called *loving-kindness meditation* or *metta* (a strong wish for the welfare and happiness of others) *meditation*. These approaches help us learn to focus on compassion for as little as 10 minutes a day, and thus change our neurochemistry and neurobiology, thereby altering how we are in the presence of animals. I provide specific techniques on p. 117.

In *Glimpse After Glimpse: Daily Reflections on Living and Dying* (Harper-One,1995), Sogyal Rinpoche writes:

> Two people have been living in you all your life. One is the ego, garrulous, demanding, hysterical, calculating; the other is the hidden spiritual being, whose still voice of wisdom you have only rarely heard or attended to. If you can come to such an awareness, and integrate it into your life, your inner voice, your innate wisdom of discernment, or "discriminating awareness," is awakened and strengthened, and you begin to distinguish between its guidance and the various clamorous and enthralling voices of ego. The memory of your real nature, with all its splendor and confidence, begins to return to you.
>
> You will find, in fact, that you have uncovered in yourself your own wise guide, and as the voice of your wise guide, or discriminating awareness, grows stronger and clearer, you will start to distinguish

between its truth and the various deceptions of the ego, and you
will be able to listen to it with discernment and confidence.

One of the key foundations of becoming a Compassionate Equestrian is to be able to more clearly differentiate between the two beings living inside you: Your *ego* and your inner *wise guide*. Training yourself to be able to differentiate when your actions are coming from ego and when they're coming from your inner wise guide, and nurturing that inner wise guide, enables you to be happier. Then, everyone you interact with will also be happier and healthier. When we are compassionate, we work better together, and that includes both people and animals. May this become a clear guiding light for you. Listen and respond to your inner wise guide.

Questions to Consider
BASED ON PRINCIPLE 1

1 Once I realize the sentience of all beings, how does that make me feel?

2 Based on the awareness of the sentience of all beings, how would I treat others differently?

3 How do I feel when I get in touch with that deep, inner wise guide?

4 How does that feel compared to when I am coming from an egoic place?

5 How do I plan on integrating these awarenesses into my interactions with my horse, with everyone at the barn, with everyone in my daily life?

CHAPTER TWO

Treating Animals as We Would Like to Be Treated

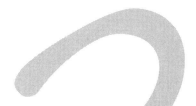

We treat animals as we wish to be treated ourselves,
with respect and compassion, to the best of our abilities.

Susan Gordon:

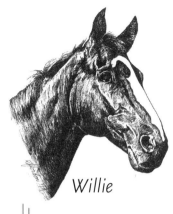

Willie

Horses, much like people, enjoy being paid a compliment. We appreciate someone who makes us feel good, and so do horses. They respond to having their talents validated with a kind word or gesture, which tends to be something a lot of riders overlook.

Willie was not able to convey his story to the inexperienced riders whose rough hands and unbalanced seats he had been subjected to. His only language was that of physical responses to pressure, and he was screaming as loudly as he could with every buck, pitch, nose-wrinkle, and pin of his ears.

Willie was a horse who needed to remember he was once treated like royalty, so I made sure to tell him in every way I could that he was the most special horse in the world. He responded to my compliments and praise, quickly turning into a different animal than the horse I'd ridden around that hardened track only short time before.

Unfortunately, my human relationship was challenged by the roller-coaster-like ride of the early dot-com days. Due to irregular cash flow, it was decided that we would move to a less-expensive townhouse that improved our commute. After less than a year with Willie at home in my backyard barn, we had to leave. I was thankful the hefty chestnut and I had been given the opportunity bond in a private setting and get to know each other as he began his healing process. By the time I moved him to a boarding stable—a relatively small operation with open-air pipe-rail stalls and pasture—he was starting to look like a show horse once more. I believe he was feeling quite proud of himself again too.

Watch a herd of horses turned out together. Their interactions are dynamic and fascinating. They are constantly tuned in to one another, even if they do not outwardly appear to be paying attention to anything other than grazing or lolling about.

Willie had been through the wringer, from life as an upper-level show jumper to the skin-and-bone, post-injury state I found him in as an 18-year-old. His early training reemerged in his inherent straightness and responses to aids, or cues, that he was given, and even though a bit slow to warm up and damaged from athletic injury in past years, he became bold and animated when even the smallest of jumps was placed in front of him. Somewhere in the back of his mind was a horse that obviously loved to jump, and he was very good at it. It was a thrill to ride him over fences as he reminded me of that old lesson horse—aptly named "Grouch"—on which I first learned to jump. Mutual joy is a great exchange between two beings.

Willie also managed to use his ability to levitate to pull off some rather interesting moves, and he was good at embarrassing me, usually in front of other professional horsemen or students. On the other hand, our rides caught the attention of a well-known hunter-jumper trainer who was training a Warmblood mare for the owner of the boarding stable we had moved to. His eventual invitation to have me work with him was what drew me out of my hiatus from the horse business. It wasn't too long afterward that Willie and I left the quiet facility for a busier show barn. By that time, we had come to mutual agreements over our "differences of opinion" and were ready for a return to a more professional setting.

Horses, too, seem to benefit from a supportive, caring community.

I respected Willie's wisdom and the many years of training, "detraining," and compromising circumstances he had lived through on his journey into my hands. Further down the road in our relationship, he confirmed he was so reliable and steady in his personality that I frequently turned him out with scared, sick, or very young horses to keep them calm and help them recover from trauma. He also seemed to be a genius at creating a supportive community for himself amongst equally old pasture mates. He was a quiet, contemplative leader, peacefully organizing and convincing the other horses to follow him wherever he wanted to go. One day, for example, I found him wedged into a tight spot between fences with the other horses lined up behind him, likely wondering what they were supposed to do next. It was an odd sight! As I stood there scratching my head, trying to decide how to get them all out safely, everyone agreed to back out once their leader decided to change gears to "reverse." They were out of trouble without a problem and nonchalantly returned to grazing.

It is very common for two pasture-buddies to stand face to tail with each other, making use of the other horse's perpetually swishing tail as a handy fly deterrent. Willie's tail was not particularly effective given that it had been chewed to his hocks by another horse and never grew back to full length. Yet every warm day in the pasture, there was my big old gelding parked in the middle of *two* horses with full tails as they dutifully kept the flies out of his eyes, nose, and ears. They did not receive much benefit from the arrangement themselves, and I wondered how he convinced *two* horses to help with his situation, whereas everybody else had one. Finally, one day I watched in fascination after turning him out in the field. He walked over to the big tree under which the rest of the herd was standing. Two of the other horses lifted their heads as Willie approached and quickly moved into position on either side of him. Willie decided one of them wasn't close enough, so he broke formation, walked to the outside of the errant horse, nudged him closer, and then promptly moved himself back into the middle so the mutual fly-swatting could proceed.

What was the deal they had made? Whatever it was, each horse seemed quite content with their arrangement. I can tell you for certain that Willie was kind to other horses. He was a *healer* of sorts, and as I've mentioned, was a popular companion for other horses when they needed a soothing buddy. While I could not ask Willie if he was feeling empathy and compassion toward others horses, somehow I think I was observing it in this gentle fellow. Interestingly, he did not put up with unkindness in humans he encountered.

In my experience, a horse senses when he has been "rescued" but still responds in subtle ways to different kinds of people. He might be cynical and suspicious; he may take some time to warm up to another human (especially if the person reminds him in some way of someone who may have been abusive to him in the past). While I feel that Willie and I understood one another, he had his likes and dislikes and was not shy about expressing his opinion. He was not inclined to bite or kick at another horse, but he would certainly let a human being know whether his or her attitude was acceptable or not—for example, cow-kicking at the fellow I had purchased him from. From the day Willie arrived in my backyard, however, I never did see him take another sideways jab at a human being. At first I was concerned over introducing a new farrier to him, but as it turned out, he really seemed to love the exceptional horse-shoer who produced small miracles with Willie's neglected hooves. When he *did* decide he didn't like someone though, he would often "make faces" and display other kinds of behavior that relayed his aggressive state of mind, depending on who or what was triggering the attitude. (For example, he once tried to bite the foot of another trainer who was giving me a hard time!)

HOW DO HORSES COMMUNICATE WITH EACH OTHER?

According to Karin Appel in "The Secrets of Equine Body Language" (Behaviour Canadian Horse Annual, 2008) horses are necessarily brilliant at picking up visual cues. As a social (herd) animal, horses have a vast repertoire of body movements, which are crucial to keeping the individual and the herd safe and fed and organized. Vocal communication, of which they have remarkably few variations, can attract predators and is not necessary in a closely-knit group of grassland herbivores with nearly a 360-degree field of vision. Unlike people, a horse's body language will always reflect his emotions and intentions. Some examples of how horses communicate include:

- *Posture* (stance and presence)

- *Orientation* (proximity of one horse to another)

- *Voice* (whinnies, nickers and snorts)

- *Ears* (positioning forward, backward, and "half-mast" or relaxed)

- *Eyes* (expressions such as "soft," "fearful," or "angry")

- *Head and Neck* (may position high or low in response to behavior of another horse)

- *Muzzle* (touching and nuzzling; feeling with sensitive, long whiskers; blowing through nostrils)

- *Legs* (striking out or kicking)

- *Tail* (switching from side to side or clamping)

Does a horse really think about how he would like to be treated? How do we translate his language to ours?

When we think of treating horses as we ourselves wish to be treated, it may feel like an awkward translation. I might love the gift of a spa treatment, for example, while my horse can't wait for a roll in the dirt, especially right *after* I have given him an equine version of the spa treatment! Yes, I speak a different language: When we witness a lot of activity in a group of horses, it may take us a minute or two to figure out whether they are arguing or playing. They play rough! They bite at the thin skin on each other's faces, or squeal and strike at each other, then take off at a gallop, bucking, and kicking with enough power to do some damage if they make contact. Sometimes, too, they are genuinely aggressive with each other and there are personality clashes that can end in injury.

The one thing we cannot do with horses is what we are trying to do with each other in this book—teach them how to have compassion for their fellow beings. It is up to us as their watchers and keepers to help them stay out of trouble in such regard. They are like a class of small children who never grow up. One may always be more of a bully than others. One may be so passive he always ends up being the one who gets short-changed on group feedings or has to wait to have a turn at the watering trough. Others are like Willie—benevolent leaders.

How do you wish to be treated? Do you find that you often remember *how people made you feel*, more so than remembering *what they said*? Have you noticed how much of your relationships with both people and horses are reliant upon nonverbal cues? Think about how good it feels to be loved and feel safe with another person, or cared for and supported by a community, and then imagine your horse and how he feels about the protection, care, and close bonds with his herdmates...including *you!*

Dr. Allen Schoen:

We qualify Principle 2 with "to the best of our abilities" because it is easy to forget to come from a place of tolerance and forgiveness all the time in a busy barn situation. There can be a tendency to lack mindfulness in the moment.

Being mindful in *every moment* and coming from a place of compassion *at all times* for the benefit of *all beings* is a simplistic definition of the term *Bodhicitta* in Buddhist philosophy. It means "the awakened heart." There are various interpretations of *heart* and *mind*. Here I relate to both what we conventionally consider the *mind*—being *mindful*, meaning being attentive to the present moment without thinking of the past and future—as well as the *heart-mind*, the feelings and senses and wisdom that reside in our heart, as well as the integration of these.

Wikipedia states: *Etymologically, the word is a combination of the Sanskrit words bodhi and citta. Bodhi means "awakening" or "enlightenment." Citta derives from the Sanskrit root cit, and means "that which is conscious" (i.e., mind or consciousness). Bodhicitta may be translated as "awakening mind" or "mind of enlightenment."* For me, as a veterinarian, Bodhicitta can be a continuous challenge as well as a continuous opportunity. When I drive up to a barn, and I've just been in traffic and people have been cutting me off, driving too fast on the highway and distracted by their cell phones, I am not always coming from a place of mindfulness, nor am I in the present moment. I see clients waiting to talk to me right away. I can either not be in the moment, still thinking about the guy who cut me off and being irritable as a result, or I can *change my thoughts* as I did on p. 33, come into the present moment, and decide to be mindful of the situation I am facing *right now* rather than continuing to be affected by moments that are *past*.

Does thinking about those to-do lists put you in an irritable state of mind? Coming back to the present moment with your breath can make a world of difference in how you feel.

The reason I recognize Principle 2 and promise to follow it "to the best of my abilities" is because I am a human being. My presence has repercussions. It is one stone thrown in to a pool of water, and all the ripples from that one stone affects every person and all the horses I am about to encounter. In each moment we can be "awake" or "not awake" when it comes to mindfulness. From my limited perspective at this moment, it isn't so much that "once you're awake, you're awake," and from there on out you are always mindful—it is more of a moment-to-moment opportunity. When I experience moments of *not* being mindful or awake, it offers me a chance to experience the contrast. When we do not take that moment to regroup, however, and become *present* in the moment, and our minds are still back in the traffic or on the to-do list and we are irritable, we bring that energy with us into our next experience, whether it is with a horse,

Simple Quiet Focused Intention (QFI) Before Entering a Barn

To get you started with a simple practice to relax and clear your mind prior to working with your horse, try these steps. I describe aspects of this meditative practice in more detail in chapter 6 (p. 133).

1   Once you have turned off your car's engine and quieted the car (this happens quickly if you drive a Tesla or other electric car!), sit in your car and quiet your own engine.

2   Gently close your eyes and take in a slow breath through your nose, inhaling deep into your chest, lungs, and filling your abdomen.

3   Allow the breath to "sit there" for a comfortable moment.

4   Then slowly exhale out through your chest, throat, and mouth.

5   Repeat this full breath at least three times.

6   If you like, visualize the in-breath as a calming, loving, white light permeating your entire body.

7   Visualize, sense, and feel all the tension leaving your body through your out-breath.

8   If you feel it to be beneficial, "shake off" any lingering tension by moving your hands and feet and "sigh out" any inner tension through your mouth.

9   Then perhaps say to yourself, "I am *here*, *now*, in calm, loving presence, for the benefit of my horse and for all beings in the barn."

10   Sense how this statement feels, how it changes your body.

11   Repeat as needed.

12   Create your own variation, using a theme that resonates with you.

groom, trainer, rider, or someone at work or at home. We can all recount numerous examples of what has happened in situations when we were not present mentally. Think of that ripple from the stone: it disturbs the water bug, distracts the fishing bird, and steals a little sand from the shore. If we can simply learn to *catch* ourselves as we fall prey to the human weakness of dwelling on the past and consciously switch to being in and focused on the present moment, it will prove to be better for all of us.

The Principles of Compassionate Equitation offer an opportunity to teach yourself to take a certain amount of time, whether it is one minute, or 10 minutes, whatever is necessary, to make sure that when you walk into the barn, you're coming from a place of open-hearted kindness and tolerance for all creatures. We introduced this idea of Quiet Focused Intention (QFI) as one of the three components of our foundation on p. 8.

What I personally try to do when I arrive at a barn is take in a few deep breaths, slow down, and become more *centered* (redirecting my energy to my physical center of gravity), because mindfulness *is all in the breath*. As I breathe slowly, in and out, I go ahead and recognize that I may have just been in traffic, I may be a little irritable, I may be an hour behind, people may be waiting to talk to me, I may be coming in for a second or third opinion and everyone has their agenda of what they want from the horse and everyone's agenda for the horse is different. *Whatever* the situation, I breathe, and recognize the events that are unfolding. As we've already discussed (p. 3), there are numerous universes or "*you*niverses," depending on any particular moment at any particular barn.

I simply close my eyes, take a few deep breaths in, and I exhale, releasing all that frenetic energy.

When I pull up to a barn and turn off the engine of my Jeep—because even the engine has a vibration that has an impact on the body and mind—I close my eyes, take deep breaths in, and I exhale, letting all that frenetic energy from the drive release. As I breathe in and out, I say to myself either, "Relax and release," or "Let go," and then, "May I be of benefit to all beings, here and now." Or simply, "It is all good now." Or whatever feels right at the moment. This shifts my *neural wiring* from the past moments of tension to the present moment of being right where I am in loving-kindness and compassion. The neural wiring is the way our brain, our neurons, are wired from past *programming* or habits. The neuroscience cliché, "You wire what you fire," means that whatever neural pathway we keep on triggering ends up getting "hardwired" in our brain, and that is where we tend to go, how we tend to react in a triggering situation, unless we catch ourselves and consciously change that habit or neural pattern. This is part of *neuroplasticity*, our ability to change our previous programming, allowing us to consciously choose to respond differently to a particular situation. Once I consciously catch myself, through my breathing and QFI I can shift from a habitual pattern or reaction to a more calm, more present, mindful state. Then I am ready to walk into the barn and really *see* everyone who wants my attention. As I do so, I repeat to myself, "May I be of benefit... may I be of benefit," and then let go of that focus so I can see to the job at hand.

This process seems to help bring everyone else around me into a calmer state as well. Oftentimes, my clients say, "We just feel a sense of peace when you walk into the barn," or, "The whole energy shifts when you walk in." As I hear others sigh deeply and feel my calm reflected back to me, I recognize it as the *Transpecies Field Theory* that I propose and describe in this book for the first time (see the sidebar as well as p. 7 for more on this). There is an energetic field all around us, and it is impacted by each and every one of us and our thoughts.

INTRODUCTION TO THE TRANSPECIES FIELD THEORY AND COMPASSIONATE FIELD THEORY

My *Transpecies Field Theory* (TSFT) proposes that there is a dynamic, continuously interactive, behavioral, energetic *field* (the surrounding flow of energy) that impacts all living beings involved. If everyone in the field behaves in ways based on their various *past programming* or habitual behavior patterns, they will have certain effects on all others in the field. Once we recognize this field exists, the next exciting step is that we realize we can actually have a conscious impact on this field by focusing our intention on a particular positive thought or emotion, such as compassion. This is the basis for my Compassionate Field Theory (CFT), as well as the Compassionate Equestrian Approach and this book. Personally, once I realized the potential impact of these insights, I was so excited that this new awareness was the stimulus for me to write this book. This is the next step in my search, asking the question, "What is *Ultimate Healing*?" Perhaps training our hearts and minds to be more compassionate could impact the health and happiness of not only our horses, but all of *us*, as well as the world we share. I examine these ideas more closely in chapter 2, p. 17.

We have a choice: "React-ability" or "Response-ability."

In every scenario, we have a choice between "React-ability" and "Response-ability." We have an opportunity to *not react* from a place of irritability about *what just happened*. Rather, we can shift our awareness to the *now* and choose to *respond* from a calmer, more centered space within ourselves. Whether the trainers are arguing in the barn, or the grooms are being moody, or the horses are cranky, or we find ourselves in the middle of other energetic, emotional baggage people carry with them, instead of reflexively *reacting* to the situation, we can tell ourselves to take a moment to breathe, release, and *respond* in a thoughtful and forgiving manner. By simply *being aware* of our ability to shift our own internal response to all manner of scenarios, we then can help shift the feeling of everyone else to a calmer, happier place, inside and out.

We must first treat ourselves as we wish to be treated by others. Try not to chastise yourself.

It seems that before we treat our horses as we would like to be treated by others, we need to first treat ourselves in a kind and compassionate way. If you are always "on your own case," upset about this or that, and tense and angry, obviously you are chastising yourself. We tend to be our own worst self-critics. Sometimes, if not too harsh, this tendency can support us in our efforts to become the best we can be. But it can also be quite destructive to our inner peace and contentment. It all depends on *how* that inner voice is speaking to us and *what* it is saying. Where is it coming from? From old *con*structive or *de*structive imprints on our *neural nets*? Our *neural nets* are formed of repeated thoughts and emotions from previous experiences embedded into our brains. Each of life's experiences can leave a *neural imprint* or "etching" in our brains; these can be either beneficial or decidedly less so. One *de*structive example of this is known as Post-Traumatic Stress Disorder (PTSD).

The good news is we can change that self-critical voice to be more understanding, nonjudgmental, and compassionate. Would we not feel much better if we chose a more tolerant and generous inner voice? Modern psychology has, in fact, integrated these concepts into many different therapeutic fields, including cognitive emotional therapy, positive psychology, and neurolinguistic programming, to name just a few.

Loving-Kindness for the Self

The concept of *self-compassion* or loving-kindness for the self is *not* about being narcissistic, but rather being forgiving, gentle, and sympathetic with yourself when viewing your thoughts or actions.

1   Learn to acknowledge, "I am being irritable because such and such happened."

2   Simply recognize the fact that irritability is showing up, without allowing yourself to identify with it.

3   Then, breathe in and out, and *release* the irritability, asking yourself, "Do I want to treat everyone else like that? Do I want to treat myself like that? Look at the way I am treating myself. I am beating myself up!"

4   Next, say to yourself, "Let me be compassionate with myself. I understand I have had a rough morning, or a rough day...I understand I am doing the best I can at this moment."

5   Breathe in and out again, recognize any tension, or irritability, and then release it.

6   Say, "I have the ability to relax and be compassionate with myself."

7   Shake it out. Let go. Relax.

I choose to be compassionate with myself and to not bring "baggage" to the barn with me because I do not want to treat anyone else in a manner that makes them feel irritable or unhappy.

If I am being compassionate with myself and extending loving-kindness to others, then I can see the groom, the trainer, or the client as also doing the best *they* can. If they are upset and stressed, I can say, "Wow, you've had a really hard day, I understand. Can we take a moment to quiet our hearts and quiet our minds so we can be who we really want to be with our horses?"

We hold tensions related to our experiences not just in our minds and our hearts, but in various other parts of our body, as well. Pent-up emotions manifest as *somatic contractions* (control functions under conscious voluntary control, such as skeletal muscles and sensory nerves) throughout our body. Horses may then sense these contractions when we get on them. It is not uncommon to hear a client say, "My horse doesn't want me near him!" One client confessed to me that her horse was biting her, but not anyone else. "Do you think it's me?" she asked.

It was good that she even thought to ask the question. That was a good start. My recommendation to her was to look at herself and take a deep breath in. She needed to come to her horse from an open-minded, gentle, and forgiving place. She needed to not bring all her own "stuff" to the barn and see what a difference there might be in the way her horse reacted around her. This is true for everyone. We have the ability to be aware of our "baggage," set it aside, and choose to say, "I will be compassionate and loving to everyone I meet in the barn today, just as I will be to myself."

The choice is ours: rudeness or kindness.

These days we often hear reports in the media state that "rudeness is the new normal." The blame is placed on politicians, media, youth, and popular culture for a shift in values and how people choose to interact with each other. When you dare to disagree with anyone else, you can almost *expect* to be treated in an uncivil way by the person you do not agree with. Many people now seem to get some kind of "rush" out of being rude.

This phenomenon is essentially all *ego*. Remember what we learned about the *ego* and the inner *wise guide* in chapter 1 (see p. 37)? Today's obsession with a general lack of courtesy is due to people identifying with self-constructed neural nets of life experiences that they *believe* represent them, but again, we have a choice: Rather than declare "rudeness is the new normal," we have the opportunity to instead say, "If people have that mindset, it is their *choice* to allow it to call the shots. But that is not *my* choice." The invitation we offer with Principle 2 is to *treat horses (and others) as we wish to be treated*. We do not accept that "rudeness is the new normal." We choose to interact with all beings in a civil, respectful way, and to believe that *this* is *the* normal.

The cliché, "Think globally, act locally," relates to each horse barn we enter and each interaction we have with our horse and others. In fact, it applies even *more* locally than each interaction we have with other beings—it applies to our own hearts and minds. Rather than accepting rudeness as the new normal, we can apply the concept of "Think globally, act locally," by striving to create a *more respectful, kinder normal in ourselves first*, and then in each barn, each horse show, each equine event. Let us imagine and visualize how a global compassionate equestrian community would look if we brought consideration and civility to each and every situation.

PRINCIPLE 2 IS KEY BECAUSE IT ASKS:

Do you want to be treated rudely, or do you want to be treated with kindness and consideration?

Does your horse want to be treated rudely, or does he want to be treated with kindness and consideration?

Do the groom, the barn manager, and the farrier want to be treated rudely? Or would they like to be treated with kindness and consideration?

What would the barn feel like if you shifted your perspective and treated every being there (including yourself) with kindness and consideration?

At barns and training facilities grooms and barn staff often think they are in a subservient position. Or, if they come from a place of far less affluence than the people they work for, they may feel they do not deserve the same level of respect, tolerance, and consideration. Yet they do. I observe this situation all too often in my travels. When I work with a groom who's used to not being treated very well, and I regularly thank him or her for assistance, I see his or her eyes light up. I watch the groom smile in response to someone acknowledging him or her. When I was in South Africa treating some racehorses, the grooms who were holding the horses constantly cowered in fear, and because of this, they would hold the horses too tightly. When I said a simple "Thank you," to them, they smiled, and then held the horses differently. And then the horses stood differently. Each one of us desires to be acknowledged and loved. That really is what *all* beings want.

We have the ability to respond to, instead of react to, the old imprints in our neural net—our mental memories.

What has happened in the past—our childhood experiences imprinted from generation to generation and including various emotional, physical, and mental traumas—may impact our current moment and our current experience. Whether it is past violence, alcoholism or drug-abuse, rudeness, or some other emotional trauma, anything we "received," any acknowledgment in whatever form that came from our parents, we tend to equate with "love" going forward. So for example, if the kind of attention our parents gave us was abusive, we may equate cruel words and hard hands with love. We have the "Response-ability," though, to *not* react to our old imprints. As soon as we awaken to this idea and say, "No, I want to be treated with compassion. I want to be acknowledged and acknowledge others with kind words, not cruel," then we can break the cycle. When we no longer react from old destructive mental imprints by *choosing* to come from a new perspective, we consciously create new positive *neural wiring* (nerve pathways) and imprints in our brains.

Transforming Rude to Kind

1   Take a moment and visualize a particular situation that may have appeared as rude, hurtful, negative, or destructive.

2   How does it make you feel? What do you feel? Where do you feel it?

3   Write down your feelings.

4   Now visualize how you might be able to change that same situation and what that shift might look like.

5   How does that feel now? What do you feel? Where do you feel it?

6   Write down your new feelings and what that positive, more considerate and civil scenario looks like.

7   Now going forward, create kinder, friendlier, more courteous situations, and shift the experience for yourself and others.

When we are grateful for everyone in the barn and how they are helping, they are going to be nicer to the horses, knowing they are acknowledged, appreciated, and loved. Others in the barn might still be in a state of tension or distress based on *their* previous life imprints, yet they have the ability—like you—to shift to a place of compassion in *each* and *every* moment. After you act in a kind and considerate way toward a barnmate, he or she may then say, "Wow, so-and-so is acting so compassionately toward me, and it makes me feel good. That's how *I* am going to act toward others today." Then your barnmate's horse receives all this love and positivity from those around him, and he responds accordingly, by being less tense or fearful and being more relaxed and open to working with his rider. It becomes this big, beautiful circle of loving-kindness and open-mindedness—but it starts with each one of us.

Riders may think they have compassion for their horses, that they love their horses, but their actions and reactions to the horse, who may have significant health problems, indicate otherwise.

It is not uncommon to see situations where a horse's owner claims to love his or her horse completely. The horse has the best care, the best food, the best stabling, and fancy clothes. The horse is perfectly trained, well-bred, and beautiful. But when you get on the horse, he doesn't want to move forward, and it becomes apparent that *something* is wrong. At least to a professional trainer or veterinarian, resistance in a horse is often a glaring sign of pain—physical or emotional. Many horse owners simply translate it as a "behavioral issue." This "love of the horse" paired with an inability to appreciate the horse's physical or emotional pain is a common contradiction in the equine industry.

We know in humans that chronic pain creates imprints of resistance, such as irritability, grouchiness, defensiveness, and bitterness. The more it continues without an individual addressing the chronic pain, the more resistance there is. In Traditional Chinese Medicine, any pain is a *disruption*, a block of energy flow. Once you release and correct the flow of energy, the pain goes away.

As a horse caretaker, the first course of action when you notice any new resistance or a sudden change in behavior is to stop working or training and have the horse evaluated by a qualified veterinarian or practitioner to find out if there is a pain issue.

If you, like so many others, typically blame a horse's training or performance problems on bad behavior, choose to shift thinking and *first find out* if there is pain somewhere. Recognize that you may have to go to a few different practitioners to locate a cause. As a conventionally trained veterinarian who is also trained in acupuncture, manual therapy, chiropractic, physical therapy, and other modalities, I am prepared to provide a unique perspective and sensitivity to the possibility of pain in the horse. Oftentimes I am called when a horse owner is looking for an additional opinion after another primary care veterinarian has failed to identify pain based on conventional methods of Western medicine.

It is hard to say which form of medicine or care will ultimately best serve a horse and his particular situation. Every approach has its place, its indications, and its limitations. The key is to find out what's best for *that horse at that time*, so the care is really coming from a compassionate place. Remember to ask the question, "What is best for my horse?" A caring and generous practitioner who may not have all the expertise or right tools for the job at hand ideally should be willing to help guide you to find the right practitioner or next step to obtain proper diagnosis and treatment. A veterinarian or practitioner should not be attached to thinking his or her approach is the *only* approach.

It is not uncommon to find multiple musculoskeletal issues, treat them from my perspective, and also tell the owner the horse may need an MRI or a bone scan or other additional diagnostic techniques to elucidate an underlying problem.

If I can't correct a particular issue in a few treatments, I try to look at what is causing the underlying, recurring condition. I try to offer advice regarding the horse's saddle fit, shoeing, biomechanical rider issues, and musculoskeletal imbalances when evaluating various lameness issues, often recommending an additional workup by the owner's primary care veterinarian. Yet sometimes the cause may still be hard to pinpoint. It can be very challenging because sometimes I see the underlying cause might actually be the horse's training or how he's ridden—that is, the issue might be with the rider and her attitude. That's a very delicate situation. It goes into a "sticky area" for sure. The rider may be training her horse in the way she feels is best for the horse based on her own education and experiences, yet sometimes, the way the horse is worked with relates more to the human's *personal* life experiences (those imprints from childhood I mentioned on p. 53) and it turns out it's not the best way to handle or ride horses.

Challenging Questions to Ask Yourself

Find a moment of loving, reflective, self-inquiry, and ask yourself:

"Am I treating this horse like I was treated as a child?"

"Was I in emotional or physical pain at some point and told to just, "Get over it?" or "Push through it.""

"Am I reacting to my horse's resistance the way my parents, guardian, teachers, or other authority figure reacted to me?"

I am not a psychologist or a transpersonal psychologist, but I do have a master's degree in animal behavior and neurophysiology, and I've come to realize that animal behavior and human behavior are distinctly related.[1] Issues caused by early abuse in the animals and childhood abuse in people are similar. That is why the compassionate mindset should have you asking, "Am I taking my *early childhood imprints* and imposing them on my horse? Is that the most compassionate choice for myself? Is that the most compassionate choice for my horse?" Here we must consider a potentially deeper exploration of what Ultimate Healing for our animal friends might be—that is, it may be beneficial to look for professional assistance and appropriate health care practitioners, such as therapists and psychologists, to explore and heal *us* when necessary.

1   *In "The Cambridge Declaration on Consciousness" (2012) edited by Jaak Panksepp, Diana Reiss, David Edelman, Bruno Van Swinderen, Philip Low, and Christof Koch, the following is stated: "The absence of a neocortex does not appear to preclude an organism from experiencing affective states. Convergent evidence indicates that non-human animals have the neuroanatomical, neurochemical, and neurophysiological substrates of conscious states along with the capacity to exhibit intentional behaviors. Consequently, the weight of evidence indicates that humans are not unique in possessing the neurological substrates that generate consciousness. Non-human animals, including all mammals and birds, and many other creatures, including octopuses, also possess these neurological substrates" (http://fcmconference.org/img/CambridgeDeclarationOn-Consciousness.pdf).*

Based on these principles, determining the appropriate therapy and what treatments may be beneficial involves first asking yourself a few questions.

First of all, look at the horse's resistances as possibly originating from pain. Who are the most qualified practitioners to evaluate whether your horse is in pain or not?

I personally feel that veterinarians who have received additional training, such as advanced training and certification in acupuncture, chiropractic, and manual therapies, are the most likely to offer a more expansive, integrated, holistic perspective on possible causes of pain in the horse. I have found that such training has certainly broadened my own point of view, as well provided alternative routes to emotional and physical wellness.

Rather than waiting to evaluate the horse only when he already *is* lame or resistant, alternative therapies allow you to see issues that *precede* lameness and resistances and prevent them from occurring. These issues are what I consider "pre-clinical"—the horse is "not quite lame, but not quite right." I sometimes joke, "What you are seeing is what you are not getting." In other words, by involving preventive approaches, such as acupuncture and manual therapies, in your horse's care, you may be avoiding future lameness issues. Find practitioners who make an effort to do what is best for the animal, who are coming from the "right place" within themselves, and who are not pushing visits and treatments from a business point of view. Recommendations from other horsepeople you respect who have had positive, long-term experiences with a particular practitioner is a reasonable place to start.

Second, ask those deeper questions of yourself that I mentioned on p. 56. Are your rationalizations and justifications for "pushing the horse through his resistance" coming from someplace *inside you*? When the answer is, "Yes," then it is perhaps time to look for the source of *your* pain, whether physical, emotional, or psychological, and acknowledge that it could be preventing you from seeing that the horse's resistance is *also* coming from pain. Even when we think we are doing our best with our horses, we may be bringing our own "baggage" to the paddock, barn, and saddle.[2]

In their article "The Effectiveness of Equine-Assisted Experiential Therapy: Results of an Open Clinical Trial" (Society and Animals 15, 2007), Bradley T. Klontz, Alex Bivens, Deb Leinart, and Ted Klontz describe how EAET offers a unique opportunity for the therapeutic use of metaphors. Horses elicit a range of emotions and behaviors in humans, which can be used as a catalyst for personal awareness and growth (Zugich et al., 2002). Horses also offer a variety of opportunities for projection and transference. A horse walking away, ignoring, being distracted by other horses, sleeping, wanting to eat at the wrong time, biting, urinating, and neighing are common horse behaviors to which humans respond (https:// www.animalsandsociety.org/assets/library/736_s3.pdf).

The bottom line is physical pain, in human and horse, creates behavioral changes that manifest as resistance, anger, and depression, to name just a few. Physical pain doesn't just mean lameness. It goes well beyond joints, tendons, and ligaments. It goes beyond musculoskeletal balance, or issues such as gastrointestinal ulcers, hormone imbalance, and neurological problems.

*In treating your horse as you wish to be treated, first ask what the most compassionate and loving thing would be to do for yourself if **you** were being asked to push through pain, and then do the same for your horse.*

One book among many that I have found beneficial in exploring ways to free yourself from you own limitations and soar beyond old imprints is *The Untethered Soul: The Journey Beyond Yourself* by Michael Singer (New Harbinger Publications, 2007). As stated on the book's back cover, it is a guide to your relationship with your own thoughts and emotions, "helping one uncover the source and fluctuations of our inner energy. It then delves into what you can do to free yourself from the habitual thoughts, emotions, and energy patterns that limit your consciousness." This book helped me on my personal journey of trying to be of benefit to horses and all beings. See what you think.

Questions to Consider
BASED ON PRINCIPLE 2

1 Am I treating myself, my horse, and others as I would like to be treated? (If so, congratulate yourself!)

2 If not, why not? What is preventing me from treating myself and others as I would like to be treated?

3 Would it be beneficial for me to get professional support in exploring potentially deeper issues and my own physical, emotional, or psychological pain?

4 How does it feel when I treat myself and others with loving-kindness and compassion?

CHAPTER THREE

Building the Foundation of Compassion

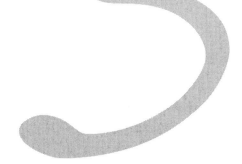

Compassionate Equitation is based on an underlying foundation of respect, compassion, and loving-kindness.

Susan Gordon:

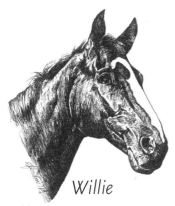

Willie

Perhaps it was a compassionate awakening of sorts that occurred, but Willie certainly taught me the value of an older horse. As a trainer, I was always looking at juvenile horses for show and investment prospects, many of which were off the racetrack, or clients would bring in younger ones for training. Old horses were on the lesson strings and expected to earn their keep.

Willie came to my backyard as a stranger, but we quickly bonded. With lots of good hay, a new farrier, and plenty of attention, he thrived and turned into a "Cinderella" of a horse.

My respect and compassion for older horses blossomed as a result of my experience with him. He taught me to appreciate and value the wisdom, experience, and steadiness of character you find in an aged horse with good training. He never lost the exceptional base he was given when first started under saddle, it was just temporarily hidden. He seemed thrilled to be allowed to "show his stuff" again. He may have lost the ability to fly over 6-foot fences or produce tempi changes, but he was still amazing to ride and eventually made an exceptional teacher for other riders.

Like Willie's quality training foundation, I think our inherent base of compassion is always present. Sometimes it is perhaps hidden, but all it takes is the right circumstance to awaken the loving-kindness in our hearts. I believe we are constantly seeking that loving-kindness, even though our present circumstances, or issues such as the childhood imprints Dr. Schoen mentioned in chapter 2, might be preventing us from outwardly displaying the tolerant, caring person we know exists within us.

How, when, and where is the foundation instilled for extending love, mercy, and respect for all beings? Kind and attentive parents who possess such qualities and are generous toward others set an example for their children who tend to mimic that behavior. Some children even grow up in war-torn parts of the world and still demonstrate the kind of compassion that can only come from a pure heart and genuine empathy, preserved and encouraged in the home.

Observing an animal's reaction to a particular person may reveal the true nature of that person more than he or she realizes. Some people are unaware of how exposed their intent is when placed in the company of a horse. As a professional rider, my daily activities were very physically and mentally demanding, as they are for most people working in equestrian facilities. In the usual crunch to get all the barn chores completed, every horse ridden, and handle unexpected injuries or health problems with those in the stable, I sometimes tended to overlook the fact that every extreme and every corner of my persona was pulled to the surface at one time or another. My moods and reactions were frequently exacerbated by situations in the barn with other people or trainers, and the horses picked up on those moods. The challenges to remain diplomatic and in control of oneself are enormous, especially when riding professionally, but you can't hide what you're feeling inside from a horse! You want to help everyone, but sometimes it is impossible to do so in spite of your best intentions. You start to rush, miss details, become grouchy, and before you know it, everyone in your path, including your horse, is grouchy too!

Horses have a way of revealing who we really are.

It is easy to become caught up in the world of luxury, material goods, wealth, and influence that is the atmosphere at many types of horse shows, or to long for a stunning barn and indoor that could rival a five-star resort. To some outside observers, much of the horse industry certainly appears to be an exclusive subsection of society far removed from those who are not so fortunate. As a professional rider and trainer, you put most earnings back into your horses and show expenses. Most of us in that category become used to providing our services to much wealthier clients. Our job is another's recreation, and most of us are in the industry simply because we *love* horses. However, we are not always able to outwardly exhibit this due to the sheer intensity of working with and around horses, perhaps under the watchful eye of a demanding trainer or owner. Even with a good foundation of compassion, this kind of stress can test the most loving hearts and kindest intentions.

Horses are not machines, but individuals with minds of their own, and true to that can choose to perform as we expect or completely surprise us! Clients and owners can become very stressed and edgy during competitions or tough lessons. Add to these facts weather issues, early mornings, late nights, and lots of waiting around for classes, test times, or rounds, and we may find Principle 3 somewhat challenging! At large, multi-week horse shows I've often heard the arguments coming through the walls from neighboring stalls or barns.

At clinics, expos, and demonstrations, it always seems as though differences in opinion tend to arise. No matter how innocently conversation begins, tensions can escalate around everything from training solutions to gossip about clinicians to breed preferences.

Compassion takes practice and tends to be most difficult when circumstances arise that challenge our desire to be kind and loving toward others.

As mentioned, the conditioning of such a foundation of kindness and respect ideally comes from familial or other guiding influences at an early age, and it is then reinforced by a system of education.[1] There are many schools of spiritual and philosophical thought that aim to promote peace and respect toward *all*. Why then, do we have so much violence in the world and people who seem to show little respect or love for others, or who are selective as to whom they show respect and love? What is it about human nature that allows us to cause the amount of suffering we know to be prevalent around the world?

1

On the website Transcendental Meditation (www.tm.org), Dr. Christopher Clark writes: "Children can start the Transcendental Meditation technique at the age of ten. There are no side effects—research has found only positive benefits, such as greater focus, clarity of mind, improved grades at school, higher intelligence, more creativity and self-esteem. Children younger than ten can learn a special walking technique, which has been found to have a harmonious and stabilizing effect" (http://www.tm.org/benefits--childhood--and--adolescent--disorders).

Remember the definition of compassion itself. It goes beyond having empathy for another being. Compassion is derived from a Greek word meaning *co-suffering*—it is a deep desire within yourself to alleviate the suffering of others. It is the reason why common bonds are formed amongst survivors of disasters and those who have experienced similar traumas.

Once we have affirmed the inherent foundation of loving-kindness within ourselves, we realize we have the opportunity to build on that foundation, furthering our tolerant and loving nature. It may be a challenge to do so, but when we realize the benefits to our own health and that of our animals, we can understand the motivation for cultivating our foundation of kindness.

Find a method that works for you.

If we develop compassion as our base from which to function, we will continue to grow in our capacity for extending respect, consideration, and forgiveness to others. You really *can* transform the way you interact with horses and other people, at all times and in all equestrian venues.[2] When we develop the ability to maintain a steady nature, it has a positive impact on all beings that find themselves in our presence.

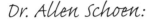

> *Neuropsychologist and bestselling author Dr. Rick Hanson presents a free, online, eight-part video series called The Compassionate Brain that explores effective ways to change your brain and heart and life (http://live.soundstrue.com/compassionatebrain/).*

Dr. Allen Schoen:

The key is QFI—taking 10 minutes of contemplative time, breathing slowly, and focusing your intention on being compassionate to all beings, prior to working with your horse.

As described in the three foundation components (p. 8) and in chapter 2 (p. 46), a deep breath is integral to putting yourself in the moment. When is the best time to take 10 minutes to focus your intention on compassion? Can it be done while grooming your horse, or sitting on your tack trunk?

I honestly feel there is rarely a bad time to practice breathing and find your compassionate place, although I think by the time you are in your tack room or with your horse, it may not be as beneficial as doing it *before* you get to the barn. You want to bring inner peace into the barn *with* you. The goal is to quiet your *mind traffic* and not be preoccupied when with your horse. Ideally, I try to practice QFI for 20 minutes in the morning before work, and then as I described on p. 35, I renew that for a few minutes sitting in my car before I go into a barn.

In a University of Wisconsin-Madison study by researchers at the Center for Investigating Healthy Minds, it was found that adults can be trained to be more compassionate. According to one of the researchers, Helen Weng, "It's kind of like weight training... we found that people can actually build up their compassion 'muscle' and respond to others' suffering with care and a desire to help."

Within two weeks researchers found alterations in the brain function of the participants. After only seven hours total of guided audio instructions, there was increased activity in the *inferior parietal cortex* of the subjects. This part of the brain is a region involved in empathy and understanding others. Compassion training also increased activity in the parts of the brain involved with emotion regulation and positive emotions.

The study concluded that compassion, like physical and academic skills, appears to be something that can be enhanced with training and practice.[3] We expand on this idea in subsequent chapters. Developing a more compassionate mind and heart is one of the keys to the Principles of Compassionate Equitation. It is exciting to realize that you can develop a kind, tolerant and forgiving nature through appropriate guided instruction and "brain-muscle training."

Jill Ladwig wrote in her article "Brain Can Be Trained in Compassion, Study Shows" in the University of Wisconsin-Madison News *(May 22, 2013): "Our fundamental question was, 'Can compassion be trained and learned in adults? Can we become more caring if we practice that mindset?'" says Helen Weng, a graduate student in clinical psychology and lead author of the paper. "Our evidence points to yes." (http://www.news.wisc.edu/21811).*

If a quiet space could be made in every barn to be used for 10 minutes of QFI before riders and trainers interacted with horses, that would be ideal. If such a space did exist, I feel more people would be likely to use it than not. Kind of like, "If you build it, they will come." I would make it a room or empty stall away from the noise and activity of tack rooms and grooming areas if possible. This 10 minutes dedicated to quiet and becoming self-reflective is extremely effective at making changes in the human heart and mind in a very short space of time. It really is one of the components of our foundation for developing compassion. It all goes back to illustrating the old neuroscience cliché that states we "wire what we fire" in our brains—in other words, we literally change the functioning of our brains with our thoughts. We work on that by continuing to practice compassion, and practice makes perfect.

Thank you for taking time to get in touch with your loving self and choosing to radiate that loving kindness to your horse and all beings you meet.

WHAT IS COMPASSION?

The wonderful online resource *Greater Good: The Science of a Meaningful Life* (greatergood.berkeley.edu) defines compassion as follows:

> *Compassion literally means "to suffer together." Among emotion researchers, it is defined as the feeling that arises when you are confronted with another's suffering and feel motivated to relieve that suffering.*
>
> *Compassion is not the same as empathy or altruism, though the concepts are related. While empathy refers more generally to our ability to take the perspective of and feel the emotions of another person, compassion is when those feelings and thoughts include the desire to help. Altruism, in turn, is the kind, selfless behavior often prompted by feelings of compassion, though one can feel compassion without acting on it, and altruism isn't always motivated by compassion.*
>
> *While cynics may dismiss compassion as touchy-feely or irrational, scientists have started to map the biological basis of compassion, suggesting its deep evolutionary purpose. This research has shown that when we feel compassion, our heart rate slows down, we secrete the "bonding hormone" oxytocin, and regions of the brain linked to empathy, caregiving, and feelings of pleasure light up, which often results in our wanting to approach and care for other people.*

Reprinted by permission from *Greater Good*:
(http://greatergood.berkeley.edu/topic/compassion/definition).

What follows are sample meditations to assist you in deepening your connection with your horse as well as other horsepeople. The meditations, which can be used to establish your Quiet Focused Intention (p. 8), are meant to help you get in touch with the loving-kindness and compassion that is already within you.

These meditations are here to quiet and nurture your heart and mind.

These meditations may help you communicate with your horse at a deeper level.

They may help you create a more compassionate and kind atmosphere within yourself and at your horse barn.

They can possibly help you create a field of compassionate and kind energy wherever you are with your horse, as well as wherever you are in each moment.

These meditations are just suggestions. Feel free to change the visualizations, the words, or whatever you need to resonate with who you are. The goal is simply to assist you in connecting with your true, loving compassionate self, as well as with your horse and all beings.

My intention and wish is that these meditations be of immense benefit to you, your horse, and all beings!

Do not use any of these meditations while driving or operating equipment or riding on your horse. Sit in a comfortable position, for example in a chair or in your car—when the latter the motor should be turned off. These are not meant to replace medical or veterinary advice. They are simply offering options to assist you in finding ways to be more at peace with yourself and to possibly create a happier, healthier relationship with others.

HOW TO CULTIVATE COMPASSION?

The website Greater Good explains that compassion isn't something you're born with or not. Instead, it can be strengthened through targeted exercises and practice. Compassion training programs, such as those out of Emory University and Stanford University, are revealing how we can boost feelings of compassion in ourselves and others. Here are some of the best tips to emerge out of those programs, as well as other research:

- Look for commonalities: Seeing yourself as similar to others increases feelings of compassion. A recent study shows that something as simple as tapping your fingers to the same rhythm with a stranger increases compassionate behavior.

- Calm your inner worrier: When we let our mind run wild with fear in response to someone else's pain ("What if that happens to me?"), we inhibit the biological systems that enable compassion. The practice of mindfulness can help us feel safer in these situations, facilitating compassion.

- Encourage cooperation, not competition, even through subtle cues: A seminal study showed that describing a game as a "Community Game" led players to cooperate and share a reward evenly; describing the same game as a "Wall Street Game" made the players more cutthroat and less honest. This is a valuable lesson for teachers, who can promote cooperative learning in the classroom.

- See people as individuals (not abstractions): When presented with an appeal from an anti-hunger charity, people were more likely to give money after reading about a starving girl than after reading statistics on starvation—even when those statistics were combined with the girl's story.

- Don't play the blame game: When we blame others for their misfortune, we feel less tenderness and concern toward them.

- Respect your inner hero: When we think we're capable of making a difference, we're less likely to curb our compassion.

- Notice and savor how good it feels to be compassionate. Studies have shown that practicing compassion and engaging in compassionate action bolsters brain activity in areas that signal reward.

- To cultivate compassion in kids, start by modeling kindness: Research suggests compassion is contagious, so if you want to help compassion spread in the next generation, lead by example.

- Curb inequality: Research suggests that as people feel a greater sense of status over others, they feel less compassion.

- Don't be a sponge: When we completely take on other people's suffering as our own, we risk feeling personally distressed, threatened, and overwhelmed; in some cases, this can even lead to burnout. Instead, try to be receptive to other people's feelings without adopting those feelings as your own.

Reprinted by permission from *Greater Good*:
(http://greatergood.berkeley.edu/topic/compassion/definition).

A Foundational Meditation Practice

Gently close your eyes.

Take in a slow deep breath through your nose, into your throat, chest, and abdomen.

Hold your breath in your abdomen for a comfortable brief moment.

When you are ready, gently exhale from your abdomen up your spine and out your mouth.

Repeat this breath three times.

With your next inhalation, visualize your breath as a pure, white, healing light that penetrates each and every cell.

With each slow exhalation, visualize any negative thoughts or emotions leaving your body through your mouth.

Repeat this visualization and breath three times.

With your next three breaths, as you visualize the in-breath as a white light, say to yourself, "May I be of benefit to all beings."

On the out-breath visualize loving, compassionate thoughts radiating out from you to all others.

As you finish, gently open your eyes, let out a gentle sigh, and when you are ready, may you be alert and calm in each moment as you enter your barn, stall, or wherever you are in time and space with your horse.

Blessing for the Well-Being of You and Your Horse

Sit in a comfortable position, in a chair or in your car, for example. Gently close your eyes.

Take in a slow deep breath through your nose, into your throat, chest, and abdomen.

Hold your breath in your abdomen for a comfortable brief moment.

When you are ready, gently exhale from your abdomen up your spine and out your mouth.

Repeat this breath three times.

Slowly and gently, with your next inhalation, visualize your breath as a pure white healing light that penetrates each and every cell.

With each slow exhalation, visualize any negative thoughts or emotions leaving your body through your mouth.

Repeat this visualization and breath three times.

With your next breath, slowly inhale and visualize your horse being calm, peaceful, and happy.

With your exhalation, visualize your horse being surrounded by a field of loving, peaceful energy.

Repeat this visualization and breath three times.

With your next slow inhalation, visualize you and your horse in an interconnected field of healing white light, sharing your ideal, happy, and safe moments together.

With your next slow exhalation, visualize that loving, kind interconnected field surrounding both of you and flowing between you.

As you finish, gently open your eyes, let out a gentle sigh, and when you are ready, may you begin your day with your horse alert and calm. May your heart and mind be clear and lucid.

Blessings for the Well-Being of You, Your Horse, and All Beings in Your Barn, Home, or at Events

Gently close your eyes.

Take in a slow, deep breath through your nose, into your throat, chest, and abdomen.

Hold your breath in your abdomen for a comfortable brief moment.

When you are ready, gently exhale from your abdomen up your spine and out your mouth.

Repeat this breath three times.

With your next inhalation, visualize your breath as a pure white healing light that penetrates each and every cell.

With each slow exhalation, visualize any negative thoughts or emotions leaving your body through your mouth.

Repeat this visualization and breath three times.

With your next slow inhalation, visualize that loving, compassionate, white, healing light permeating everyone in your barn or at your show or event.

Visualize all beings present enveloped in a kind, compassionate loving light-field.

With your next slow exhalation, visualize a white, loving light radiating out to everyone in your barn or at your show or event, filling them with kind, compassionate thoughts and feelings.

Repeat this visualization and breath three times.

May you and your horse be present in the moment, alert, happy, and calm.

May you and your horse enjoy each and every moment together.

As you finish, open your eyes, let out a gentle sigh, and when you are ready, may you begin your day being alert and calm. May your heart and mind be clear and lucid.

For You, Your Horse, All Beings You Meet Everywhere and All That Is

Gently close your eyes.

Take in a slow deep breath through your nose, into your throat, chest, and abdomen.

Hold your breath in your abdomen for a comfortable brief moment.

When you are ready, gently exhale from your abdomen, up your spine, and out your mouth.

Repeat this breath three times.

With your next slow inhalation, visualize the breath as a pure white, healing light that penetrates each and every cell in your body.

With each slow exhalation, visualize any negative thoughts or emotions leaving your body through your mouth.

Repeat this visualization and breath three times.

With your next slow inhalation, visualize that loving, compassionate, pure white, healing light permeating everyone, everywhere that you meet.

With your next slow exhalation, visualize that loving, compassionate, pure white, healing light radiating out to everyone, everywhere you go today, and filling them with kind, compassionate thoughts and feelings.

Repeat this visualization and breath three times.

May you and your horse be present in the moment, alert, happy, and calm.

May you and your horse enjoy each and every moment together.

As you finish, gently open your eyes, let out a gentle sigh, and when you are ready, may you begin your day with your heart and mind clear and lucid.

Enter your barn or wherever you are with your horse.

Join the movement toward a more compassionate world.

It has been a joy over the past few years to see the beneficial outcomes from the pioneering work of religious historian Karen Armstrong, who through her award-winning TED talks has developed the Charter for Compassion (charter-forcompassion.org). I would encourage all readers to visit the website and social feeds and consider joining the movement toward a more compassionate world. Because of Armstrong's work to begin a "compassion revolution," many universities and research institutions have supported recent studies of the science behind compassion. In the next chapter we'll review this science.

Let us create a paradigm shift by creating a prize for The Most Compassionate Equestrian at every level of horse show and competition, from Pony Club to the Olympics.

One of my visions for this book is that everyone who reads it supports the creation of a new ribbon or award at every horse show or sporting event. This award will be for The Most Compassionate Equestrian, and it is presented to the exhibitor who demonstrates compassionate training, compassionate care and treatment of his or her horse, and compassion for everyone on the competition grounds. By creating a ribbon for The Most Compassionate Equestrian, we begin to change the entire horse showing world, heart by heart.

We are all co-creating this journey. Each one of you can send photos to contribute to The Compassionate Equestrian blog and website, with a description of how you are integrating kindness, tolerance, and forgiveness into the care of your horse, and into the treatment of everyone you work with and meet in horse circles. We would like to create a Compassionate Equestrian "support system" to give us a way to percolate, process, and pass on our acts of gentleness and consideration, as well as check in with each other. By doing all of this—a ribbon, a social network, horse lovers explaining their connection to a Compassionate Equestrian lifestyle—we learn things, see what works for others, and spread our ideas for a more just, more humane, more civil horse industry.

First we study, then we experience, then we share. Thomas Merton, Trappist monk and author wrote, "The whole idea of compassion is based on a keen awareness of the interdependence of all these living beings, which are all part of one another, and all involved in one another."

WHY PRACTICE COMPASSION?

Better relationships. Better health. A more fulfilling life. The *Greater Good* website gives us many good reasons to practice compassion:

Scientific research into the measurable benefits of compassion is young. Preliminary findings suggest, however, that being compassionate can improve health, well-being, and relationships. Many scientists believe that compassion may even be vital to the survival of our species, and they're finding that its advantages can be increased through targeted exercises and practice. Here are some of the most exciting findings from this research so far.

- Compassion makes us feel good: Compassionate action activates pleasure circuits in the brain, and compassion training programs, even very brief ones, strengthen brain circuits for pleasure and reward and lead to lasting increases in self-reported happiness.

- Being compassionate—tuning in to other people in a kind and loving manner—can reduce risk of heart disease by boosting the positive effects of the Vagus Nerve, which helps to slow our heart rate.

- One compassion training program has found that it makes people more resilient to stress; it lowers stress hormones in the blood and saliva and strengthens the immune response.

- Brain scans during loving-kindness meditation, which directs compassion toward suffering, suggest that, on average, compassionate people's minds wander less about what has gone wrong in their lives, or might go wrong in the future; as a result, they're happier.

- Compassion helps make caring parents: Brain scans show that when people experience compassion, their brains activate in neural systems known to support parental nurturance and other caregiving behaviors.

- Compassion helps make better spouses: Compassionate people are more optimistic and supportive when communicating with others.

Continued ➡

(Cont.)

- Compassion helps make better friends: Studies of college friendships show that when one friend sets the goal to support the other compassionately, both friends experience greater satisfaction and growth in the relationship.

- Feeling compassion for one person makes us less vindictive toward others.

- Restraining feelings of compassion chips away at our commitment to moral principles.

- Employees who receive more compassion in their workplace see themselves, their co-workers, and their organization in a more positive light, report feeling more positive emotions like joy and contentment, and are more committed to their jobs.

- More compassionate societies—those that take care of their most vulnerable members, assist other nations in need, and have children who perform more acts of kindness—are the happier ones.

- Compassionate people are more socially adept, making them less vulnerable to loneliness; loneliness has been shown to cause stress and harm the immune system.

Reprinted by permission from Greater Good: (http://greatergood.berkeley.edu/topic/compassion/definition).

Questions to Consider

BASED ON PRINCIPLE 3

1   How can I integrate a minimum of 10 minutes of Quiet Focused Intention—compassionate mind training—into my daily routine?

2   How do I feel once I have integrated this 10-minute training into my life?

3   How do I see this impacting my horse, everyone at my barn and in my riding circle, and in the rest of my life?

CHAPTER FOUR

The Science in Support of Compassion

Compassionate Equitation is based on the latest in neuroscience and equitation science and the benefits of a compassionate brain and heart for all interactions.

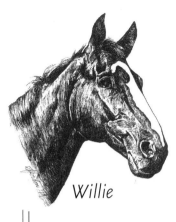

Willie

Susan Gordon:

Something had happened to Willie that caused him to almost completely shut down. What was going on in his head to make him behave as he did the day I first tried him? His expression was dull: eyes sullen, nose wrinkled, lackluster gaits. It was like he was someone affected by constant, long-term stress. When pushed past his comfort zone, he became aggressive and went into attack mode. Once he regained his strength, he attempted to pitch me off at the beginning of every ride. This went on for months, and I had to come up with a forgiving, yet firm and consistent method to handle him. Willie had obviously gotten away with bucking off quite a few riders—I was able to confirm this hunch when I met people who recognized him, through friends and at shows. Gradually, I was able to piece together his history. As the story went, he would dump his rider, and then get to leave the arena.

He had also been badly injured in a fall over a cross-country fence at an event in Florida, according to one woman, splitting his neck in a large wound from throatlatch to chest. It may have explained some of the lumpy scar tissue.

My evaluation, based on experience, told me his bucking probably originated with him being ridden while injured and hurting, and being forced to keep working through his pain until he had finally had enough.

Getting a horse like Willie to trust humans again and accept leadership is not easy. His brain and body had likely been flooded with stress-response chemicals so many times it would instantly switch to fight mode whenever he felt provoked. In humans this could be compared to a psychosis, which can include symptoms such as sudden changes in mood and behavior. It's possible that his perception of how he was going to be treated set off the extreme resistance. Fortunately, he had been so well started as a youngster his violent pitches went straight up and straight down, and I was able to stay in the saddle.

When I put my leg on to request that Willie go forward, he would quickly flip his powerful hindquarters almost vertically, kicking his right hind leg to the side. If he was still hurting, he certainly retained the ability to perform a very acrobatic move! For most horses this type of behavior does indicate pain, but I thought that if he had a rib out of alignment, or a sore back or withers, I would have generated some kind of reaction by grooming, tacking up, or scanning his acupressure points, as best as I had been taught to do. I had gotten no such indications from him, although the kicking out under saddle continued. A call to the vet to ensure that my assessment was right was the next step.

Even when it has been determined that a horse acting out like Willie is not hurting at the time you are riding him, if he has memories of pain, you have to make sure you are not creating a scenario that makes him think he is experiencing the actual pain all over again. This was a classic example of the complex decisions a trainer has to make when determining the causes of training or behavior problems and reschooling a horse's body and mind. The fact that Willie also turned and charged me when on the longe line or in the round pen added to my assessment of his aggression-related issues. In those instances, there was no equipment on him that might have been causing soreness in pressure-sensitive areas, so it appeared the aggression was more related to memories that had been triggered by a particular level of activity, or possibly by the activity and visual cues of a nearby proximity to jumps and a dressage arena.

Given my experience with previous reschooling projects, I could tell Willie had been previously whipped and spurred and jerked on simultaneously. It is a tactic typically based in fearful riding, and it makes horses very angry and confused. To resolve the problems embedded in a horse that has been ridden this way, timing is critical so as to make the associated aid the issue and not create an additional problem by mis-timing the correction. Every time Willie pitched I would drop the reins and tap behind my leg with the dressage whip to reinforce the leg aid that he wasn't correctly responding to. The tap was absolutely not intended to hurt him, but a single flip of the wrist sends the signal through the "artificial aid" right at your boot's contact with the horse's side, reminding him that "leg means go forward." He knew precisely what was wanted of him with the leg aids, but something in his mind reacted with a blatant, "No." And I knew he was sound enough that the "No" part didn't match with the level of resistance.

I didn't attach emotion to the request, but repeated my response every time Willie kicked out, until he went forward. I was still waiting for him to simply move off into an active walk without the effort he put into pitching, as he was actually building muscle and becoming more supple, leading me to continue thinking much of this behavior was related to painful memories, plus the fact that he had been able to relieve himself of riders in the past, and not his present physical condition. Then one day, it happened.

We had the usual start to the ride. Leg. Pitch. Tap. Leg. Pitch. Tap. I left my reins loose, always providing the "open door," even if it was at a dead run. I *didn't care what he did, so long as it was forward and not upward. I had to get through Willie's barrier caused by long-term stress, and "change his brain" to cue a new response. Keeping him out of the riding arena and letting him face a big open field was one tactic I used to solve the problem. All of a sudden, Willie took off across the pasture at a gallop. Surprised, I came up into two-point position and let him go. I let him gallop as fast and as far as he wanted. His ears pricked. I gave him a hearty scratch on the neck and a lot of, "Good boys!" He ran across the pasture, through the water jump (he loved the water jump), into the arena, and we had a lovely ride.*

That was the last time he planted his front feet at the beginning of a ride, refusing to take a step forward. Something in his mind had finally been freed. I would love to know exactly what changed that day. Did the effect of his long-term stress finally dissipate? Was his state one of euphoria? Was it a permanent result? All I knew at the time was that we'd had a major breakthrough and could finally have a lot more fun together. Challenge Number One with Willie had ended, reaffirming my feelings about at least part of the reason behind his bucking. It appeared my hunch concerning his behavior was actually related to how he had been ridden in the past. Even though I had always given Willie an invitation via loose reins, he did not accept that as an opportunity to go forward, until one day the concept clicked, and off he went.

It was as though his behavior had now been "reframed," much like human behavior following trauma is reframed around an inciting experience. Willie had become completely resistant to the leg either with or without the presence of a dressage whip. While many would say, "Forget the whip," he would "plant his feet and pitch" regardless. I brought in the extra tool, figuring that was part of the situation that incited the original behavior, which had become compulsive. You repeat the triggered sensation with predetermined variables in order to enact a different response. In this case, it was loose reins and a single, precisely-timed tap. When desensitized to the fact that neither the leg nor the whip was going to make him hurt and further confused, he "let go" of the block, and we never had to go back to that situation again. There are likely other methods for working with a horse that is "stuck" in a mental scenario such as Willie was, but at the time, this technique ended up being successful for both of us. Of course, it would really be ideal to never have to reschool any horse or reenact these kinds of triggers.

The benefits and practices of compassion and *Equitation Science* (defined on www.equitationscience.com as an objective, evidence-based understanding of the welfare of horses during training and competition by *applying valid, quantitative scientific methods that can identify what training techniques are ineffective or may result in equine suffering*) are complementary and practical when applied to both horses and humans.[1] Principle 4 correlates the compassionate brain and heart with the qualities of correct riding and training techniques that use research to determine what does and does not cause distress in a horse. We have defined compassion and determined the beneficial effects of a foundation in compassion to be established in the human being, and the necessity of treating animals as we ourselves would wish to be treated. Being attentive to current studies regarding the mechanisms responsible for compassion, and merging that information with equitation scientists' findings about sentience in horses, it is possible to determine how science is supportive of learning to ride and train to the best of our abilities *and* in consideration of the horse's welfare. We have the capacity to self-regulate and approach our horses with a positive state of mind.

> *According to the International Society for Equitation Science (ISES) website (www.equitationscience.com), equitation science promotes an objective, evidence-based understanding of the welfare of horses during training and competition by applying valid, quantitative scientific methods that can identify what training techniques are ineffective or may result in equine suffering. Equitation science uses a multidisciplinary approach to explain horse training, for example from a learning theory perspective that removes anthropomorphism and emotiveness.*

When we talk about bonding with an animal—especially with a horse, as we sit on his back and direct his movement—all our thoughts, moods, and emotional responses translate into signals. Sometimes these signals are almost imperceptible, yet the horse, being as sensitive as he is, will register those subtleties at a level that is often more finely tuned than our own. If the horse has experienced trauma, and possibly has "blocks," such as Willie's, it is the consistent state of mind and non-emotional, but necessary, repetitive actions on our part that will help him recover and reconnect with more positive, natural behavior.

Stressed or happy? There is a chemical basis for feelings and emotions.

Horses have most of the same mechanisms in their bodies responsible for emotional responses as human do. Understanding this, it stands to reason that we can connect the process of neurotransmitters and the role they play in the basic, instinctual behaviors of both species.[2] The barrier to clear communication between humans and horses is that of language, and it seems possible to bridge that gap as well, as seasoned horsepeople will attest to having "learned by osmosis" or having been with horses long enough to have the capacity to interpret their form of conveying information.

2

It's amazing to think of our glands, organs, tissues and cells as storage places for emotion and memory, yet this was given explanation through the scientific research of Dr. Candace Pert, a neuropharmacologist who worked at the NIH and Georgetown University Medical Center. Dr. Pert famously stated, "Your body is your subconscious mind. Our physical body can be changed by the emotions we experience" (http://candacep-ert.com/where--do--you--store--your--emotions/).

Humans and other living beings are a mass of chemicals that are somehow infused with life and the ability to think. The horse has a cerebral cortex, and we have a cerebral cortex. We have the same senses, and many physical parts that have the same names. With such similarities, how could we *not* notice and respond to horses in much the same way we do with other humans?

Besides the mental and emotional connection we have with horses, our physical touch, especially when grooming, has a distinct impact on the chemical processes relating to sensory pleasure experienced by the horse. And think about how delightful it is when you receive a soothing massage or loving touch from your human partner. When horses mutually groom each other, using their teeth to scratch around the withers and neck, they release *beta-endorphin*, a brain chemical that causes relaxation and promotes a feeling of well-being. Some horses love to be curried, and the same kind of pleasure-response may be generated as you give your horse a thorough grooming. You can always tell by his expressions—how he stretches his neck and curls his lip when he is enjoying your touch.

Horses have pressure-sensitive points on their body, just as humans do. Excessive pressure on certain areas can create the release of pain and stress chemicals—exactly the opposite of what pleasurable touch produces. This can cause the horse to associate the equipment or the rider with that pain, and create memories that remain long after the cause of the pressure is removed.

THE IMPACTS OF STRESS VS.
PLEASURE/LOVE/COMPASSION

According to an article by Salam Ranabir and K. Reetu in *The Indian Journal of Endocrinology and Metabolism* (2011), in the modern environment we are exposed to various stressful conditions. "Stress can lead to changes in the serum level of many hormones, including glucocorticoids, catecholamines, growth hormone, and prolactin," the authors write. "Some of these changes are necessary for the fight or flight response to protect oneself. Some of these stressful responses can lead to endocrine disorders. Stress can also alter the clinical status of many preexisting endocrine disorders."

Compare this to the findings of Tobias Esch and George B. Stefano, who wrote "The neurobiological link between compassion and love" in *The Medical Science Monitor* (March, 2011). "Love and compassion exert pleasant feelings and rewarding effects," say Esch and Stefano. "Besides their emotional role and capacity to govern behavior, appetitive motivation, and a general 'positive state,' even 'spiritual' at times, the behaviors shown in love and compassion clearly rely on neurobiological mechanisms and underlying molecular principles. These processes and pathways involve the brain's limbic motivation and reward circuits, that is, a finely tuned and profound autoregulation. This capacity to self-regulate emotions, approach behaviors and even pair bonding, as well as social contact in general, i.e., love, attachment and compassion, can be highly effective in stress reduction, survival and overall health."

I believe Willie's resistance was due to his memories and a firm belief that the moment a rider mounted he would face excessive, uncomfortable pressure. The horse's response to physical pressure is indicative of how the horse is feeling, which is of concern to the rider, and can be useful in helping make decisions that support the horse's well-being. This includes being aware of weight in excess of the horse's carrying capacity, poorly fitted tack, and misuse of aids, all of which could contribute to the release of stress-hormones in the horse's body.[3,4,5] Consistently causing uncomfortable physical pressure to the horse ultimately results in long-term stress effects—such as those exhibited by Willie—that are directly related to the release of *cortisol, epinephrine (adrenalin)* and *norepinephrine*. A repeated state of stress wears down a body's defenses, and chronic ailments, such as depression and agitation can occur. According to "Need to Know: How Stress Affects a Horse's General Health" provided by the Alberta SPCA (2013), "Stress can cause health issues in horses. However, stress can often be identified and controlled. Stress will trigger a 'fight or flight' reaction, caused by the release of the cortisol hormone. Frequent release of cortisol can affect the horse's digestive, reproductive, immune and cardiovascular systems, and can cause diarrhea, gastric ulcers and colic. It can also affect the horse's behavior."

3,4,5

In "How Much Weight Can a Horse Carry?" on www.horsesciencenews. com Liz Osborn writes, "When carrying 15 and 20% of their body weight, the horses showed relatively little indication of stress. It's when they were packing weights of 25% that physical signs changed markedly, and these became accentuated under 30% loads. The horses had noticeably faster breathing and higher heart rates when carrying tack and rider amounting to 25% or more of their body weight. A day after trotting and cantering with the heftier weights, the horses' muscles showed substantially greater soreness and tightness. Those horses that were least sore from the exercise had wider loins, the part of a horse's back located between their last rib and croup" (www.horsesciencenews.com/horseback-riding/how-much-weight-can-a-horse-carry.php).

The 2008 article in the Journal of Equine Veterinary Science *by Debra Powell, MS, PhD, et al, explains further: "Muscle soreness and muscle tightness scores were determined using a subjective scoring system 24 hours before and 24 hours after exercise. Heart rates remained significantly higher when the horses carried 25 and 30% of their body weight. Plasma lactate concentrations immediately and 10 minutes after exercise differed when horses carried 30% of their body weight compared with 15, 20, and 25% weight carriage. Horses tended to have a greater change in muscle soreness and muscle tightness when carrying 25% of their body weight, and a significant change in soreness and tightness scores was found in horses carrying 30% of their body weight" (http://www.j-evs.com/article/S0737-0806(07)00413-3/abstract).*

According to the Fédération Equestre Internationale (FEI) Code of Conduct for the Welfare of the Horse, welfare must take precedence over all other demands at all stages during the preparation and training of competition horses. This includes good horse management, training methods, farrier and tack, and transportation, as well as encompassing the use of medication, surgical procedures that threaten welfare or safety, and the misuse of aids (http://www.feicleansport.org/welfare.html).

Put some "pressure" on yourself to help gain a more effective understanding of the horse's biomechanics and responses to exercise.

I noticed a marked difference in the results my students were obtaining from their horses after we began a twice-weekly Pilates class. We would ride in the morning, then the Pilates instructor would come to the barn in the afternoon. We put yoga mats on top of saddle blankets and went through an intense core workout with lots of active stretching and appropriate breathing techniques. It took about two months, but then aids such as half-halts that previously just weren't coordinating correctly suddenly became *really* effective. Riders increased suppleness in their hips, were able to maintain a taller, more elegant position in the saddle and the horses became lighter in their frames. It was exciting to see the changes in almost everyone who took the classes—they looked and felt more confident—and had a very positive influence on their horses.

A controlled, educated seat can remain in balance and follow the horse's movement through more effective timing and coordination of aids. This allows for more freedom in the horse's gaits and results in less pressure on the horse's back. When a horse can move freely and without discomfort, he is much happier. It is wonderful when horses respond as though they have had a massage by the time you finish a workout! Even if they are tired, they are happy and relaxed with no visible signs of stress. It is nice to have pleasure-related chemicals flooding the horse's brain and body by the time you leave the arena, much like the feeling a human athlete has following a productive workout combined with a proper cool-down using appropriate recovery techniques. You can still periodically push the horse to his physical limits during a workout, and you actually *have* to do so sometimes to reach a sufficient level of development, but the reward comes when you drop those reins, back off the intensity, and the horse immediately offers you a relaxed, swinging back and a long, loose frame, releasing any tension that has accumulated.

Riding with a light, following seat (the rider's seat bones are not fully weighted in the saddle, made possible by the correct alignment of shoulders, hips, and heels, and a relaxed, supple back) has been found to be most conducive to

Mounting with Intention

One of the purposes of yoga is to cultivate compassion and feel empathically for others. We want to become gentle and soft in our connections, finding peace and serenity. The beginning of a ride offers the perfect chance to practice a bit of yoga, extending the QFI meditation exercise you began before interacting with your horse (see pp. 70–73 for sample Guided Meditations).

Tadasana, or Mountain Pose, is usually the starting position for all standing poses. It is a posture-toning position and brings you into full body awareness just before mounting your horse. This exercise is an adaptation, since your partner—your horse—is standing with you for the duration. If you are new to yoga, you may want to practice *Tadasana* without your horse at first. This also assumes your horse is patient enough to stand for mounting. If he isn't, perhaps becoming more mindful of your mounting practices will be helpful. This exercise will help you become aware of your breath and movement, and how you could be affecting your horse. Watch for subtle changes in your horse's breathing and posture as you go.

With practice, this will become a fluid and simple exercise, taking no more than a few breaths to complete.

1   Bring your horse to the mounting block (using a mounting block helps prevents "torque" on the saddle and unnecessary pressure on the horse's back when mounting) and stand on the block, facing the saddle as you normally would prior to mounting. Keep your reins in your left hand with the excess over the horse's neck to the off side. Your toes are pointing forward, heels slightly apart, weight evenly distributed.

2   Firm your thigh muscles and lift your kneecaps slightly, then lift your inner ankles to help strengthen the arches of your feet. Imagine a column of energy flowing upward along your inner thighs, continuing through your body and out through the crown of your head. Turn your thighs slightly inward. Lengthen your tailbone toward the ground.

3   Push your shoulder blades into your back, then widen them across your back and release. Lift your sternum without pushing your ribs forward. Widen

your collarbones and relax your arms. If your horse moves, gently apply the reins to stop him or reposition him and begin again if he has stepped away from the block.

4   Balance your head directly over your pelvis, with the underside of your chin parallel to the ground, and keep your throat soft. Soften your eyes. Take a deep breath, feeling your abdomen expand with the inhale.

5   Mount correctly from the block according to the type of saddle you are using, lowering yourself slowly and lightly onto the horse's back. Maintain the good posture you've just established, take another deep breath, and begin your ride, grateful for the experience and time you are spending with your horse.

maintaining a sound, healthy back in the horse. This is actually very reflective of yogic practice, as a correct seat requires focus, balance, symmetry, and good control of both body and mind, as does many forms of yoga. You will feel better physically and mentally riding in this way, as will your horse.

New research provided by organizations such as the International Society for Equitation Science is leading to a clearer picture of what causes stress to horses and what doesn't. Researchers are investigating exactly how the interactions of tack, pressure, and riding techniques affect horses' levels of comfort and their ability to focus on what's being asked of them. If you have ever tried to perform a task while in pain, not only does it affect your mood, but also the capacity of the rest of your body to respond as well as it would if it were pain-free. There is no reason why horses would be any different under the circumstances.[6] Utilizing this valuable data will help us determine if the choices we make for our horses are, in fact, compassionate ones.

In HIPPOH (Horse Industry Professionals Protecting Our Horses) "Naked Truth" symposiums, attendees are taught how to develop their abilities to listen to and understand what their horses are trying to tell them, particularly when it comes to pain or discomfort manifested as behavior or performance issues. HIPPOH is "a global network of equine professionals dedicated to providing trustworthy information based on science, research, and years of experience to keep your horse safe, sound, and sane. The emphasis is on helping horse owners build their 'Circle of Influence,'

6

which consists of united equine professionals who understand that the best care for your horse involves the cooperation and collaboration of every equine professional who tends to your horse. This involves your veterinarian, farrier, saddle fitter, trainer and body workers—it is important they work together to supply a total whole horse approach." Educational resources include online videos and live symposiums. Check out www. hippohfoundation.org.

Dr. Allen Schoen:

In *The Art of Happiness: A Handbook for Living* (Hodder, 1998), the Dalai Lama says, "The systematic training of the mind, the cultivation of happiness, the genuine inner transformation by deliberately selecting and focusing on positive mental states and challenging negative mental states—is possible because of the very structure and function of the brain."

Current research in neuroscience indicates that when you focus on compassion during meditation, areas of the prefrontal cortex—the part of the brain responsible for personality, decision-making and social behavior—light up with activity. Even after 10 minutes a day for two weeks, people develop more compassion as a result of their meditation practice.[7]

Led by world-renowned neuroscientist Dr. Richard J. Davidson, the Center for Investigating Healthy Minds is located at the Waisman Center, University of Wisconsin-Madison. The Center's founding in 2008 marked a personal and professional triumph for Dr. Davidson, who in 1992 had been challenged by His Holiness, the 14th Dalai Lama, to use science to study positive qualities of mind. Dr. Davidson has since devoted his life to uncovering scientific discoveries that can help people live happier, healthier lives through mental skills training (www.investigatinghealthyminds.org).

In the July 2013 issue of *Psychological Science*, Helen Weng, et al, published the article "Compassion training alters altruism and neural responses to suffering," describing the first study to investigate whether training adults in compassion can result in greater altruistic behavior and related changes in neural systems underlying compassion. Compassion training was compared to a control group that learned cognitive reappraisal, a technique where people learn to reframe their thoughts to feel less negative. Both groups listened to guided audio instructions over the Internet for 30 minutes per day for two weeks. Researchers found that people trained in compassion were more likely to spend their own money altruistically to help someone who was treated unfairly than those who were trained in cognitive reappraisal. The researchers measured how much brain activity had changed from the beginning to the end of the training, and found that the people who were the most altruistic after compassion training were the ones who showed the most brain changes when viewing human suffering. They found that activity was increased in the inferior parietal cortex, a region involved in empathy and understanding others. Compassion training also increased activity in the dorsolateral prefrontal cortex and the extent to which it communicated with the nucleus accumbens, brain regions involved in emotion regulation and positive emotions. Compassion, like physical and academic skills, appears to be something that is not fixed, but rather can be enhanced with training and practice.

As touched on in the previous chapter, a foundation of proposed contemplative quiet time (QFI) prior to interacting with all people and animals is fundamental to the development of the Compassionate Equestrian. We've described ways to create a program of meditative practice that focuses the intention of, "May I be awake and compassionate to all beings here, including myself so that I can be of benefit to all." When people bring this intention to their simple meditative practice, they "wire what they fire" (see p. 47). The more of that intention they "fire" the more easily the related neural pathways become wired as a program in their brains. This is the way the intention becomes a pattern and the pattern becomes habit.

This process applies to the good, the bad, and the ugly of our habits. For example, if you are "firing" anger, short-temperedness, or irritability much of the time, then that is what you "become." If you consciously choose to focus and "fire" mindfulness, attentiveness, and compassion, along with intentions of tolerance and humane action, then that is what your mind creates. We *become* and *act out* our repeated thoughts and emotions. And, the way you are with other beings is the way they will begin to interact with you. The characteristic of *mirror neurons*—neurons that fire both when you act *and* when you observe the action performed by another—is that people start mirroring behaviors back, so it can become a very positive cycle, or potentially a negative one.[8]

8

In "The Mind's Mirror," Lea Winerman's American Psychological Asso-ciation Monitor on Psychology *October 2005 cover story, what was then a "new" type of neuron—called a mirror neuron—was said to potentially help explain how we learn through mimicry and why we empathize with others. Neuroscientist Giacomo Rizzolatti, MD, who with his colleagues at the University of Parma in Parma, Italy, first identified mirror neurons, said they made it possible to begin to understand how and why we "read" other people's minds and feel empathy for them. If watching an action and performing that action can activate the same parts of the brain in monkeys, then it makes sense that it could also elicit the same feelings in people (http://www.apa.org/monitor/oct05/mirror.aspx).*

From what I understand, much of our neural substrate is similar in most species.

It does not seem unreasonable for us to assume horses have mirror neurons, too. That would explain how foals *imprint* from their mothers, as well as how horses commonly imprint behaviors. If we *do* have an appreciation for mirror neurons in the horse, and if the horse senses *we* are being compassionate, then we need to believe that horses can *also* demonstrate compassion. Likewise, where destruc-tive emotions are present, we can presume they will be mimicked back, as well.

In addition, the horse's amygdala, being that of a prey animal, reacts from fear. If a horse has had negative experiences with one person, let's say a guy with a beard, he will extrapolate that experience to *any* guy with a beard and may react defensively. That defense can mean avoidance, resistance, or it can mean *attack*. Simply put, the fight or flight mechanism can generalize, characterizing one experience as similar to another, and then repeat related behavior.

Considering the impact our own behavior has on the horse, it is not unreasonable to consider that some destructive behaviors in horses may stem from what I call the mirror neuron effect.

I suspect that some destructive behaviors in horses are caused by our own destructive emotions, reflected via the *mirror neuron effect*. When owners and trainers and riders are irritable and angry, then the grooms are, too, and every-one is quite rough with the horses. Then the horses are angry and defensive, and they become more dangerous and protective of themselves because they are prey animals. All of this snowballs into an avalanche of negativity. The flip side of this is that the mirror neuron effect applies to *constructive* behaviors as well. When constructive behaviors have developed through interactions with a compassionate veterinarian, trainer, barn manager, and staff we can see the difference it makes in horses, from the top down. In such a barn, *every being* is compassionate, as one positive behavior ripples into the next.

SUBSTANCE ABUSE AND ITS IMPACT ON THE HORSE INDUSTRY

Susan and I have a common voice on this issue as we have both experienced situations in barns and at shows where people affect others and their horses as a result of the use and abuse of alcohol and other drugs.

Unfortunately it is not uncommon to see horse people who have a problem with alcohol and/or other drugs. This makes it difficult to create a positive environment. Horses are confused by the unpredictable and aggravated behaviors of people under the influence of psychoactive substances (which can include not only alcohol, but illegal drugs and legally prescribed medications that are used inappropriately). The horses then react to these behaviors.

This becomes a matter of recognizing the neuroscience of how alcohol and other drugs affect the human brain, understanding those patterns, as well as how they in turn affect the horse. This is not about judgment. This is reality. In some percentage of the horse world, substance abuse issues impact behavior of both humans and horses, especially in competitive circles, and unfortunately they go largely unaddressed.

One of our hopes with the 25 Principles of Compassionate Equitation is to make people aware that if they *do* have trouble controlling their interaction with alcohol and/or other drugs, they might consider, first of all, to be honest and compassionate toward themselves and admit to their problem with substances. The first step is having people recognize they have an issue.

Continued →

(Cont.)

Second, there must be recognition that substance addictions can result in a lack of attentiveness, mindfulness, compassion, and empathy toward themselves, other people, and their horses, as well exacerbating impulse-control disorders. When horses are pushed in order to "qualify" or to "win at all costs," it may be due to personality and behavior that has been modified by alcohol or drug consumption. Under the influence, riders or trainers may also be verbally abusive to students and staff.

The equestrian show world—like other competitive realms—tends to be driven by ego and the desire for success. Healthy egoic tendencies are not necessarily destructive and may have many self-esteem-building benefits. However, tendencies that may in fact hurt others, as well as the use of psychoactive substances can fuel a negative form of competitiveness that needs to be acknowledged and understood. *Everyone* suffers when addiction is a problem, including the horses.

The third step after recognizing there may be an issue and its effect on all interactions is finding appropriate, professional health care to help resolve the problem, enabling the person suffering from addiction to lead a healthier, more attentive, lucid, and happier life.

As those committed to the 25 Principles of Compassionate Equitation must remember, even at the worst of times, it is important to show compassion to those who have a problem with substance abuse. This can be a very challenging situation for everyone involved. Please seek professional help if you, or someone you know, appears to have an alcohol or other drug addiction issue.

Neuroscience is revealing what destructive emotions and addictions do to our minds.

As we can become addicted to alcohol, drugs, food, and other sources of stimulation, we also can become addicted to behaviors that create inner stress. *Chronic stress can create an adrenaline addiction.* Are you always running 5 or 10 minutes late, or more? This can actually create a subconscious addiction to an "adrenaline rush." We "self-medicate" by creating situations—like being chronically late—to keep stimulating our stress hormones, such as adrenaline and cortisol. A chronic release of cortisol bathes the neurons in our brains, causing a "brain fog," an actual inability to think clearly, decreasing our ability to make decisions. Some postulate that this chronic bathing of neurons in cortisol may possibly be one cause of dementia and cause further nerve degeneration. This can eventually result in adrenal burnout, chronic fatigue, and exhaustion.[9]

> *The National Institute of Mental Health (NIMH) July 2014 Science Update "How Might New Neurons Buffer Against Stress?" discusses studies run by Dr. Heather Cameron, Chief of Neuroplasticity at NIMH, in which her team of researchers inhibited the development of new neurons in mice. These mice were prone to stress-related behavior and prolonged increases in stress-hormone levels (www.nimh.nih.gov/news/ science-news/2014/how-might-new-neurons-buffer-against-stress.shtml).*

Early in my veterinary career I was taking additional training in mind-body medicine and working the "graveyard shift" in an emergency clinic once a month. I realized I tended to be 5 to 10 minutes late for everything, inadvertently creating spurts of adrenaline release, and that in many ways it was *this* that was keeping me going. I reflected on my veterinary journey up to that point and realized that my "adrenaline habit" was not healthy. I began to retrain myself, actually trying my best to be early or at least on time. While I felt I was for the most part "healthy"—I did not drink or smoke or have any other addictions—I did not completely appreciate how unhealthy that adrenaline addiction of tending to be late was. Experience turns knowledge into wisdom, and I eventually began to look at how to manage stress better in my life overall. Since then, I have done better at times and then experienced the contrast at others. I just constantly remind myself that I will have another opportunity to rebalance my work with the rest of my life.

It all comes back to energy fields.

If this resonates with you at all, perhaps this is an invitation to explore your own work-life balance. I find that when you have many interests in many different areas, as I do, that you must continually readjust this balance. It does not seem like the biological term *homeostasis* (a state of balance) is quite accurate—instead perhaps *homeodynamics* is more appropriate, whereby there is a continuous change and constant activity. As we have already learned, we need to be compassionate to ourselves as well as others. By allowing ourselves work-life balance, we have the ability to create a calm, smooth flowing, centered energetic field within us, around us, and surrounding everyone nearby.

According to the Transpecies Field Theory we create an energetic, electromagnetic field with all the other beings we are around (see p. 7). What's radiating from our hearts is impacting our horses' hearts and minds. We can create a healthy field of compassion, awareness, and mindfulness, and the horses will respond. The Institute of HeartMath Director of Research, Rollin McCraty, writes: "The heart is a sensory organ and acts as a sophisticated information encoding and processing center that enables it to learn, remember, and make independent functional decisions."[10]

The heart, like the brain, generates a powerful electromagnetic field, Institute of HeartMath Director of Research, Rollin McCraty explains. "The heart generates the largest electromagnetic field in the body. The electrical field as measured in an electrocardiogram (ECG) is about 60 times greater in amplitude than the brain waves recorded in an electroencephalogram (EEG)." HeartMath studies show this powerful electromagnetic field can be detected and measured several feet away from a person's body and between two individuals in close proximity (http://www.heartmath.org/free-services/articles-of-the-heart/energetic-heart-is-unfolding.html).

The neuroscience of the human-animal bond addiction offers another interesting perspective. What happens when people ask themselves, "Why am I choosing to be with a horse?"

If horses can be a vehicle to the opening of consciousness, part of the process is asking *why* you have a horse. The reasons may be all good and noble, so asking the question may simply be an affirmation of your intentions. This is a very deep question due to the potential addiction and control factors involved with the ownership of an animal. Sometimes the need is due to a "lack of love," as seen with the "hoarding" of small animals. It is as though there is never enough of anything you desire. You are trying to fill an empty hole with something from the outside. When this is the case, if you do not work on loving yourself, then there is never going to be enough, even with one horse or several horses.

Some researchers suggest that animal hoarding can be better understood using an addictions-based model, as these individuals share many characteristics with substance abusers, including: a preoccupation with animals, denial of a problem, excuses for their behavior, claims of persecution, and neglect of personal and environmental conditions.[11,12]

In the article "Animal Hoarding: Structuring Interdisciplinary Responses to Help People, Animals and Communities at Risk" on the Cummings School of Veterinary Medicine at Tufts University website (edited by Gary Patronek, et al, 2006), animal hoarding is described as a misunderstood and under-recognized community problem that is responsible for substantial animal suffering and property damage. "Often associated with adult self-neglect, animal hoarding can also place children, elders, and dependent adults at serious risk and can be an economic burden to taxpayers" (http://vet.tufts.edu/hoarding/pubs/AngellReport.pdf).

Amanda Reinisch's "Understanding the Human Aspects of Animal Hoarding" (The Canadian Veterinary Journal, 2008) defines an animal hoarder as someone who has accumulated a large number of animals and who: 1) fails to provide minimal standards of nutrition, sanitation, and veterinary care; 2) fails to act on the deteriorating condition of the animals (including disease, starvation, or death) and the environment (severe overcrowding, extremely unsanitary conditions); and often, 3) is unaware of the negative effects of the collection on their own health and well-being and on that of other family members (http://www.ncbi.nlm.nih.gov/pmc/articles/PMC2583418/).

If you own or ride horses strictly to compete, you may realize there may never be enough ribbons, because to you, the ribbons likely equate with love and attention, as well as satisfying the ego. Even if you don't show, attachment to a horse may also indicate unhealthy attachments to other material goods, or another person, for example, and the possibility that you are acting out all the same emotional issues with your horse. This, again, is an opportunity to really look at yourself and ask if there is something that needs to be healed. Many people do own horses for the *right* reasons and theirs is not an unhealthy form of attachment. Some people in the horse world, however, choose to have horses for the unhealthy reasons, which affects both the horses and themselves.

What are your feelings and emotions behind your desire for receiving unconditional love from your horse?

Perhaps you truly do love your horse, and you want to give him a good home, and you provide him his best chances to stay sound and healthy—and you do all this *unconditionally*. That is absolutely great, *but* here again is another opportunity to reflect and ask yourself: If you want to give the horse unconditional love and you think of the horse as an extension of yourself, could it be that it is *you* who desires to receive unconditional love? There is nothing wrong with this, but there is strength to be found in awareness.

If your horse is a rescue horse, and you think, "I want to rescue this horse," could it be that one part of you is thinking, "I want to be rescued?" With everything you say or think about your horse, play a little mind game and reflect it back on yourself. Some people believe that the whole world is a projection of each individual's own inner mental screen, so perhaps taking the opportunity to ask yourself, "Why do I want a horse?" can help you identify and project a compassionate "reality." Make an exercise of it by writing it all down.

Your horse can be a reflection of your inner self. It can be a valuable and productive exercise to look into your mirror for answers.

Replace the horse in the questions you just asked yourself...with *you*. Ask, "Why do I want *me* in my life?" Is it for unconditional love? Can you be everything to yourself that you wish to give your horse? It is when you have fulfilled all your desires and needs from a source inside yourself that your neural wiring changes, and you realize you have everything you need *within*. From this new place of awareness, you will see you do not *need* anything from your horse. You can simply *be* with him. He is, after all, just a reflection of *you*.

I believe in the *hundredth monkey effect*, where a new behavior or idea spreads rapidly when a critical number acknowledge it. I have seen it happen firsthand with acupuncture and natural medicine. Back in the 1980s, once a core number of people saw my (then) unique approach combining acupuncture and chiropractic with musculoskeletal alignment, and they noticed horses getting better with as few as one treatment, word spread quickly through the horse world, and everyone wanted my services. And so, I believe that once a critical number of people know why they have horses in their lives, and can treat them as they would compassionately treat themselves and other humans, everyone will want

The Horse as Your Reflection

Ask yourself:

"What's the most compassionate way to be with myself?"

"Do I want to push myself physically until my tendons and joints are so sore they need to be injected with steroids?"

"Do I want to lock myself up alone in a tiny room with one high barred window?"

Now remember that your horse may be a reflection of you. Treat him as you would choose to treat yourself.

to mirror that behavior and before long, every barn will want to be known as a Compassionate Barn and every trainer will want to be a Compassionate Trainer. This movement may stimulate more people involved with the horse business to look at their own personal "baggage" and destructive neural imprints, and choose to become involved in positive personal growth programs or to seek professional health care support. To me, as a veterinarian who wishes to help and heal all beings, I believe this process of acknowledging which areas of one's self may benefit from exploration to be an important key.

One Health: We are exquisitely and elaborately connected, and we must address our own health, the health of our animals, and the health of our planet as if this is so.

In veterinary medicine, and medicine in general these days, there is much discussion of a *One Health Approach*. According to the American Veterinary Medical Association (AVMA) One Health Initiative Task Force: Final Report (2008), the term *One Health* is defined as the collaborative efforts of multiple disciplines, working locally, nationally, and globally, to attain optimal health for people, animals, and our environment. "Achieving the end point of One Health is truly one of the critical challenges facing humankind today," the Report says. "The convergence

SCIENCE AS PART OF POSITIVE CHANGE

In some parts of the world there are signs of positive change in the care of horses with the enactment of ever-evolving standards of equine welfare. In 2002, the *Equine Welfare Compendium* was first published by the National Equine Welfare Council in the UK and has since been regularly updated. The entire document and current information can be found at: www.newc.co.uk.

In addition, Equine Canada ("the dedicated national voice working to serve, promote, and protect the interests of horses and Canada's equestrian community") released "The Code of Practice for the Care and Handling of Equines" in 2013. The entire broad spectrum of equine care is covered: shelter, feed, freedom of movement, companionship, veterinary care, emergency preparedness, hoof care, and end-of-life considerations. One of the key features of the Code's development process is the Scientific Committee. It is widely accepted by stakeholders that animal welfare codes should take advantage of the most current and best available scientific research.

of people, animals, and our environment has created a new dynamic in which the health of each group is inextricably interconnected....We need to adopt an integrated, holistic approach that reflects both our profound interdependence and the realization that we are part of a larger ecological system—exquisitely and elaborately connected."

I believe the foundation for a *One Health Approach* needs to be based on creating healthy minds, hearts, thoughts, and emotions based on the Charter for Compassion and a compassion-based decision process, as we have already discussed in this book. The interconnectedness of One Health for humans, animals, and the environment supports and is supported by the Transpecies Field Theory (see p. 7).

We are beginning to see others exhibit this belief, as well: some veterinary schools and medical schools are offering training in mindfulness and mindfulness-based stress reduction (MBSR) to students as part of their curriculum. The idea is to produce veterinarians and doctors who can address both physical health and emotional well-being.

The concept of compassion is often challenging to champion successfully because people have different perceptions of what compassion is.

Nowadays, as I make my rounds to various barns, I discuss the 25 Principles of Compassionate Equitation with clients and others, and I see that so many people can identify where they *already are* compassionate in their lives. This is quite hopeful: when compassion is brought to your attention, then you can begin to nurture the habit more in your heart and mind.

In addition, I am fascinated by the many views individuals have regarding what they consider to be *compassionate*. What compassion *is* differs for every person because it is understood through his or her "filters" of life experience. It is unique to almost every individual. I admit there have been times when someone was describing what they thought was compassion, and I caught myself being a bit judgmental, thinking, "Really?" I must remind myself to continue to be open to others' experiences in order to help them, help horses.

For example, some may feel that riding without a bit or without a saddle is somehow a more compassionate act than riding *with* a bit and saddle. First of all, this depends on the type of bit and the saddle fit. Second, the FEI Code of Ethics has stated in the past, "In the interest of the horse, the fitness and competence of the rider shall be regarded as essential." So while on one hand training techniques that involve removing bits or saddles may be thought of as "more compassionate," the lack of bit or saddle can potentially put more stress on the horse if the rider is now not riding correctly or competently. The "act of compassion" ultimately causes more harm than good.

One of the awarenesses inherent in the 25 Principles of Compassionate Equitation is that what qualifies as *compassion* or *compassionate* can vary, as well as be misconstrued, misinterpreted, or manipulated—consciously or unconsciously—to fit a certain riding school of thought or training approach. When striving to be compassionate you should, as the Dalai Lama says, "Never trust anything… look and see if it is true for yourself." Ask yourself, "Even though some say this act is compassionate, kind, or humane, is it *truly* just for the good of the horse?"

Questions to Consider

BASED ON PRINCIPLE 4

1   Do I have a better understanding of how my thoughts and emotions impact my relationship with my horse and my riding?

2   Based on recent findings in neuroscience, are there ways that I can improve my relationship with my horse? With others around me?

3   Are there ways I can create a more healthy, compassionate *mindstream* or am I doing great just as I am?

CHAPTER FIVE

The Benefits of Self-Reflection

We make time for a period of self-reflection and re-evaluation of various areas of horsemanship. Do our choices meet basic humane standards of respect for all life?

Susan Gordon:

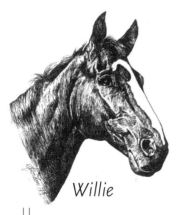

Willie

With an old show horse like Willie I had to ask myself if riding him was helpful to his well-being or if he needed permanent retirement. Initially, we were just hacking around in my backyard after all, and his competitive days were behind him. There was no pressure on me as a trainer or on him as a performance horse. I had to really think about how and what I would ask this horse to do. As with people, horses are designed to move, and some are far healthier when given a carefully chosen protocol of exercise to maintain muscle and body condition. Determining exactly what to do with an old horse limited by past injury and poor handling can be a bit of trial and error to finding the limits of his desires and ability to work. Certainly, you want to do everything you can to minimize the "errors" part of this picture though, and it is always best to have your veterinarian confirm whether or not some form of exercise is actually best or if your retiree would benefit more from pasture turnout, with regular attention, and good care.

Besides putting together the pieces of Willie's background as best I could, I also dug into my own past to try to understand why I had decided to purchase this horse. I had "left the business" so far as I was concerned and didn't have a burning desire to ride recreationally. Yet, here I was, all of a sudden finding myself with the kind of horse I would have enjoyed immensely when we were both in our showing heyday. What, exactly, was the meaning of this?

Apparently neither Willie nor I was ready to completely throw in the towel. What was needed was a compassionate, humane adjustment to the situation in which we found each other. If left "doing nothing" and retaining the disdain for humans he had arrived in my hands with, he might have been bored and uninterested in life. I felt he was more the type of horse who wanted to engage with people and activity when given a safe and productive opportunity. Willie could no longer jump huge fences, nor did I have a desire to jump huge fences. He needed the chance to remain supple and conditioned as much as his body would allow, so I decided to put him on a joint supplement, while incorporating a program of slow rehabilitation with very short rides and hacks into the open desert. We eventually had to work through those "blocks" as I described in the previous chapter, but the process was beneficial for me, too.

I was riding just enough to keep muscle memory alive and well, and enjoying it enough to remember why I loved horses so much in the first place.

Self-reflecting, examining why we ride, why we have a horse, and how we can provide that horse with the most humane form of horsemanship, is an opportunity to offer the horse the respect he deserves. We seem to have a purpose in serving each other.

In the article "Neural Correlates of Self-Reflection" (*Brain*, 2002), Sterling C. Johnson, et al, write, "The capacity to consciously reflect on one's sense of self is an important aspect of self-awareness. A sense of self is a collection of schemata regarding one's abilities, traits and attitudes that guides our behaviors, choices and social interaction. The accuracy of one's sense of self will impact one's ability to function effectively in the world."

Through our self-reflection, we explore the "abilities, traits and attitudes that guide our behaviors, choices and interactions with *our horses*." My choice from a very young age was to work with animals and train them. Like my co-writer Dr. Schoen, who, ever since he can remember, knew that he wanted to be a veterinarian, I had a deep desire to make my life's work with animals.

My fascination was with trying to understand how an animal's personality could merge in harmony with a human's. Perhaps for many years I was simply trying to use animals as a "cover." When at home, it wasn't unusual to have a dog, a cat, and my pet rat, surrounding me as I sat and did homework. I put them between me and the expectations of other people, especially my parents. It was likely quite a shock for them to see their "dainty" little girl go from frilly dresses and dance costumes to grit-covered boots and a wheelbarrow full of manure, not to mention wrestling 1,000-pound animals full speed over solid cross-country fences. Maybe I just did not want to seem too fragile and dependent on anyone. Whatever the reason, I felt great joy and gained a lot of self-confidence on the fastest, most powerful horses I could get my hands on.

What turns a shy, reclusive child into someone who feels most at home on the back of a "hot," bold, Thoroughbred?

My first two training projects were as "green" as I was. I had a two-year-old, barely-broke Appaloosa filly at the age of 14, and then a yearling Appaloosa colt as a 17-year-old. A cowboy had started the filly by throwing a saddle on her and riding her across the fields until she stopped bucking. She was forever a "hair-trigger" and would explode at the slightest provocation. Determined to get things right and turn out a better horse, the young stallion was my pride and joy, and the eventual product of my own intense study of classical traditions of riding and training. My high school allowed a course self-designed by the student, and I was granted a "special project" for credit—and so my training program for the colt was born! Both horses reflected my developing self and sense of identity as a young woman, and they also reflected the moodiness of a typical teenager. There are many moments I remember when I handled both horses in ways that I am not proud of, but they were inevitably my teachers, as well as a form of therapy, through those difficult growing-up years.

EXERCISE IN COMPASSION

Who You Were, Who You Are

Can you relate your own personality and experiences with horses to your behaviors, traits, and attitudes as a child? Think back about who you were and how it might connect to your decisions and actions as a horseperson today. Write down *who you were* and *who you are*, and then consider *who your horse needs you to be*.

The bulk of my professional training career involved reschooling off-the-track Thoroughbreds. I was 19 when I had the chance to ride one for the first time, and I loved the feel of such an athletic horse. I realized even then, it takes a long time to learn how to handle large animals that have been taught to run full speed when a bell goes off and gates fly open in front of them. Thoroughbreds leave the racetrack for various reasons. By the time they reach a trainer capable of starting them in a second career, the plethora of problems they come with reads like a gourmet menu.

While I loved my Appaloosa horses and admired many other breeds at the barns where I rode, it was these racetrack rejects that taught me the most about myself and which skills were needed to help horses and people with training challenges. Every horse presented a tremendous learning opportunity, as the only way to *learn* how to ride through bucking, rearing, and spooking is to *actually* ride through bucking, rearing, and spooking! I gained invaluable insight as to how to remain calm and focused in spite of tense circumstances and poor behavior caused by race training and time in the track environment.

Handling ex-racehorses requires developing a tough exterior and particular skillset. You learn to be as alert as they are, move as quickly as they can, and be prepared for them to "play up" in a way that could cause injury to both of you. Off-the-track Thoroughbred personalities require certain kinds of human personalities to get along with them. Do they suit you? Or do you feel like a different breed and personality suits you better? What inspires you to be with a particular type of horse?

Thoroughbreds are sometimes subjected to training techniques that could be construed under some lenses as inhumane. In North America, they are started under saddle while very young and immature. Many colts are not gelded in the hope they will become winners and subsequently moneymaking sires. The fact that they are so young, and many remain as stallions, requires that handlers maintain control of fresh and unruly horses at all times. A horse that is badly misbehaved on the track is frowned upon and may cause problems for other horses and track personnel if excessively disruptive. I have had Thoroughbreds come from the track that were known to buck their rider off, flip over in the starting gate, spook at just about everything, rear, bolt, you name it. Truthfully, by the time a horse is "retired" from the track, separating his *behavior-modified issues* from his *pain-related issues* becomes a bit of a challenge. He's been handled with lip and nose chains, led by his sensitive ears, shoved into starting gates, and generally enervated by the shouting, clanging, and constant noise of life at a race track. When he finally breaks down—either physically, mentally, or both—he either meets a fatal ending or is lucky enough to find his way to a new owner, willing and able to help him adapt to a new lifestyle. Unfortunately, there are not as many ex-racehorses retired to green pastures as we would hope.

" ...when there are things too powerful or too difficult to accept about ourselves, we project them onto the world around us, usually onto those who help us and love us the most—our teacher, the teachings, our parent, or our closest friend."

Sogyal Rinpoche, *Glimpse After Glimpse: Daily Reflections on Living and Dying* (HarperOne, 1995)

Besides my personal experience with this type of horse, I am writing about off-the-track Thoroughbreds because of the extreme highs and lows they experience. They present an excellent opportunity for the trainer to reflect and evaluate him- or herself as a compassionate horseperson while determining which techniques are most humane in the course of reschooling. The environment these horses originated from and their resulting conditioned behaviors require careful thought and planning as to how they will be transitioned to pleasure or show use. I really enjoyed the rewards that came with the turnaround of a difficult, traumatized horse, transforming him into a safe, well-schooled show hunter or jumper suitable for kids or amateurs to ride.

TINY BUDDHA®: SIMPLE WISDOM FOR COMPLEX LIVES

A message from "How to Come Home to Yourself" by Julie Hoyle:

On a subconscious level, we are afraid that if people (or the community) "knew the truth," we would be judged, reviled, rejected, or worse, thrown out.

As a consequence, we try to hide what we believe is unacceptable. This pattern of behavior begins from the moment we are born. A normal aspect of growing up is that we are taught what constitutes appropriate social behavior and what does not.

However, on a subtle or not so subtle level, we might also learn from our parents or caregivers that "being creative" is unacceptable, or that expressing moderate anger or frustration is going against the norms of society.

When we internalize these messages, we form beliefs about what is "wrong" with us and repress them so deeply they become unconscious. What we do not realize is that these aspects of who we are must find expression, and so we project them onto other people, organizations, or the world at large.

Read more at: http://tinybuddha.com/blog/how-to-come-home-to-yourself/.

Looking back, I believe working with off-the-track Thoroughbreds was a pathway to building self-esteem and confidence, and instrumental in my recovery from the trauma of growing up with an alcohol-addicted parent.

Horses allowed me to uncover the generous, kind, talented aspects of their personalities, and by doing so, I was able to *reveal myself* in a better way. When my mother recovered from alcoholism, her more generous, kind, loving, and compassionate nature was revealed, too, and she in turn helped other alcoholics find balance. Perhaps dealing with challenging horses like Thoroughbreds was a mirror for what I went through dealing with the challenges of an alcoholic mother. I now see how our subconscious fears can be exposed through our relationships with horses *and* how their *authentic* personalities can be revealed when we help *them* heal from their own traumas.

If a horse falls into the wrong hands for training or reschooling and is pressured or forced in any way that is inhumane, traumas will only be exacerbated, not resolved, and the horse may potentially become dangerous. This is one of the reasons it is important for someone taking on a reschooling project to be very clear and honest in his or her self-reflective analysis. If there is going to be a problem, the horse will ultimately *mirror* the difficulties of the rider, and a traumatized horse seems even *more* acutely aware of human issues than a non-traumatized horse.

When riding, ask yourself, "What is it about me that wants this horse to perform a certain way, right now? Is it for me, or is it really in the best interest of the horse?"

The post-trauma behaviors exhibited by off-the-track Thoroughbreds can be challenging to the most seasoned of trainers. They are programmed to run about 10 minutes after leaving their racetrack stalls, and the routine does not leave their heads for a long time. As we learned earlier in this book, *they* also—like us—"wire what they fire" in their brains (see p. 47). On many occasions I've been forced into what I call an "*over*-ride." If an ex-racehorse decides to go from "zero to launch" upon hearing that imaginary bell go off in his head, or a particular sound or sight triggers an extreme reaction, it is necessary for the rider to respond quickly but not provoke further reaction either—that is, the horse's behavior and excitement may force you into using stronger aids than you would prefer to use in order to keep the horse under control.

The most humane response in such situations is one that is based on your ability to avoid an emotional reaction to the horse's behavior. *Over-reacting and over-riding are not the same.* If the horse decides it is time to run and finds he's not allowed to, it is not unusual for him to go upward instead of forward. Riders do not like to end up on the ground, so when the horse displays a strong reaction, we usually scramble in the moment to do anything we can to stay in the saddle *and* not let the horse get away. A Compassionate Equestrian doesn't *want* to pull on the reins and put excessive pressure on the horse, but sometimes it is an absolute necessity. The compassionate key in such situations is: *do not let your emotions get the best of you*. Do not punish the horse for misbehaving in these moments—as in repeatedly striking the horse or jerking the reins in anger.

If you need to "shut a horse down" for "playing up," bolting, or spooking, enlist the help of someone who can teach you how to utilize the *pulley rein*, also known as a *one-rein stop*, and consider the exercise in the sidebar below as well. Rearing is rather different and can be exacerbated by *any* kind of rein or poll pressure, so enlist professional help if your horse gives any indication as to having such an issue. This should include the help of a veterinarian who can evaluate for a potential pain-source, as well as a period of self-reflection. In all cases of unwanted behavior with a horse, look carefully at yourself and what might be behind *both* the horse's behavior *and* your response to it.

EXERCISE IN COMPASSION

Resisting Compromising Behavior

This isn't a "how-to" horse-training book—there are other manuals out there that go into great detail regarding techniques. That said, I do want to mention one method that produces a change in behavior based on a relatively simple concept: resistance/yield. I also refer to this as a "block" followed by a "release." There are *mental* blocks—which may manifest in a horse in the form of physical resistance (think of Willie's case)—as well as your own capacity to enact *physical* blocks, which you can use to regain control of a horse engaged in an activity that may compromise both your safety and his. Resistance/yield is exactly what it sounds like: You essentially set up a strong resistance to unwanted behavior, then immediately yield to the horse when the behavior stops. Please note this is strictly in reference to an "in the moment" correction, perhaps involving excessive exuberance or an unexpected spook, and not a long term "fix." In addition, every horse-and-rider situation is different, and many require specific evaluation, first for potential soundness issues in the horse, and then for the lengthy list of potential causes stemming from how the horse has been handled and ridden.

1   Make the best effort possible to determine the cause of your horse's behavior and what needs he has that may be going unmet. If his issue is pain-related, address that first. Note that this doesn't mean simply blaming a single piece of equipment, such as the bit or the saddle—evaluating proper tack can provide further insights when incorporated as part of a comprehensive search for solving the problem, which may be part of a multifactorial issue.

2   If your horse is declared sound, and the unwanted behavior continues, consider other possible needs the horse may have that are not being addressed. Does he need to be longed before you ride? Does he need more turnout? Does he need less grain? Does he need a companion? Does he need desensitization schooling? You may want to do some self-reflecting here and ask what you are looking for from this horse, and perhaps even if he is the right horse for you.

3   Following your explorations of the questions in Step 2, if you can confirm the behavior is "learned" and a result of your horse having gotten away with something repeatedly so he has become "spoiled"—say, for example a trail horse that repeatedly tries to turn around and run back home—consider his behavior a "resistance," and resist back. Your reaction should be similar to how one horse treats another horse until the leader, or more dominant personality, emerges the "winner." You want to emerge the "winner" in this case, and your horse will be a safer ride as a result.

4   A lot of being successful with a reschooling ride is having done your groundwork and established a system of progressive, gymnastic exercises in the arena under saddle—such as correct circles, changes of rein, and other

Continued →

(Cont.)

school figures—so you have good directional control over the horse's shoulders and haunches. Effective groundwork also tells you a lot about the horse's baseline personality, and you can watch how his expression changes under varying circumstances and exercises. In the case of the unwanted turnaround on the trail, as you can feel the horse's body "set up" underneath you (when he's preparing to use his strength to ignore more subtle cues and override your aids), remember all the fundamentals of good equitation: eyes up, heels down, elbows at your side, and weight evenly distributed in the saddle. Close your fingers, flex the muscles of your arms, and keep your legs on, matching or even being stronger than the amount of pressure the horse is putting on you. You literally are physically "blocking" the unwanted behavior and preventing the horse from turning around. Your strength and reaction-time actually does count, so your level of fitness is a factor in responding to a horse in this manner.

5   By simply blocking the horse from getting his way, you are not, in effect, punishing him. You are not doing anything outside the context of what the horse already understands if he was correctly schooled in the arena before you began riding him on the trail. And you are not escalating the situation by becoming angry or over-reactive. Your horse resists, you resist back, and you put up the "block" *until you have gotten the desired response from your horse*. While it is critical that your resistance be immediate in relation to the horse's errant action, it is equally important that you time the "release" just as well. The horse's reward comes as part of a *mutual yield-yield response*: He goes forward (yielding to your resistance), and subsequently, you take the pressure off (yielding to his more appropriate response to your cues).

As mentioned, this isn't a one-time fix, and depending on the situation and background of both you and your horse, you may have to repeat the resist/yield sequence regularly, or whenever the horse's resistance reappears. At some point, as with Willie's story, the extreme behavior may vanish altogether, but that's never a guarantee when it comes to working with a horse. The questions you ask yourself throughout the process are of the utmost importance, both in determining your next step forward and ensuring your and your horse's safety, as well as being a valuable exercise in self-reflection. Both you and your horse have the opportunity to learn if you come to the issue with compassion and an educated seat.

You only have a split second to correct a misbehaving horse so he will understand what he is being reprimanded for. If your response is too late, he won't associate it with the behavior. This is a true test in compassion and horsemanship: Withhold the correction if you know it is too late.

We all love a happy horse, but sometimes his exuberance and need to "play" can be disconcerting. Our version of fun doesn't necessarily correlate with that of the horse! "Play" can also mean "fresh" to some horsepeople, as it denotes a horse that has been stall-bound for a day, for example, and has a lot of extra energy. Several barns I worked at had a "closed" policy on Mondays to give staff and horses a complete rest, but it also meant the ex-racehorses stayed indoors—I used to refer to Tuesdays as "Terrible Tuesdays" because some of the fitter Thoroughbreds were a bit wild after a day off!

Some horses—and this can be any breed—just have a playful personality, and this can make them either quite entertaining, or just frustrating, depending on how well they nick with the personalities of their riders. The playful horse is different from one that worries and spooks frequently out of anxiety. The latter can be even *more* challenging due to the reasons behind their spooking—which may include inherent fear, conditioning, or trauma.

What goes in the arena has to come out of the arena. And then go back in again the next day. How would you like your horse to feel about the training session you just shared?

Always make time for additional moments of quiet and reestablishing a normal heart rate and breathing rhythm following a workout. That goes for both the rider *and* the horse. As human athletes, we do this when we include a recovery period between harder intervals. Not all sessions with a horse will end on the "best" note, but it is worth it to get to a point of calm regrouping before leaving the arena. The horse you leave the ring with is the horse that will come back into the arena the next day. The wisest riders finish a session with a relaxed horse. The cool-down period of a workout is *as essential* as the warm-up for both mental and physical aspects of athletic conditioning. Allow enough time at the end of your ride for recovery processes to occur. This is also a good time to reflect and clarify in your mind what the most positive moments were and where you possibly could have made improvements, as well as identifying where you perhaps let aspects of *your* behavior and personality affect the ride.

The next time you enter the arena to work with your horse,
what memories of the previous session will you take with you?
What memories will he bring with him?

Know yourself, and know your horse. Take the time to practice exercises in self-reflection that will identify the aspects of yourself that you may be projecting onto your horse. As we discussed, there are reasons why we are attracted to a particular type of horse and why we find our greatest sense of self-confidence and

COMPASSIONATE SKILLS FOR RIDING "PLAYFUL" AND "SPOOKY" HORSES

- *Patience.* This is part of your exercise in self-reflection. If you are not able to treat a horse with patience, *ask yourself, "Why?"*

- *Curiosity.* Try to understand how the background training of the horse may have led to extreme behavior.

- *Confidence.* A strong, independent seat learned on safe horses will help a lot when difficult moments arise.

- *Focus.* The ability to concentrate for long periods of time is a benefit to a horseperson. A horse knows exactly when you have taken your attention away from him. The sensitive ones will choose that moment to over-react or "play up."

authenticity with a certain breed or personality. When we identify and overcome the sources of our own aberrant behaviors, we can help horses with theirs, and find a compassionate, humane pathway to healing.

Dr. Allen Schoen:

Are you taking your stress and tension into the barn and literally "spooking" your horse?

One of my clients, Serina, was concerned that her horse would not let her near him whenever she would run to the barn after a hectic day in New York City at her stressful job. She usually got caught in traffic heading north out of New York—this would happen almost every day she rode—making her at least 10 minutes late for her training session, tense from "road rage," and inevitably, like the rabbit in *Alice in Wonderland* looking at her watch and saying, "I'm late, I'm late, for a very important date."

Serina is the representation of so many of us who try to fit too much in our days. I see the habit of overachieving and "self-taskmastering" over and over again, and I also see how horses respond. The horse picks up on the tension of the person as part of the Transpecies Field Theory (see p. 7). There are different levels to this theory: Part of the Transpecies Field is *the horse watching the human.* The visuals and the sounds he observes in a person have an effect on him, and he gets tense because of the human's tension. Then there is the electromagnetic field that surrounds our body as described by the Institute of HeartMath (see p. 94). This is an energetic field, and when a being feels tension, he *literally* vibrates. You actually can *feel* this reaction in yourself (see the sidebar for an exercise to pinpoint and change this feeling).

You are putting that whole, vibrating energy field on top of the horse. How would *you* feel carrying a tense, anxious child piggy-back? Watch the horse's ears. Are they tense? Are they pinned back? Has his body tightened in general? Is he tighter under the saddle? In his neck and shoulders? Is he resistant to your contact? Is he resistant to moving? Are his eyes tightened up and showing signs of anxiety? While in the saddle, do a First-Aid Self-Reflection *body scan* to pinpoint where tension has gathered in *your* body (see sidebar). Then, practice breathing as I describe at the end of the exercise. Do you *feel* the difference in your body? Do

First-Aid Self-Reflection

How do you feel when you're feeling rushed and behind?

Do a simple *body scan,* beginning with the top of your head, and ending at your toes, progressively checking in with each area of your physical self. *Where* are you feeling it?

What are you feeling? What does it feel like? (Think of another similar sensation to help quantify what you're feeling.)

Take a slow, deep breath in, and exhale. Repeat this three times.

Do you feel a difference in your body? What are you feeling now? Where do you feel it? Do another body scan.

Now, *what choice do you want to make* regarding how you feel? The power to change how you feel when you are rushed, tense, or anxious is in your thoughts, your breath, and your heart.

you *see* a difference in your horse? As you teach yourself to take the time to notice the difference with your horse, depending on your state of mind, and, become familiar with the pros and cons of the Transpecies Field Theory first-hand through experience, you gain a very valuable tool for self-reflection and determining what you *want* to bring to your human-horse experience.

Now let's return to Serina and her concern because her horse was always anxious when she rushed to the barn to fit in a ride after work. She had her regular veterinarian evaluate the horse, and he could not find any obvious issues. She also had me evaluate him, and I didn't find anything either, but I noticed how tense and nervous *she* was when she came into the barn. I suggested she try *First-Aid Self-Reflection* (see sidebar above) and *centering* (see p. 10) and that did the trick. Once Serina took time to slow down, breathe, and become calmer, centered, and more present in the moment, her horse calmed down and her lessons were more pleasant and rewarding for both of them. Serina and her horse were more in touch with each other, interconnected in a much quieter energetic field. Her friends and the barn staff were all much happier around her, her horse, and each other, and a few moments of quiet self-reflection ended up being the talk of the evening when their horse group got together socially!

If you always over-stack your day with more to-do lists than you have time for, begin to set time aside that cannot be filled as a period for deeper self-reflection.

When I teach seminars I always joke, "I teach what I most need to learn." My assistant will often say, "Oh, this barn called and said they only had x-number of horses, but they just added three or four more." Well, this adds a couple of more hours to my visit. Then all of a sudden I'm late, and it is only nine o'clock in the morning. Or my assistant will say, "You're going to a barn in this area, can you fit in one more?" I'll think, "Oh, sure," and then the next thing you know I am running behind, and I may not always be *in the moment* with the horse I am with, unless I catch and remind myself, that my energy is everyone else's energy (see sidebar). I then breathe and center myself as quickly as I am aware of my anxious state.

EXERCISE IN COMPASSION

Recognizing Your Energy Is Everyone's Energy

As soon as you have identified your state as one of anxiety or tension, ask yourself:

How often do I do this to my horse?

How often am I like this in other parts of my life?

How does this energy impact my life?

How am I impacting everyone else in my life by being in this constant state of, "I'm late, I'm late for a very important date"?

Recognizing that *your* tension, *your* energy, impacts the energy all around and the world as a whole, can help you take steps to breathe and center, as needed throughout your day.

Over time, I've learned from having survived in an environment like that, so I now estimate how my day will go based on a certain amount of time each horse will take. I'll allow for things like traffic and factor in an extra half-hour of buffer time. If I happen to arrive somewhere early, and my clients are ready for me, then great. If I arrive early and they are not ready for me, it gives me a few spare moments for self-reflection or to catch up on the rest of my to-do list. I found that it is much healthier to have a little spare time than to always be running behind.

MINDFULNESS AND MINDFULNESS-BASED STRESS REDUCTION (MBSR)

"It is not the potential stressor itself but how you perceive it and then how you handle it that will determine whether or not it will lead to stress," says Jon Kabat-Zinn, Founder of the Stress Reduction Clinic and the Center for Mindfulness in Medicine, Health Care, and Society at the University of Massachusetts Medical School. Kabat-Zinn is also the founder of Mindfulness-Based Stress Reduction (MBSR), which is described as follows:

Mindfulness is a way of learning to relate directly to whatever is happening in your life, a way of taking charge of your life, a way of doing something for yourself that no one else can do for you—consciously and systematically working with your own stress, pain, illness, and the challenges and demands of everyday life.

In contrast, you've probably encountered moments of "mindlessness" —a loss of awareness resulting in forgetfulness, separation from self, and a sense of living mechanically. Restoring within yourself a balanced sense of health and well-being requires increased awareness of all aspects of self, including body and mind, heart and soul. Mindfulness-Based Stress Reduction (MBSR) is intended to ignite this inner capacity and infuse your life with awareness (http://www.umassmed.edu/cfm/stress/index.aspx).

Remember: when we are always rushing, we are self-medicating.

As discussed in chapter 4 (p. 92), we can become addicted to the adrenaline rush that occurs when we are always racing to get somewhere or get something done.

This happened to me and I ended up "burning out" and experiencing "adrenal exhaustion." Now as a form of preventive medicine, I create those spaces in my day where I can be ahead rather than behind. This helps break the destructive pattern of adrenaline addiction, preventing the long-term physiological damage that occurs with adrenal exhaustion and resulting chronic fatigue.

Try creating space in your day, and as the laws of nature go, it will likely get filled! It is still nice to have that space and be able to consciously choose what to do with it. You can ask yourself if you *literally* want to smell the roses. Look at flowers, groom your horse, or take the time to self-reflect, to stop, breathe, and come into yourself, and *be here now*. Or, you can also say, "All right, I have x-number of phone calls, text messages, or emails to return, and this space gives me some time to do that." What the space gives you is the *presence of the moment*. It is a gift.

Jon Kabat-Zinn's Mindfulness-Based Stress Reduction program (see sidebar) teaches a method referred to as "The Body Scan" with the purpose of "catching" and identifying stressors and sources of anxiety. Not unlike the simple body scan we used in the sidebar on p. 114, Kabat-Zinn's technique is a powerful way to reconnect with your body by directing your breath and focus. (A full script for the classic body scan technique for passive progressive relaxation is available at http://im4us.org/Mindfulness--Based+Patient+Handouts.) Once you get in touch with that deeper part of yourself and can relax your body and your mind, you can then explore and experience many of the exercises in this book, such as these simple meditations for yourself and others:

1   *Metta*, loving-kindness meditation, says, "May I be happy, may I be safe, may all beings be happy, may all beings be safe." Find a quiet space and surround yourself with this intention of universal goodwill (see also our discussion of this on p. 36).

2   Or you can practice a meditation on gratitude. For example: Gently close your eyes, breathe slowly in and out three times, and then say to yourself, "I am so grateful that I 'caught' myself and that I am able to slow down. I am so grateful for this moment. I am feeling gratitude in my heart. I am feeling gratitude for myself, my horse, and for all beings."

Check in with yourself after practicing a simple meditation such as these. How does it make you feel?

The exercises in this chapter and throughout this book can change your biochemistry, your neurochemistry, your heart, and your mind. You can become much more peaceful within and ultimately much happier. You can then share and extend that inner peace and happiness with your horse, your family, everyone else you encounter today, and everyone else in your world. This can lead to compassionate, humane standards of respect for all life. Before we can help our horses, we need to help ourselves. As Confucius said 2000 years ago, "To put the world right in order, we must first put the nation in order; to put the nation in order, we must first put the family in order; to put the family in order, we must first cultivate our personal life, we must first set our hearts right" (from Lama Surya Das' book *The Big Questions*, Rodale Press, 2007).

From the perspective of the Compassionate Equestrian, we might add: "To put our horses in good health and happiness, we must first set our own hearts and minds right."

Questions to Consider
BASED ON PRINCIPLE 5

1   What am I sensing and feeling as I create time for self-reflection in my life?

2   How does this period of self-reflection impact my relationship with my horse? With other people?

3   What do I notice when I do a body scan on myself on the ground? From the saddle?

4   What do I notice in myself when I do *metta* or loving-kindness meditation? Gratitude meditation? (see p. 117)

5   How can I benefit my horse and others as I integrate these exercises into my life?

CHAPTER SIX

Slow Down, Center, Relax, and Release

We take a few moments of silence to become heart-centered, allowing for the release of any destructive emotions, prior to working with any horse in any way. This allows both the individual and the horse to interact from a place of inner calm, peace, awareness, and mindfulness, thereby allowing for the most positive, constructive outcome from all interactions between humans and horses.

Susan Gordon:

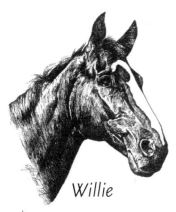

Willie

I hesitatingly knocked on the door of one of Willie's previous owners. At least she was willing to meet with me and offer her insights on Willie's background. The woman was slight, quiet, and conservatively dressed. She seemed like the last person who would have ever been aggressive with a horse or taken her frustrations out on him.

She explained she had purchased Willie after his show jumping career ended—or rather, after Willie himself had ended it by refusing to jump at all at a show one day. The woman had thought it would be appropriate to have him continue in the dressage arena, where his advanced eventing skills would still be useful, but without the demands of jumping. Unfortunately, Willie was not going peacefully into any arena by this time! I was told he regularly exploded when asked to lengthen stride across the diagonal in the dressage test, leaving her sitting in the dirt as a result. This helped explained why Willie had decided he could get away with obstinate behavior to get what he wanted.

The woman said she had sold him but had no idea how he had fallen into the hands of a dealer.

Having compassion for what had happened to Willie, and even for the riders and trainers who worked with him in the years before I found him, helped me face his behavior with more tolerance. Meeting aggressive behavior such as his with more aggressive behavior has the same consequences with horses as it does with people. A battle likely ensues and there is a win-lose situation. On the other hand, an aggressor who is always allowed to be a bully is also likely to repeat the behavior over and over again, even gaining in confidence and strength if his tactics enable him to get what he wants. Sometimes it is hard to remember that bullies become that way for a reason. Often they have been bullied themselves, and their behavior comes from a place of fear. Willie decided he was going to "get" his rider, before the rider could "get" him. I had to remember this every time he attempted to eject me from the saddle.

I have no doubt that Willie was genuinely hurting at one time and may have even sustained permanent musculoskeletal damage, especially after learning of the fall he had on the cross-country course in Florida. Even in the 1990s it was very difficult to find a veterinarian who could help horses in *regards to "upper-body lameness" and spinal issues. I really had to just feel those horses out and figure out "how to ride" in a way most conducive to maintaining soundness, relieving their spines of as much pressure as possible, while still furthering athletic development. In Willie's case I knew I was pushing him, but based on my assessment, to the best of my ability and background knowledge, it was appropriate under the circumstances. If he continued to lag and buck it was going to be more painful for him than what I was actually asking for. Horses that hang behind your leg are often dangerous—they are the ones that will suddenly put all their power into an unexpected launch. Not only that, but Willie had already proven his bucking prowess, unloading a series of riders that came before me. I had to find a way through the issue.*

Willie never did get over his dislike for dressage. Later in his reschooling, he somehow always seemed to know in advance when we were going to a dressage show, becoming progressively more violent as it got closer to show time. I tried everything to fool him. I stayed out of the arena, backed off the training, practiced tests on a different horse, and even tried not riding at all the week before a competition. Nope. He knew. He kicked a hole in the arena fence at a simple request for a canter one day. Jumping though, was a different story altogether. Once he was physically comfortable—and I was no longer attempting to take him to dressage shows!—and the bucking episodes had subsided, he was more than happy to get in a trailer, go to a show, and pack kids around low hunter courses.

It's possible this horse never would have come around had he not been treated calmly and consistently, and if I hadn't strived to quell all negative emotional responses to his behavior. You have to be ever so mindful, aware of your emotions, and always prepared to come back relaxed, calm, and centered when dealing with this kind of horse. Willie and I met in the middle, so to speak, and the end result was extremely positive for us both, as well as for everyone else who had the opportunity to learn from him.

Agitation. Stress. Shallow breathing. Increased heart rate. Upset stomach. How do you feel when you are in such a state? How do you feel in the presence of an irritated, stressed-out person? Probably not so good. As we touched on in chapter 4, the release of stress hormones such as cortisol in the body can cause a lot of damage if the stressful state is severe or recurring.[1] Health problems caused by chronic stress are only preventable when we can eliminate, or at least reduce, the cause of our stress and make a conscious attempt to rebalance and regain wellness.

While most horse people might say they find just being around horses soothing and calming, sometimes the strain of affording and managing a horse and a horse facility, or of being part of situations at boarding and training barns with staff, trainers, or other boarders, actually *amplify* stress and agitation. And ultimately, this has a detrimental effect on the horses, as well.

STRESS CAUSES ULCERS IN HUMAN AND HORSE

According to the Equine Performance Institute in Oregon (www.equinepi.com), horses get stomach ulcers just like people get stomach ulcers, and generally speaking, they are primarily due to stress.

When performance horses are subjected to intense training, competition, transport, and confinement, the accumulated stress can promote inflammatory symptoms in the equine gut. Exercise increases pressure in the abdomen, collapsing the stomach, forcing acid gastric contents upward. When this highly acidic fluid comes in contact with the lining of the upper part of the stomach, inflammation and potential erosion occurs. In addition, the overuse or misuse of non-steroidal anti-inflammatory drugs (NSAIDS) is also known to result in gastrointestinal injury that may cause stomach ulcers.

Adult horses with ulcers may exhibit symptoms of abdominal discomfort (colic), poor appetite, mild weight loss, poor body condition and attitude changes. Ulcers can also develop secondarily due to stress from other problems relating to ill health or hospitalization.

If you suspect your horse has gastric ulcers, confer with your veterinarian to ensure proper diagnosis and treatment. (See more on this subject in chapter 16, p. 279.)

There are steps we can all take to prevent stress-related health problems in ourselves and in our horses. We've already discussed a few ways in previous chapters. Taking the ideas of self-reflection and 10-minute QFI meditation a step further, consider this: Before you approach your horse, take just a few moments to check in with your feelings and emotions, ensuring you are in an appropriate state of mind for working with him. Athletes may recognize this pause to clear the mind as "Getting in the Zone." "The Zone" is a state of calm and unclouded thinking that allows for optimal performance and quick decision-making. Many top sports professionals prefer to spend time in quietude and silence before their events to center themselves and find their focus. Consider making this a regular habit before getting on a horse's back, as well.

As riders, we tend to be chatty when in the presence of others who are grooming and tacking up. Each of us can choose to be mindful of those who might wish to be quieter during the process. Some use this time to slow themselves down after a busy day. Some just enjoy being quiet with their horses. I like to remain reasonably silent during my ride as well. When a rider is in deep concentration with a horse, it is best not to disrupt him or her unless it is really necessary. My focus stems from having had horses that would blow up the moment my attention was taken off them. That is how sensitive horses can be—they know when our minds wander!

Athletes also know that nutrition and mood are connected. Are you getting enough of the right foods and hydration? Riding is exercise. Food is fuel. When you feel agitated without knowing why, ask yourself if you've had enough to eat or drink before working with your horse.

When we acknowledge the horse as an athlete, the state of his athletic partner— which is you, the rider— becomes even more important. I have seen horses that are obviously in discomfort and distress being ignored by a distracted handler or rider. Or worse, a person aggravated by something *other* than the horse consciously or unconsciously placing the horse in an uncomfortable situation. In these scenarios, riders may be taking out their frustrations and problems on their horses without even being aware of it. The key to avoiding a situation that sacrifices the well-being of the horse is to "Get in the Zone": *slow down, breathe, settle into a calmer state,* and *release* whatever emotion is preventing you from having an enjoyable ride. *Let it go,* at least for now, in the best interest of your horse. Focus on *what you are doing* and the best thing you *could be doing* for your horse in the moment.

There are ways to ensure you gain the time and place to "Get in the Zone" before you get on your horse.

Try to arrive at the barn early enough to allow yourself enough time after grooming your horse to sit quietly, breathe deeply, and monitor your thoughts and feelings before tacking up. Encourage quiet zones in the barn where conversation is only out of necessity. Quickly disperse arguments and differences with diplomacy and calmness. Become aware of techniques for calming both agitated horses and humans.

Whatever your routine, however little time you know you have, *slow down, take a deep breath.* It only takes a minute or two. Soften your gaze, give your horse a pat on the neck, and be kind to both of you. If this is quite different from your usual groom-tack-up-and-get-to-the-arena routine, just give it a try and then hopefully over time, make it a habit. If you have been rushing throughout your day, this is a chance to return yourself to the natural mind state—where you are not anxious, worried, analyzing, or planning—and tune in to your horse as much as he is tuned in to you. If you sense that he is tense as well, then the two of you can take a moment to relax together before heading into the arena or out on the trail.

Once mounted, continue your *soft eyes*—a method first created by Sally Swift in the book *Centered Riding* (Trafalgar Square Books,1985)—to help maintain the relaxed state you created in the grooming and tacking up process. By widening and softening your gaze, you open to a greater awareness and sense of connection to your horse, and your surrounding environment. Swift said, "Using soft eyes is like a new philosophy. It is a method of becoming distinctly aware of what is going on around you, beneath you, inside of you. It includes feeling and hearing as well as seeing. You are aware of the whole, not just separate parts."

The routine of grooming, cleaning tack, feeding, and even cleaning stalls can be mesmerizing and calming. The aroma of the horses, clean bedding, polished leather, and fresh hay embeds in our psyche and rarely fails to return us to the happiest of thoughts. Well-meaning friends and family members used to ask me why I didn't do something else besides the horse business. Why didn't I pursue my artistic passion? Why didn't I do something less expensive? Why was I cleaning stalls for a living if I was smart enough to do a hundred other things? The answer was only explicable to like-minded souls who felt the same

"My Timing Is Perfect"

1   Next time you are late, in a rush, and starting to panic, take a deep breath and say to yourself, "My timing is perfect."

2   Repeat this over and over until you feel your anxiety ebb as you actually begin to believe it. These four words can restore calm by convincing you that all will be well.

way about horses as I did. Even though the day-to-day aspects of running a barn are demanding and rarely turn a big profit, there is a very deep connection to horses that's hard to just release and walk away from.

Walk away, I have done, however, and I spent many months considering why I withdrew from the love of my life, and what it was that eventually brought me back. Horses have witnessed the most fragile times in my life, from pre-teen years, through two marriages and divorces, and years of unsettled living arrangements combined with volatile finances—definitely *not* the kind of scenarios that encourage you to slow down, center yourself, and release pent-up emotions. In situations like the ones I've lived through, you have to consciously take stock of what is causing you to lose sight of the peace in your life, and work hard to regain a sense of stability and relative calm.

When I brought Willie home, I believe it was a subconscious attempt to rekindle the sense of being centered and connected through contact with horses. It seems many people these days are searching for that same kind of reconnection to nature and a slower, more peaceful way of life that interaction with horses can provide.

I've had to ride horses while also on emotional roller coasters, and when relationship issues and unstable clients were tormenting my heart. Getting on a horse, especially one I knew was going to be a potentially troublesome ride, provided an outstanding opportunity to learn how to put a distraught mind aside. I had to focus on the "now" and whatever was necessary to make that session as productive and progressive as possible. I had to be careful not to let my ego allow me to make a training error in an attempt to impress an owner. No matter how I felt inside, it was still important that the horse left the arena feeling relaxed and perhaps better than when he entered it. Riding horses for clients at a show barn is a great lesson in the importance of self-control and "Getting in the Zone." Loss of self-control can have serious consequences if you can't slow down and take some deep breaths, catching yourself in a state of mind that is not conducive to a good relationship with anyone, least of all yourself.

Sometimes the darker days of one's life are necessary so we know the light when we see it.

Accepting the impermanence of everything, especially in our youth, is not easy to assimilate. As children, growing up with a lot of animals in the house, my brother and I learned about the cycles of birth and death. As with all life, it is far too simple...one day we're here, and then we're not. Realizing all sentient beings are related by this common fact is a good starting point for the release of emotions, especially long-term feelings of guilt, anger, and regret. We are all in the same boat regardless of immediate circumstances and surroundings.

When it comes down to it, we're all just "walking each other home."

If we have acted out on destructive emotions, we put ourselves into a state of suffering as we start to wonder, "What if?" What if I hadn't said those angry words? What if I hadn't ignored that horse in distress because I was in such a hurry? By asking "What if?" we can put ourselves through all kinds of mind games. We tend to create negative situations in these moments of self-talk. Our instincts tell us to look for the worst in a situation. We look for the negative so we can protect ourselves from potential danger. It is a *default mechanism* that we are born with, but we can train ourselves to respond differently when the situation is not as threatening as our instincts may initially perceive it to be. Observe the situation without attaching judgment or blame, and have empathy for all those involved, rather than immediately addressing it from a negative viewpoint. This is why compassion takes practice—the more tension that has arisen in a given circumstance, the more challenging it becomes to exercise mindful awareness and tolerance.

My background is comprised of a blend of traditional religious practice and spirituality, having learned prayers, rituals, and meditations particular to more than one tradition. I keep my practices personal and very low key. It is all too easy to offend people with perceived differences and worldviews. Differences in philosophies and theologies may be viewed the same way we compassionately view differences in horse training methods. We see others as needing and deserving relief from suffering, therefore boundaries of beliefs and practices are transcended. In meditation and contemplation you find answers coming to you as you become mindful of your breath and your stillness. Thoughts come and go, and the best technique is to just watch them come and go, without placing judgment or trying to analyze anything. If you see your anger, *keep breathing*. If you see how stressed you are, *keep breathing*. Place your hands on your horse for a minute, and *keep breathing*. Be grateful for your breath and grateful for the present moment with your horse. Be grateful that you are alive and have the opportunity to be with this wonderful animal.

Taking deep, slow breaths and engaging the abdomen encourages full oxygen exchange. This slows the heartbeat and can lower or stabilize blood pressure.

Think of the most positive, inspiring moments you have had with horses. There is a story for each one of them. To some of my own mounts, I owe an apology. I have attempted many times to resolve in my mind the circumstances that may have led to my having to leave them behind or find them a new home. It is comforting to know how some concluded their lives, and that they were lovingly cared for until they passed on. But there are many who came and went that I did not keep track of, and it bothers me that I do not know how their lives played out once they left my barn.

Early in my life, in the long, busy days at the barns, I did not always take the time to become heart-centered. Nor did I take time for both myself and the horse I was about to get on to properly connect and check on my emotional state in the moment, and his. I could have managed my stress better had I learned meditation techniques, such as those presented in *The Compassionate Equestrian*, a bit sooner than I did. In addition to the physicality of working with horses, sometimes trainers take on the brunt of emotional stress conveyed by other trainers, clients, and boarders who express themselves in an insensitive way, coming from their own "filters" and conditioning. I know many trainers try very hard to maintain decorum through exhaustion and quite often, they do a wonderful, caring job of putting others ahead of themselves. Good self-care is important for a professional in any field who has spent a considerable portion of their day taking care of others' needs.

Atonement

A beautiful method of atonement and practice for correcting errors of our past actions comes through a simple mantra from the Hawaiian practice of *Ho'opo-nopono*. The mantra is:

"I am sorry, please forgive me, I love you, and I thank you."

Say this to yourself, your horse, and anyone else in your life who may need to hear it.

In appropriate situations, Dr. Schoen suggests this approach to his friends and clients based on his own personal experience with its benefits. Joe Vitale's *Zero Limits* (Wiley, 2008) examines this practice in more detail.

Over-protecting every detail of a horse's life, or on the other side of the spectrum, leaving him to virtually fend for himself, is not a balanced way to approach horsekeeping. Either has consequences for the well-being of both horse and humans. Both extremes are related to depression and other disorders.

In the days of my self-assigned "removal from horses" after experiencing burn-out, I would gravitate to other activities I enjoyed, such as painting, playing drums, hiking, and even a stint in fashion advertising. I did volunteer work for youth substance abuse programs and medical organizations, and studied various modalities of holistic health, trying always to be absorbed in learning something new. At some point I would meet a horse, sometimes in the most unexpected place, and we would stare at each other eye-to-eye for a while. In one instance it was with a police horse in Washington, DC, in September 2000. I had been on hiatus for several months and was enjoying exploring the Capitol area. The horse and I looked at each other, and I just wanted to hug the big gray. He tugged on the officer's reins pulling him in my direction.

Meeting "a horse" was usually the first sign I was ready to come back to the equine industry, refreshed and a little wiser. With every return I added another dimension to my training program. Much of it just good, old-fashioned, basic horsemanship, but with mindfulness and more *spaciousness*—an *ease* of mind—between the tasks of horsekeeping and riding. It took a long time, but eventually I was allowing the horses to tell *me* as much about them as they could, and I was taking better care of my own needs.

Compassion means thinking of others and their feelings. It is all about the *other*—which means first of all giving compassion to ourselves so that we can calm ourselves, approach the horse with clear intentions, and understand his needs in relation to the situation at hand. We *can* learn how to focus on the horse's well-being while letting go of our own problems through breathing and visualization. We *can* release negativity *before* doing any kind of work with the horse. The results are worth it.

ALTERNATIVE THERAPIES IN BRIEF

Whenever I came back to horses after taking a break, I would take lessons learned during my "hiatus" into the barn. For example, I spent some "down time" studying applied light therapy, therapeutic touch, and breathwork, and these transitioned wonderfully to the stable and riding arena.

- *Applied Light Therapy:* Also referred to as *phototherapy*, this method applies light directly to the skin for a variety of health benefits. In particular, monochromatic red wavelengths in the 660 nanometer range are used effectively for the relief of pain and sports injuries.

- *Therapeutic Touch:* In this non-contact energy therapy, the practitioner places his or her hands close to the patient's body with the intention to help or heal pain and anxiety.

- *Breathwork:* A method or combined methods of using breathing patterns to establish relaxation and a peaceful sense of mind, as well as for therapeutic reasons and "journeying" (attaining higher states of consciousness).

Dr. Allen Schoen:

By integrating your mind and heart, you create an intention to be compassionate to all beings at home, at the barn, and in your life. Visualize yourself doing this as you go into the barn each day and you go about all your usual activities. This exercise is based not only on ancient traditions that transcend all spiritual belief systems, but it confirms results obtained from the latest research and advances in contemplative neuroscience, quantum physics, and interpersonal neurobiology, as well as other evolving interdisciplinary fields of study. Our goal is to meld information from current studies and ancient traditions into all of our interactions with horses, and then expanding this to all animals and society in general.

Visualize your thoughts as actual, physically present "bubbles" that envelop everyone in your presence, including your horse.

In quantum physics there is acknowledgment that everything is a *wave*, a vibrational frequency and resonance, and *when intention or a thought is attached to that wave it actually has an effect in physicality*. It is almost like we create "thought bubbles" with our mind and these thought bubbles then either bounce off or penetrate everyone else we interact with. How do we control the quality of thoughts we put into the thought bubbles, shifting the waves into a more harmonious resonance? What might that look like?

Let's go back to our earlier scenario in which you drive up to your barn, and it seems to be one of those days where nothing is going as planned. Your to-do list is longer than the week, you're worried about an unidentified health issue with your horse, there are certain individuals in the barn that you are not looking forward to seeing...and this is creating a somewhat chaotic, possibly anxious feeling throughout your body and mind. In one moment of mindfulness you can go from a *reaction* to a *response* when you catch yourself and say, "Wait a minute, yes, all this is going on in my mind, but I *consciously choose to change what is going into my 'thought bubbles,'* and I am *not* going to bring that into the barn and impact everyone else there. I am going to take 10 minutes and just remain in my car, simply being quiet and calming my thoughts so my 'bubbles' can help create harmony rather than further discord." Recognizing that you have the ability to change your *emotional reactions* into more *compassionate responses* is the "Response-ability" we discussed on p. 49.

THE ROOTS OF COMPASSIONATE EQUITATION

The ideas espoused in this book are based on concepts found in a number of innovative, interdisciplinary fields of study such as:

- *Contemplative Neuroscience*: In a lecture at the Center for Compassion and Altruism Research and Education at Stanford University, Richard Davidson, PhD, described contemplative neuroscience as a multidisciplinary field that to some degree overlaps with the study of neural mechanisms of mindfulness meditation. It examines neurological, physiological, epigenetic, behavioral, social, and cognitive manifestations or consequences of a state of mind. I am extrapolating and expanding this field to include the impact of the effects of contemplative neuroscience between different species—here, between humans and horses specifically. This provides one foundation for my Transpecies Field Theory (see p. 7).

- *Quantum Physics:* A simplistic definition from Wikipedia states that "quantum mechanics is the science of the very small: the body of scientific principles that explains the behavior of matter and its interactions with energy on the scale of atoms and subatomic particles." In this book, the term is used to refer to the behavioral interactions between matter and energy.

- *Interpersonal Neurobiology:* In his book, Lloyd W. Davis describes this field as "a developing biopsychological approach to understanding the human condition based on scientific evidence about the mind, brain, and relationships. An important implication from this interconnected system recognizes that change in one evokes change in the others." Interpersonal neurobiology emphasizes the influence of the social world in the construction of the individual. Dr. Dan Siegel, author of *Brainstorm* (Tarcher, 2014) and *Mindsight* (Bantam, 2010), among others, offers one popular perspective in this area of study. In this book, I propose that this interdisciplinary approach is related to the human animal bond, how we all interact with each other, and is therefore one component of the Transpecies Field Theory.

Sometimes in life, we need to take more time to slow down, heal, regroup, reflect, and rejuvenate. That is what certain types of vacation are for. After my first book for the mass market, *Love, Miracles and Animal Healing* came out, I was sent on a 16-city book tour, my already busy practice took another enormous leap, and I found it quite challenging to keep up with all the demands on my time and energy. I had two veterinarians helping me out with the small animal section of my veterinary practice, but I desperately needed additional support as my equine natural medicine practice blossomed. One veterinarian I had trained was kind enough to cover for me while I took some time off to regroup and reflect.

Like I say to my small animal clients when their dogs need time to recover from injury or illness, "Stop, sit, heal!" That is what I needed to do for myself.

I chose an unusual journey for this period "away" spending some time trekking in the Himalayan mountains, exploring different cultures, being in solitude in nature, and meditating in high-altitude monasteries while wondering where the next steps on my life's journey might lead. One afternoon I was sitting on a small bench along the trail that led up to the highest monastery on Mt. Everest, looking up at the blue skies, appreciating the vastness and the quiet. "Out of the blue," so to speak, one of my greatest teachers approached and sat down beside me. I never knew his name or who he was, though he was dressed in the maroon and saffron robes of a Tibetan Buddhist monk. We sat there in silence for quite a while before he then, oddly enough, asked me a question in English: "What are you doing here?"

I was shocked to hear the English language, and even more so, the question. I pondered my response, as there were different levels from which I could answer. I simply chose to say I was sitting, asking that same question, and doing some Tibetan chanting that someone taught me. "Why not chant something in English?" suggested the monk. "Like what?" I responded, curious as to what he'd recommend. "Why not say something like, 'May I be of benefit to all beings.'" He then quietly stood up and disappeared over a rocky knoll back into the mountains, never to be seen by me again.

I decided to try his recommendation, and with each step up and down the steep Himalayan mountainsides, I chanted to myself, "May I be of benefit to all beings." Combined with the physical action of hiking, it slowly became a part of my subconscious, wiring my brain with that mantra. To this day, I continue to bring that intention into my mind each morning and throughout each day. It has changed the entire way that I look at my life and all other beings. I returned from that trek a different person with a more expansive perspective on my veterinary practice and the animals and humans under my care.

I am forever grateful to my unknown teacher.

Once when I shared this experience with some veterinarians who were participating in a mind-body medicine workshop I was teaching, one of the veterinarians suggested that perhaps I expand the phrase to say, "May I be of benefit to all that is." I have played with that and it has led to even more expansive experiences. Find a phrase that resonates with you, and incorporate it into your daily routines. See how it feels for you and your horse.

Heart-centering is finding a calm, silent space in the middle of your heart. The below meditation is a variation on a theme from the pioneering work of Dr. Herbert Benson, Head of Mind-Body Medicine at Harvard Medical School (see the sidebar on p. 135) and also an extension of the simple QFI practice I introduced in chapter 2 (p. 46).

Before you interact with any being, make time for *Self-Calming, Heart-Centering*:

1   Remain in your car with the engine off, find a nice quiet place outdoors, or a peaceful corner in the barn.

2   Sit comfortably with your back straight and your eyes closed.

3   Take a slow, deep breath in through your nose. Feel that breath slowly being inhaled into your throat, your chest, and your abdomen.

4   After a moment, slowly exhale that breath, visualizing it going back up your spinal cord then out through your mouth.

5   Repeat this three times.

6   On the next inhalation, visualize the breath as a calming wave of light that permeates all your cells, enters your heart and your mind, causing a sense of peaceful relaxation through your entire body.

7   Repeat this visual as you breathe in three times.

8   On the next inhalation, visualize your breath filled with loving-kindness and compassion for yourself.

9   Repeat this three times.

10 On the next inhalation, visualize sharing the intent of loving-kindness and compassion with everyone you meet today at the barn.

11 Repeat this three times.

12 On the next inhalation, say a phrase that resonates with you, such as, "May I be of benefit to all beings here at the barn today." As you make the statement, visualize yourself *being* the words you say. You might choose to add, "May all beings be happy, may all beings be free of suffering, and may all beings be blessed with a loving, kind, compassionate heart."

13 Slowly, on your last exhalation, open your eyes, and check in with yourself. If you feel ready, go into the barn with the visualization and clear intention of being of benefit to all beings within.

When you are *really* feeling frustrated or angry or anxious, *Shake, Relax, Release* is beneficial, again *before* you enter the barn to be with your horse or other people. It is important you do this exercise in a quiet place by yourself so as not to inadvertently impact anyone else around you. While *Self-Calming, Heart-Centering* (see above) focuses on the *inhale*, this engages the *exhale* to help you release destructive emotions and thoughts.

As you practice this *Relaxation Response* and the variations of it, there are physical benefits to your body that are well documented. In her article "Learn to Counteract the Physiological Effects of Stress" (*Heart and Soul Healing*, March 2013), Dr. Marilyn Mitchell writes that the Relaxation Response is "your personal ability to encourage your body to release chemicals and brain signals that make your muscles and organs slow down and increase blood flow to the brain. In his book *The Relaxation Response*, Dr. [Herbert] Benson describes the scientific benefits of relaxation, explaining that regular practice of the Relaxation Response can be an effective treatment for a wide range of stress-related disorders" (see more about Dr. Benson in the sidebar on the next page).

1 Close your eyes, take in a slow deep breath, and gently exhale.

2 Repeat three times.

3 On the next inhalation, feel your emotions—whether anger, stress, anxiety, tension, whatever—wherever they are "sitting" in your body.

4 With your exhalation, feel yourself slowly releasing them out. Visualize your destructive emotions dissipating into the air.

5 Repeat three times.

THE RELAXATION RESPONSE

After studying the commonality of experience from numerous, traditional, ancient belief systems, Dr. Herbert Benson, chairman of the Department of Mind-Body Medicine at Harvard University, came up with the term the *Relaxation Response*, which he describes as "the opposite of the fight or flight response." He explains how to elicit the Relaxation Response on his website (relaxationresponse.org), and The Benson-Henry Institute for Mind-Body Medicine at Massachusetts General Hospital teaches patients ways to counteract stress via these techniques. I completed a training workshop in mind-body medicine with Dr. Benson years ago and so have applied some of the Relaxation Response exercises to the development of *The Compassionate Equestrian*.

6   As you get in touch with where you're feeling tension in your body, on the next inhalation, focus on your awareness of the tension.

7   On the exhalation, physically "shake out" your arms and your legs as you blow out through your lips in an exaggerated fashion to get rid of all that frustrating emotional energy pent up inside.

8   Repeat shake, relax, and release as often as you need to until you feel your inner tension is truly gone and you're relaxed. Note: A variation of this exercise is to say, "Relax" on each inhalation and "Release" on each exhalation.

In the article "Everything You Need to Know About Meditation" on HuffPost Healthy Living (April 2014), Jancee Dunn explains the positive changes that occur in your body when you meditate:

- Blood pressure drops (And the effect isn't just temporary: A long-term study from the Medical College of Wisconsin showed that people who meditated twice a day for 20 minutes lowered their blood pressure by 5mmHg.)

- Your brain releases happy chemicals (You get a boost of serotonin, dopamine, and endorphins, all linked to a good mood.)

- Digestion runs more smoothly (Stress triggers that stomach-churning fight-or-flight instinct, shutting down digestion. Relaxed, the body reboots the parasympathetic nervous system, which gets digestion flowing.)

- Pain diminishes (The practice appears to change activity in key pain-processing regions of the brain—in one study; meditators experienced a 40 percent reduction in pain intensity.)

- Inflammation subsides (Meditation can reduce stress-induced inflammation, offering relief from inflammatory conditions such as arthritis and asthma.)

After meditation, it is important not to give in to our tendency to solidify the way we perceive things.

When you do re-enter everyday life, let the wisdom, insight, compassion, humor, fluidity, spaciousness, and detachment that meditation brought you pervade your day-to-day experience. Meditation awakens in you the realization of how the nature of everything is illusory and dreamlike. One great master has said: "After meditation practice, one should become a child of illusion." (Sogyal Rinpoche, *Glimpse after Glimpse: Daily Reflections on Living and Dying*, HarperOne, 1995).

See if this principle of slowing down, becoming heart-centered, and releasing destructive emotions through the exercises introduced in this chapter may be of benefit to you and your horse. And then carry what you have discovered into other moments of your life.

Questions to Consider
BASED ON PRINCIPLE 6

1   How do I "slow down" in my life?

2   How would practicing the Relaxation Response help me in my life?

3   How does the Relaxation Response feel when I achieve it through simple meditations?

4   When focusing on the intention, "May I be of benefit to all beings," in my daily routine, does this phrase resonate with me? If not, which phrase do I feel best suits me and my life with my horse and others?

CHAPTER SEVEN

Joy, Respect, and Gratitude

Compassionate Equitation accelerates the evolution of joy, respect, and gratitude between humans and horses, and allows for a more expansive, conscious interaction between humans and equine companions.

Susan Gordon:

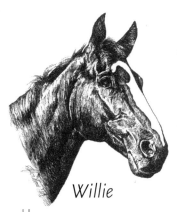

Willie

Can you relate stories about how your horse has comforted you in times of trouble? Horses often seem willing to listen, and some even seem to make conscious attempts to make us feel better.

I sat in front of my backyard barn one night, sulking. The air was crisp, but the night was clear, typical of January in the desert. In fact, it was New Year's Eve. The man I was in a relationship with had left me at home alone while he went to a party. I could hear other people celebrating all around the neighborhood. Willie parked himself as close to me as he could without being in the chair himself. I found myself staring eye-level at his midsection. My two dogs, Kisha, the Shepherd-mix, and Doc, a Welsh Corgi, were at my side, and one of the cats was playing around the barn door.

At first I was upset about being abandoned on such a special evening. But then I realized what a gift it was to have the experience of just sitting quietly with these animals. Nobody was moving, save for the playful cat who was trying to cheer me up in her own way. The horse and dogs had formed a literal barrier around me—similar to those my pets used to build around me when I was a child. My tears dried and I couldn't help but smile at the "support team" in my presence. I started to breathe more deeply and relax. What had begun as a very unhappy evening turned into one full of joy and gratitude. How many times had animals come to my emotional rescue? How many times has this happened to you?

Willie, for all the naughty, puzzling things he would do, had a heart of gold when it came to comforting me, and as I later discovered after we moved to the boarding barn, he had a gift for comforting other horses, too. In those quiet moments of interaction with this horse, we were able to exchange all of the ideals of Principle 7...at least that's how it felt to me. Joy, gratitude, and respect.

As we discussed at the end of the last chapter, there are measurable, physiological changes that take place in the mind and body when the *Relaxation Response* is activated both in people and in horses.[1,2] When this state is achieved, there is a sense of joy and a kind of happiness that cannot be derived from material goods. As the practice of relaxation and *release* becomes more spontaneous, there is an acceleration of those moments of joy, and we tend to feel very grateful for all the wonderful things in our life. The feelings begin to extend throughout our day, with less and less to distract us from that "happy place." We find fewer reasons to be angry or agitated. Everyone around us seems to be in a better mood, and our horses, too, sense the calming energy. "Good energy" produces more respectful interaction between humans and horses, and also in human-to-human relationships. It is the positive result of compassion emanating from a conscious being.

In 2009, Jeffery A. Dusek, PhD, and Herbert Benson, MD, published "A Model of the Comparative Clinical Impact of the Acute Stress and Relaxation Responses" in the award-winning journal Minnesota Medicine. *Their article examines the physiological and biochemical changes that take place during exposure to acute stressors (what they term the Stress Response) or elicitation of the Relaxation Response and the relationship between the two. As we learned in the previous chapter, the Relaxation Response "can be voluntarily elicited and is associated with decreases in oxygen consumption, respiratory rate, and blood pressure, along with an increased sense of well-being" (http://www.ncbi.nlm.nih.gov/pmc/articles/PMC2724877/).* [1,2]

Measurements in horses were tested in a 2012 study reported by Clarence E. Ferguson, PhD, Harry F. Kleinman, DVM, and Justin Browning, MS in the article "Effect of Lavender Aromatherapy on Acute-Stressed Horses" (Journal of Equine Veterinary Science, 2012). Results of the study demonstrate that lavender aromatherapy can significantly decrease a horse's heart rate after an acute stress response and "signal a shift from the sympathetic nervous control from the parasympathetic system" (http://www.j-evs.com/article/S0737-0806(12)00218-3/abstract).

Simply by being in a place of joy, you will naturally have the ability to relieve other people and animals of some level of suffering. They will appreciate your presence.

Exercise itself is known to boost the mood, and we certainly get plenty of it being around horses. As little as 10 minutes of walking back and forth from barn to pasture can make you feel more uplifted, and other equestrian activities such as grooming, tacking up, cleaning stalls, and feeding all engage muscles and pump more oxygen to the brain. As your heart rate increases with added activity, leading up to and including your ride or barn chores, be aware of how you are breathing and how your mood or energy might be shifting. Try not to let your breathing become shallower as your heart rate increases. Even when a runner is working at top speeds, the key to performing well is to stay relaxed and monitor the breath.

What part of being around horses makes you feel the most joy?

Most of us are very happy when around horses. It is understandable that life's circumstances can pull us out of a joyful state, and sometimes into deep grief. Then it becomes more difficult to lift us out of the suffering that comes with fear, sadness, or anger, and sometimes "happy" seems a long ways off. We might even convince ourselves that we do not deserve to be happy, and envy those who are.

A friend tells me people call and ask if they can come over to literally cry on her horse's shoulder. There is something profoundly special about having an animal like a horse in your presence when you are not in the best of moods. When the environment in which the horse is kept promotes healing too, then the entire atmosphere is therapeutic. Therefore, why *not* create a wonderful, peaceful, and beautiful place for both humans and horses and the restorative interactions that can come between them?

Meditation helps with the ability to recognize the illusory, temporary nature of existence. The process helps release the bonds of negative thinking and reduces emotional swings. Without so many ups and downs to distract us, meditation increases our sense of delight and joy. It also helps us reduce attachments and desires, calming the overactive mind and subsequently allowing us to be relaxed but attentive and alert at the same time...much like a satisfied horse grazing in the pasture in his own version of the *present moment*. We can learn a lot by watching horses and other animals at rest or at play, simply enjoying being alive. Horses also often appear to possess a delightful sense of humor. They seem to come by it naturally. Joining in with them on a playful occasion can restore our sense of wonder at the world.[3] It may be something as simple as a tug-of-war with a stick or playing in a mud puddle that brings smiles and childlike energy to a moment.

Invoking Joy Meditation

You can consciously practice invoking a state of well-being and joy. The more you work at this practice, the more access you will give happiness in your life.

1   Get comfortable, and if you wish, close your eyes.

2   Become aware of your breath, inhaling and exhaling slowly, letting the tension go.

3   Let relaxation flow through your entire body down to your feet.

4   Let your emotions and your mind be calm, finding your way to a still, quiet, inner peace.

5   Think of a time when you experienced great joy and well-being. Was it with your horse? Was it with a friend or loved one?

6   Recall the experience with as many details as you can. Can you remember colors, sounds, or scents? How did your body feel in that moment?

7   Allow the sensations you can invoke from that previous joyful time to resonate in your body until it feels it is part of your present, in the here and now. Keep breathing deeply and slowly.

8   Practice the recall of this joyful moment any time, and try to sustain the feelings of well-being and relaxation it brings.

Use this simple meditation whenever you want to feel uplifted. You may find after a time that you can invoke the feelings of your joyful moment without even recreating the initial imagery—you can just think, "Joy!" and there it is!

Researchers at the University of Kentucky College of Agriculture, Food and Environment in Lexington, Kentucky, recently completed one of the first studies to explore how working with horses can develop emotional intelligence in humans. Read about their findings in UK Ag News *2013 article "Pioneering Research: Collaborating with Horses to Develop Emotional Intelligence" (http://news.ca.uky.edu/article/ pioneering-research-collaborating-horses-develop-emotional-intelligence).*

3

Do you think horses have a sense of humor? Can you think of an instance where a horse made you laugh?

I recall watching five of our horses playing in a puddle. It was a typically dark and drizzly West Coast day, and the pastures were too soaked for turnout. Our small herd of Thoroughbreds, my Appaloosa, and a Standardbred gelding were turned out together in one of the sandy riding arenas when one of the braver horses began pawing at a huge, muddy puddle. I believe it was the chestnut Thoroughbred mare, Ali, who started it all. She was quick, sensitive, and had all the qualities that made her a superior jumper. "Bold" was an understatement with this horse. If Ali decided the puddle needed to be dealt with, the spookier geldings were in compliance. Soon all the horses were stomping in the muck, spraying the silty mud in their faces, under their bellies, gleefully behaving like a group of kids at recess. Then the Appaloosa poked his muzzle at Dusty, the Thoroughbred gelding he loved to tease, and all the mud-covered horses galloped off to the other end of the arena in a delightful fit of bucks and leaps.

I relate horses to a kindergarten class that never grows up. I think they enjoy *us* more, too, when we approach our equine activities with childlike glee.

We tend to have a much greater level of respect for those who make us feel joyful compared to those who make us unhappy or upset.

Those of us fortunate enough to be present during group herd-play such as I just described learn how much horses really *do* interact consciously amongst themselves for more than just survival mechanisms. We quickly see that their personalities are completely individual. They exhibit distinct emotions and have likes or dislikes for other horses, as they do for certain humans. Many of us have witnessed how people who haven't spent much time around horses can't read their expressions or recognize when they are contented or annoyed, for example. Sometimes even people who have spent *a lot* of time around horses are unable to differentiate between a horse that's expressing fear and one that's expressing pain.

In film class several years ago, I presented a one-minute trailer of a documentary I had created about horse slaughter. The trailer had a clip of a horse in a pen only steps away from where he would face the end of his life with a group of other horses. It was obvious to me by the look in his eyes that he was depressed and in shock. I mentioned that the horse was "sad" to the class, which was comprised of non-horsepeople, and they all looked at me quizzically. Someone asked, "How can you tell the horse is sad?"

It likely appeared to the other students I was anthropomorphizing—that is, attributing human emotions or personality to an animal. Or perhaps past experience with horses made me quite certain I *was* seeing sadness in this horse. His low-slung head, drooping ears, and glazed eyes were the immediate visual cues that I registered from the photo. Beyond those features, however, was a feeling. Something in my gut that read further into the expression—like knowing when another human being is about to cry. Based on his behaviors and facial expression, it seemed as though the horse was showing signs we might associate with sadness.

How can you tell if a horse is sad?

Learning to read the expressions of horses comes from spending a lot of time with them on the ground, and this is the value in consistently grooming and handling them, as well as observing herd behavior. We cannot assume that just because we are in a state of joy—say, for example, having a wonderful time on a trail ride on a sunny day—that our horses are also in a state of bliss with us. We might check in with ourselves and acknowledge how good we feel in a particular moment, but we also need to keep watch, aware of the horse's expression and potential signs of distress. Being joyful in our interactions with horses but *constantly vigilant and aware of their feelings* is being mindful and compassionate toward them. They cannot "speak up" when something is causing them discomfort. Improving this awareness and respect for the horse could possibly prevent accidents and injuries that may occur if the horse reacts to pain or fear with a buck, rear, or bolt. A happy day can quickly turn into a frightening emergency if you miss a sudden change in your horse's expression or behavior. Dr. Schoen and I have discussed this many times as we wish for joy and pleasure to be part of every riders' everyday encounters with horses, yet we acknowledge the need for common sense and focused awareness as we are still dealing with an animal whose first line of defense is *flight*, and we need to have respect for that side of a horse's nature.

Acceptance and practice of the 25 Principles of Compassionate Equitation can help you have a positive effect on others, as you live in joy, and feel so much gratitude for simply being in the moment.

Dr. Allen Schoen:

In recent decades, the world seems to have become more serious, aggressive, litigious, and adversarial. Yes, everyone needs to be cautious regarding the inherent risk of equine activities, which warrants the use of release forms and prominent placement of signage that displays state laws pertaining to the statute of liability as well as other appropriate measures. All persons entering a barn must be made aware that there is, in general, 1,200 pounds of power behind every horse, and you have to be alert and cautious or he can be dangerous. Not that a horse is by nature a dangerous animal. His natural behaviors, which might put a human body at risk, relate to the predator-prey instinct, as well as each horse's past experiences. When he spooks, leaps, or kicks out, he is just "being a horse." Essentially, there are inherent risks when we choose to be around an animal such as the horse; by his basic nature of simply "being what he is," he can be harmful to us.

Being aware and compassionate and bringing joy to the barn does not minimize the seriousness of handling horses and the need for caution and vigilance around them. I do see *many* barn managers, owners, riders, and trainers who maintain a joyous, happy barn—a compassionate barn as well as a safe barn. I am blessed with clients, trainers, and managers who *want* a positive atmosphere while keeping safety a primary focus. I see happy horsepeople who can ride, get off their horses, and say what a wonderful time they had. They exude peace and gratitude. Spiritual teachers of great traditions say it is hard to have both love and fear in your mind at the same time. If there is a chronic wiring in your brain about being cautious, worried, and afraid, then that can dampen the joy in your life. Your goal is to bring a *healthy balance* of mindful alertness and awareness along with inner peace and delight to the time and space you share with your horse.

Most of us come to horses in search of joy and love...then we realize there is "the business" of the horse world: legal aspects, competitiveness, and egoic tendencies. Once we are aware of these conditions, how do we reintegrate joy and find that balance that keeps us safe and exuding compassion? We *do* need to be vigilant and aware around horses, but we can also learn to just take a deep breath and say, "Ah, I love being here with my horse. I love being in the barn." I hear so many clients say, "When I get to the barn, this is my happy time; my quiet time." We need to be reminded that our joy, our peace, is still there. We need to breathe with joy and gratitude when we get too serious.

How can we instill joy in equestrian activities and still be as cautious as we need to be around horses?

Many people find barns their social center of activity, which is much healthier, in my opinion, than a bar. Barns provide comfortable places for people to sit and clean tack or watch horses being ridden and lessons taught, providing a great setting for both quiet time and social interaction. What isn't so pleasant is when people sit and criticize other riders or their horses, or their trainers, creating an atmosphere of contention. We need to acknowledge that we might not agree with what another trainer or rider is doing, but unless it is dangerous or hurtful to the horse, what good is passing judgment? Riders should be allowed to exhibit their joy with their horse, and not be subjected to the projections of others who might be hypercritical of them. People have different tastes in humor: Some think sarcasm is funny. Others may find self-deprecation funny. Humor in a social setting such as a boarding or training barn requires being sensitive to others' perceptions.

Consider the saying of spiritual teacher Ram Dass, "Wherever you go, there you are." If you can recognize that you may be one who brings a hypercritical mind to the barn, or to the show, or to a clinic, make a choice to instead use the barn and being around horses as places where you *let go* of some of whatever it is inside that tells you to judge others. *Consciously choose* to be mindful, respectful, and grateful.

How would you integrate Principle 7 into your barn?

A lot of horsepeople say they get along better with horses than they do people. Remember that in our fundamental exercise of taking the 10 minutes of Quiet Focused Intention or Heart-Centering prior to entering the barn, we focus on compassion for *all* beings. When you are sensitive to everyone around you and have compassion, you inherently both create joy *and* support other people's joy. Neuroscience shows when we are celebrating another's happiness it brings *us* more happiness. It has a very positive, snowballing effect. Try to celebrate everyone else's reasons for joy and that will bring you *more* joy. Say something positive when you notice someone and his or her horse is happy. Congratulate another on a challenge met or a ribbon won. This is key to this Principle.

Part of being respectful toward others is celebrating the joy they may be experiencing. Be grateful to be in the presence of happy people and horses.

When one of my clients, who was also a dear friend, was diagnosed with terminal cancer, she would often say that some of her happiest moments were with her horses in the barn. Her barn was truly "Old MacDonald's Farm"—an old stone structure—housing her top endurance horses, rescue mules, her old ponies, Icelandic horses, goats, chickens, dogs, and cats as well as her son, her caring trainer, and several grooms. My client also invited another individual dealing with cancer to come and just be around the horses. This patient also shared how healing it felt to be around all the loving animals.

So often, I hear from people with various health issues that despite their pain and suffering, they find the time they share with their horses and other animals at the barn as happy and healing. Many studies document the healing effects of being around animals, who offer a deep level of inner peace and understanding to humans in their midst. I am always grateful to each and every horse and each and every animal I share time with. I appreciate and am grateful for the sense of "good" I feel when I am helping a horse, when I'm able to relieve his suffering and discomfort. This circle of joy, respect, and gratitude between humans and animals can go round and round continuously for all of us, if we simply choose to be aware of it and participate in it.

"Just as a single light attracts attention on a dark night,
action informed by knowledge attracts and awakens others,
inspiring emulation."

Tarthang Tulku, *Knowledge of Freedom*
(Dharma Publishing, 1984)

Questions to Consider

BASED ON PRINCIPLE 7

1 How can I create my own inner joy, as well as respect and gratitude for myself, my horses, and my barn?

2 How can I share that joy, respect, and gratitude with others?

3 What am I grateful for in sharing my life with my horse?

4 What am I grateful for in sharing my life with my horse community?

5 How does a feeling of gratitude feel within myself?

6 How does a feeling of gratitude impact everyone else I interact with?

CHAPTER EIGHT

Peace and Quiet

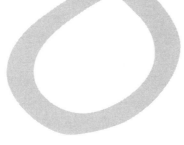

We acknowledge that a peaceful, quiet environment is of benefit. Research suggests that classical and country music are conducive to a peaceful environment for animals.

Susan Gordon:

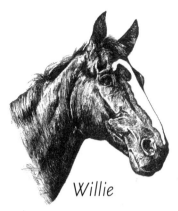

Willie

I left the house early one morning, stepping outside to a purplish, still dawn, rich with the scent of horses and irrigated pasture. It was four in the morning and remarkably hot—typical summer in the city of Phoenix. However, the blazing sun had not yet emerged, and it was as pleasant a time of day as we were going to have for quite a few months. I looked to my left, where the row of pens held four of our horses, and squinted through the semidarkness to search for the big body of the old Hanoverian.

Willie was not supposed to be let out of his pen and into the paddock area, so I snuck him out late at night and brought him in pre-dawn. It allowed him to relish a few hours of freedom before returning to his duties as a lesson horse and colt-sitter. At this time, we had moved to yet another barn, and this one was home to many upper-level dressage horses and visiting judges and clinicians, as well as FEI competitions. There was a protocol here. I was the assistant hunter-jumper trainer, and Willie, a trusted assistant in his own right.

The other horses stirred upon sensing my presence as I approached the pens, and I still could not see Willie. My heart started to beat faster. Did he somehow escape? Was he stolen? Dead? He had a habit of lying stone quiet with all four legs braced out in front. He was good at "playing dead." I quickened my steps and then came to a halt. There in the first rays of light appeared Blueberry, a strange little calico cat who showed up at the barn one day, impersonating the barn's other calico cat, Muffin. Her lithe cat-body was bouncing out of the grass, gleefully swooping at bugs that had become active with the arrival of a new day. Behind the leaping Blueberry a large ear stuck upright out of the grass, flicking away insects disturbed by the feline huntress.

The rest of Willie's massive body lay as still and flat as possible, likely hoping he wouldn't be compelled to get up and return to his stall. Wisps of the now-rising sun caught the edges of his outline and that of the happy cat, creating a scene of peace and community that had a profound effect on my soul. All was right with the world in that quiet, still moment.

We had come a long way together by then. Willie's contentment struck me as a special gift. Perhaps because contentment was something that had been missing in his life for quite some time. He had finally found a home where he *was admired and understood. If he could talk, I was sure he would have let out a big sigh and proclaimed, "Peace at last."*

When we walk into a barn we do a "sensory scan."

When I first visit a barn, farm, or horse property, I do a visual and sensory scan of the horses, people, and facility, and immediately take note of how I feel upon arrival. After meeting Dr. Schoen and developing the 25 Principles of Compassionate Equitation together, I realized he and I do exactly the same thing—we employ a technique that allows us to pick up the overall energy in the barn and surrounding area. Beyond basic observations noting cleanliness and that horses are in good flesh and health, we want to feel welcomed and absorbed in calm professionalism and order. We can usually determine fairly quickly whether or not a barn or showground is a place we would like to spend time.

There are some barns that feel like cathedrals, instilling a sense of awe. A great barn brings to mind the most wonderful aspects of our encounters with horses. This is what we refer to as a *state of grace*. Whether you have one horse in your backyard or a barn full of fancy show horses and boarders, no matter how simple or elaborate, you can make your horse's home a place of beauty. A beautiful place makes you want to linger and relax.

A large part of creating a healthy environment for your horses is to make it a quiet and peaceful one. It supports the *parasympathetic response*—the branch of the autonomic nervous system (ANS) responsible for the body's ability to recuperate and recover after stress—in people and animals. Everyone stays calmer and the atmosphere of the barn remains healthier.

To this effect, *everything* matters, and everything you turn your mind to can be affected in a positive way. When your barn is a commercial facility and you are the manager, your mindfulness is especially important to all the horses and humans who enter. *You* set the tone for the day-to-day operations and help instill a high level of trust, confidence, and ultimately, performance, from the horses and riders who enjoy their time in a compassionate environment. Kind words and a peaceful demeanor toward staff, management, and other horse owners positively affects the energy of your establishment.

*Know what's expected of you and others at your barn. A clear
set of rules and etiquette are only effective if they are posted as
visible reminders. We also encourage posting the 25 Principles of
Compassionate Equitation in a prominent location.*

Of course there will always be tense moments when associating with other individuals and when handling your own horses and those that belong to others. It is human nature. When conflicts and clashing personalities can be handled diplomatically, most problems can be quelled and mediated before reaching crisis level. Encouraging acceptance of the Principles of Compassionate Equitation by everyone who boards, trains, rides, and visits a stable is a big step to achieving a business style that brings out the best in all participants. The overall environment is more inviting if management and staff are prosocial, highly conscious, stable, and resilient.

Differences of opinions will always be part of human interaction; those differences can become a catalyst for both opening and closing of doors in regards to general social reaction and friendship. At an equestrian facility the common denominator is *horses*. Sometimes other factors bring together like-minded riders—for example, those hoping to achieve high standards within a single discipline, such as dressage. With a mixed-use facility that involves various breeds and training methods, the differing opinions and styles may cause higher or more constant tension than a single-discipline barn, especially if riding space is limited. At least that has been my own experience and observation. In these scenarios a good way to encourage compassion is to remember to see everyone, every horse, and every discipline as a learning opportunity.

*Keeping the peace at a multi-discipline barn is a challenge.
Barn rules have a positive effect if they reflect the
compassionate reasons they exist in the first place: safety,
health, and well-being of human and horse.*

Because of our human tendency to want to be accepted by and become part of a community, we can be highly influenced by those around us. This can mean finding ourselves feeling pressured or coerced to conduct ourselves in a certain way. It is important to recognize and appreciate *who you truly are* and to be able to identify the "self." Practice setting your personal boundaries both in and out of the barn. If something does not feel right to you, or you think it may not be best for your horse,

Peacemaking at the Barn

Ask yourself:

- How do I focus on creating and preserving inner calm, peace, awareness, and mindfulness?

- How could I use a compassionate mind and heart to help see all members of the horse community as connected beings, free of our usual divisions by breed and discipline?

- Why would this produce a positive, constructive outcome for everyone and especially my horse?

make your decisions from clear thinking, not emotions. Ask yourself if the barn, trainer, or situation is really the right one for *you*. Choose to be compassionate to yourself *first*, so you can be honest in your compassion for others.

Set personal boundaries and mind them when others try to influence your decisions in a way that makes you uncomfortable. Be mindful that you are not creating uncomfortable situations for others. Peaceful means a calming, safe space for everyone at a barn.

It is very easy to get pulled into the fracas of "everyday life," then drag the remnants of the stress from work, travel, finances, and relationships into the barn with you. It can be a struggle not to let other people's stress affect your focus on your horse. In my role as a professional, I always wanted everyone to be happy with the barn, their rides, and their horses, and it upset me if they weren't. It is important in situations such as mine to stay *centered*, with the "center" being the heart—the balancing point for our emotions. Our minds can easily take over and talk us into all kinds of things. This can trigger the flood of chemicals that affect moods and thoughts, which is where so much conflict and distress can arise. If this is allowed to permeate our horse time, then the ride or lesson most likely won't go as well as it could have otherwise. The saying, "Peace begins with us," is very true.

Being quiet = better ability to focus. Better focus = better ride.

Sometimes taking a few deep breaths and slowing your movements is all that is necessary to bring calmness and gentleness back into your actions and words. When small details are aggravating you, begin to ask yourself how important they really are in the big picture. Yes, if you are in a hurry and a keeper on the noseband breaks, that's annoying. If your horse spooks on the way to the arena, it might send your heart rate up. If your barnmate is angry because you didn't sweep up the mess you made in the grooming area, both you and your barnmate are likely to feel tense. If you don't *come back to center*, the tension can escalate, and not only negatively impact you and your barnmate, but your horses and anyone else you come into contact with in the hours ahead.

With all the little irritations and annoyances that add up throughout the day, it is important to put them aside and find a more peaceful state of mind before working with your horse.

As we've mentioned before in this book, for some people, the mere act of walking into the barn and taking in the aroma of horses, hay, and leather is enough to alter their state of mind. For others, it takes a conscious action to change their behavior and slow down. Beginning with 10 minutes of quiet time before entering the barn, as we explored on p. 47, is a good way to ensure the "peace is with you" either way.

Depending on whether you have already engaged in mindfulness practice or are only now just learning about it, it may take a series of small steps for your advancement, or you might be able to make an evolutionary leap once you are on the path. When you find the method or exercise that puts you in a state of peace and grace, you won't have to try so hard to get there each time. The practice becomes a part of your being. You find yourself being less angry, less irritated by small issues, and rarely coerced into another's mindset and energy if it doesn't serve your inner place of calmness.

As we learned in chapter 4, *watch your thoughts*. After all, your horse is watching *you*. He might not know exactly what you are thinking, but he will sure know how you are *reacting* to what you are thinking. Whatever is going through your mind—positive or negative—will manifest outwardly in your behavior or actions, whether you are aware of it or not.

Return to Center

When you feel overwhelmed and scattered, try one of my favorite methods for returning yourself to clarity and finding your *center*:

1 Sit or stand comfortably, feet flat on the floor or ground, about hip-width apart. Keep your shoulders back and relaxed.

2 Breathe deeply and slowly into your abdomen. Count to three on the inhale and repeat on the exhale.

3 Visualize a golden ball of energy at the base of your spine. Give the ball of energy some weight.

4 Visualize—like an anchor dropping into the water—sending the ball of energy downward through the surface of the earth, trailing a golden chain attached to the base of your spine. Imagine the ball traveling all the way to the very core of the earth, and the chain intact, connecting you.

5 Anchor the gold ball to the core of the planet.

6 Do you feel more "grounded" and centered now?

You can probably understand by now why compassion takes practice! It helps to see some of the key words we've been using in this book over and over again, and then act on them consistently to make them a habit: slow down, breathe, release, center, be calm and quiet.

One simple process could potentially lower the tension in a typical commercial boarding or training operation. If horse owners were asked by management, "Is everything all right?" on a daily basis, a lot of problems would be defused before they could escalate. Sometimes it is hard to hear complaints from your boarders or clients, but if you have taken on the responsibility of equine care and training, such is the nature of your work. It may be that those you work with and serve

Visualize the Place You Feel Most at Peace

- Is it quiet, or perhaps there's music playing?

- Is it indoors or outdoors?

- Do you find yourself taking deeper, slower breaths when you see yourself in this place of peace?

- How do you feel when it is just you and your horse in the quiet of his stall or paddock?

- How do you feel when you walk into the barn?

- How do you usually feel when you leave the barn?

- Is being with your horse or in your barn akin to being in your peaceful place? Or maybe it *is* that place?

will continue to complain amongst themselves and not be forthcoming in letting you know something is bothering them, but opening the door to discussion is a gesture of compassion. You may not be able to fill your barn with ideal boarders, but you can certainly have a policy of being very direct with your expectations of behavior, and allow others to voice their expectations as well.

Most horsepeople who turn professional do so out of a love for horses and the discipline of their choice, and ultimately want to see horses enjoying the best care and training available. They often have a difficult time dealing with the "human aspect" of the business. Like attracts like, and therefore, a well-kept barn with content, peaceful clients and horses will ultimately be a full barn and a place that provides a calming, restorative environment for everyone.[1] These are some of the benefits of creating a tolerant, considerate place for all who enter the premises.

1

A 2013 The Horse *feature by Christa Lesté-Lasserre entitled "Study: Post-Training Stress Detrimental to Equine Learning" explains how recent studies by French behavior scientists have revealed that when it comes to helping your horse retain what he learns during train-ing, you should aim to keep him as stress-free as possible—before,*

during, and after schooling (http://www.thehorse.com/articles/32080/
study-post-training-stress-detrimental-to-equine-learning).

Do you play music for your horses? What have you noticed about their reactions?

Music can be a nice addition to an equine environment, although type and volume play a role here. Because music tastes are subjective in humans, it can be difficult to convince everyone at the barn to agree to an appropriate choice of tunes. Barns that have rhythmic, instrumental music playing at all times seem to be very conducive to quiet, focused sessions with horses—at least that has been my experience and Dr. Schoen's, as well. It helps with one of the most fundamental aspects of good training, which is to instill rhythm in the horse. Riders who know music and dance seem to have an easier time establishing rhythm in their horse. Interestingly, recent research has looked at the effects of music on horses and found they actually seem to "prefer" classical and country music to jazz or rock.[2]

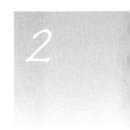

> *Kentucky Equine Research released the story "Barn Beat: What Music Style is Best for Horses?" in May of 2013 via EquiNews.com. The article states: "Results showed that horses produced the same balance of restful and alert behaviors during silent periods and when classical and country music selections were being played. They tended to eat more quietly, a behavior that is associated with calmness, when country music was playing than when no music was heard. Jazz and rock tunes were correlated to more frequent behavioral indications of stress such as stamping, head tossing, snorting, and vocalizing compared to behavior when no music was being played" (http://www.equinews.com/article/barn-beat-what-music-style-best-horses).*

Horses I've known seemed to enjoy live, acoustic instruments and the human singing voice. There once was an outdoor party at a stable I taught at, and one of the young girls brought her flute. Every horse was fixated from all around the property, ears pricked, listening intently to the instrument. I am not sure how much research has been done in working with horses and acoustic sound, but it would be worth exploring further. The effect on horses would possibly reflect similarities to effects on humans listening to specific tempos and frequencies. "Human beings have been using sound to access deeper states of consciousness, expand awareness, and heal the body for thousands of years," states Dr. Jeffrey Thompson, DC, of the Center for Neuroacoustic Research.

And Robyn Armon, et al, of the University of Wisconsin-Madison writes that "Past research reveals that types of music varying in tempo, or beats per minute, can have physiological effects on the body. It is shown that fast tempo music of 120–130 beats per minute increases anxiety observed through an increase in blood pressure and heart rate, while slow tempo music of 50–60 beats per minute has the opposite effect on the body (Edworthy and Waring 2010)" in "Effects of Music Tempos on Blood Pressure, Heart Rate, and Skin Conductance After Physical Exertion."

Dr. Allen Schoen:

One bright blue, sunny spring day I went to see a new horse at a barn that's not on my normal rounds. As soon as I walked into the barn I saw grooms with their heads down, frowning, and horses with their ears back. Loud, heavy music was playing, reverberating off all the stalls. The trainer strode in, shouting extremely critical, comments at the grooms as they cowered behind the horses. My enjoyment of the beautiful day instantly changed. My relaxed attitude that mirrored the sun in the sky quickly shifted to a dark tension that permeated my previous sense of well-being. Aware of this internal shift, I was able to catch myself and take in a slow, deep breath, fending off the negative energy present in the thick air around me.

I recognized in that moment I had a choice: either succumb to the noise and negativity that was filling the entire space, or try to change the energy to one of peace, quiet, and gentleness through my presence. I chose language that would not antagonize the trainer and grooms and mirrored back to them other more constructive, positive options and methods of interacting. This is a choice that all of us have the opportunity to make when we are confronted with similar situations.

After introducing myself, I acknowledged the beauty of the day and how it allowed everyone to be grateful for the sunshine in our lives. Instantly I found the grooms' and the trainer's energy shift. I humbly asked them if they could turn the music down, explaining that when I work on horses, I prefer a quiet, more peaceful environment. The trainer graciously accommodated me. With the noise gone, I watched as the grooms started to smile, the attitude of the trainer lightened, and even the horses' ears went forward.

Listen carefully to the sounds in your barn. Are they soothing, or are they aggravating? How can you choose to make the "sound environment" healthy for everyone?

I am grateful that the majority of barns I visit recognize the healing abilities of creating a peaceful, quiet space with soft music. I chuckle whenever I get to one particular barn as the trainer and manager play my favorite music station while I am working on their horses. The music may vary from barn to barn, some playing classical, others country, soft folk, light rock, or New Age instrumental. Whatever is calming to the humans in the barn will normally be calming for the horses as well.

One of *my* favorite times to go into barns is at dinner when the only sound you can hear is the meditative munching of horses enjoying their evening meal. That sound is like a calm wave, and soothing to the soul.

Avoid noisy equipment in barns. If it is irritating to you, it is irritating to your horse.

In contrast, today the use of machinery is often disruptive to the natural sounds of horse barns. For example, I would love to no longer see leaf-blowers used in barns and stable areas. I miss the calming sound of a broom. It seems like a sad sign of the times when the staff may put on headphones to block the noise from their machines, but the horses and riders must listen to it reverberating against everything in the barn. Everyone "tightens up" around that kind of noise and air pollution. They have has to raise their voices or even shout at the top of their lungs in order to be heard. When barns *do* go back to just using brooms (which actually seem more efficient, as well) everyone always comments how grateful they are!

While these details may seem of minor importance, they are actually integral components to creating a more harmonious barn. Sometimes you don't realize how a well-intended choice like using a leaf-blower to clean the aisle can impact negatively on well-being by creating a disharmonious sound environment. There is now more and more evidence about how the nervous system detects and reacts to chronic background noise, resulting in stress.

Reflect on which sounds bring peace and a sense of calm to you and your horses, and which sounds may be disruptive. Determine how you can modify your barn's practices to create a more soothing sound environment. There is a book co-authored by veterinary neurologist, Dr. Susan Wagner DVM, MS, DACVIM, and sound researcher Joshua Leeds, called *Through a Dog's Ear: Using Sound to Improve the Health and Behavior of Your Canine Companion* (Sounds True, 2008). Using the science of *bioacoustics*, they have discovered that certain music and tones, specifically slower tempos and simple arrangements, are calming to the canine nervous system. This knowledge has enabled them to produce a series of music CDs for dogs to listen to in situations that typically cause them stress and tension, such as loud fireworks, riding in cars or when they are staying in boarding kennels.[3] It would not seem unreasonable to try this bioacoustic research in various horse environments, too.

3   *Based on pioneering research into how the canine nervous system responds to sound, bioacoustic expert Joshua Leeds and concert pianist Lisa Spector have created music that is twice as effective as conventional classical selections for reduction of canine anxiety behaviors (http://www.soundstrue.com/shop/Through-a-Dog's-Ear/581.pd).*

Bring peace and quiet to your barn, and leave your barn in peace and quiet, as well. Take all the wonderful benefits of being present with your horses to everyone else you encounter, everywhere you go.

One of my favorite memories of quiet time with horses was when I was trekking through the Himalayas in Bhutan with a few pack ponies. I set up my tent on top of a mountain, looking up at a gazillion stars with no lights, no sound, and no motor noise. As I curled up in my sleeping bag for the night, anticipating a quiet, peaceful sleep, the yaks and pack ponies gradually, one by one, lowered themselves to the ground, surrounding my tent. Initially, there was more sound than I would have preferred with a bit of snoring, twisting, and turning. Shortly thereafter, I fell asleep to the gentle, rhythmic rising and falling of their deep sighs and breaths. As my breathing rhythm began to mesh with theirs, I could appreciate the healing resonance of "oneness" with all beings.

ZEN SWEEPING

"I actually used to enjoy sweeping the barn aisle with an old-fashioned corn broom. First I would wet the dust down using a garden watering can as I walked through the aisle. Then I would go up the middle with a rhythmic, side-to-side swishing of the broom, and down and up each side to finish off. No loud noise to disturb the horses or anyone else, and no dust blowing around. It can be a very Zen experience and provide instant gratification!"

— Susan Gordon

When we have experiences like these, we never forget them. We search for that place of oneness and calmness all the time, even in the midst of a busy day. We owe it to our mind, body, health, and to everyone we encounter, to find our way home to the one being we know as "self." Silence or healing sounds are one wave we can follow, like Dorothy in *The Wizard of Oz*, following the "yellow brick road" *home*. The exercises in this book also offer introductions to other avenues back to the place we call "self." Each one of us needs to find the one that works best for our own journeys.

Questions to Consider
BASED ON PRINCIPLE 8

1   Do I notice the background sounds in my environment? In the horse barn?

2   Do the sounds bring me peace, or do I find them irritating and disharmonious?

3   What sounds do I think my horse would like to hear?

4   What changes can I make to create a peaceful sound environment in *my* barn that would be pleasing and harmonious to all beings who enter?

CHAPTER NINE

Patience, Kindness, and Consistency

We agree to act with patience, kindness and consistency, avoiding any intentional, harmful, aggressive, violent behaviors, including actions out of anger or egoic self-interest.

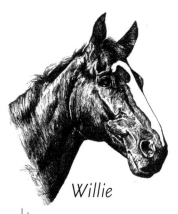

Willie

Susan Gordon:

When it comes to Willie's story as it relates to Principle 9, I have to ask, "What if the horse is the aggressive one?"

I think Willie did actually intend to do harm sometimes, although I told him it probably wasn't a good idea to "deck" the person who provided him with his meals. His aggressive outbursts ran counter to the generous and kind soul that I sensed lay beneath the surface. My agreement with Willie was that I would treat him with patience, kindness, and consistency, no matter what kind of behavior he threw at me, whether it was intentional on his part or a triggered response. In reality, I wasn't sure sometimes where the violent behavior was coming from, especially in the early days before I had uncovered more information about his history.

Who made him into the horse he became, and why? Was there an ego to blame? Had someone become so competitive that the horse's well-being suffered for it? Was Willie forced to jump even after a life-threatening fall over a cross-country fence? Was he punished for refusing in the jumper arena?

Okay, so I had a horse that may have been treated inconsistently, perhaps due to ego or anger. Maybe both. In any case, working around him at first was like dealing with a hostile person. Any confrontation only escalated the argument. He was shut down enough as it was, and an angry reaction from his handler would not have resolved anything. For a while, every day with him was like trying to make peace when one side was intent on battle.

It took a while to quell the residual anger he was holding on to, but eventually he was convinced that the human herd could be trusted again and life was comfortable. Even then, though, if I, or anybody else, ever approached him in any form of negative mood, he would exhibit an expression that might as well have been a mirror. He was a great teacher in that way. And of course my ultimate reward was when he was so content in the end—if asked to go to battle then, I think he probably would have said, "No thanks, I'm good right here where I am."

Put a tool in the hands of a kind, benevolent person, provide him or her with good training, and it will be used for the intended purpose with no harm done—short of any accidents. In the hands of an aggressive or violent person, the most benign tools can become weapons. We can all think of many examples where this has been the case. The same holds true with equipment used on horses, and the skills and intent with which it is used.

Everything we put on a horse in terms of tack or aids—for the latter both natural and artificial—applies pressure, ranging from very mild to severe. Most horse people have no intention of hurting their horses, but there are some who feel going to stronger bits, bigger spurs, or other training aids that force a horse into a desired position, is more efficient than taking the time to create a finished horse without the use of added force. When a horse came to me for training with a severe bit, allegedly for the purpose of "control," the first thing I would do is put the horse back in a plain snaffle to find out what the *real* problem was. In almost every case, the problem wasn't the horse.

A young domesticated horse is taught to move away from, or give to, pressure, which is counter to his instinct to lean into the mare for protection as a foal. With a gentle introduction to halter, saddle, bridle, and rider, the horse learns to accept our cues despite their being at odds with his nature, and respond to directions given by hands, legs, and seat, all of which must work independently of each other. Due to sensitivity of the horse to pressure—whether on the bars of the mouth where the bit lies, or the nose and poll when using a bitless bridle or hackamore, or the thin hide over the rib cage where the girth tightens and our legs are applied—we will have a more compliant horse if we are mindful of how much pressure is put on him at all times and how our use of the pressure is being received (as conveyed by his expression). Horses are generally very accommodating, adaptable animals that take kindly to consistent training and conditioning—if all goes well.

Some horses have a much higher tolerance for pain than others, just like humans.

With some horses, it is very obvious when they are hurting, while others are far more stoic and keep working until they are significantly lame. Because of this, it is necessary to *always* consider the possibility of pain when dealing with a presumed "behavioral issue." For example, I have generally found that when I am told a horse needs a stronger bit there is likely pain elsewhere in the body, often the back or joints of the hindquarters. Shooting pain from these areas can send a horse scooting forward with little warning. Many riders and trainers immediately treat this as a behavioral problem rather than searching for a potential cause of pain first. If punishment, whether through the bit, spur, or whip, is meted out while the horse is in pain, he will associate his pain with even more pain being caused by the rider, and a myriad of both physical and mental problems is the result.

As you did in chapter 4, ask yourself again, *why* you are riding this horse? For fun? For sport and competition? What are you asking the horse to do? Is *your* riding making him stiff, sore, and crooked, or supple, more athletic, and progressively stronger? Are you being patient and consistent with your requests?

Refined use of the aids is considered an art in classical horsemanship. It contributes to the beautiful, harmonious picture of horse and rider melded together in their dance. Repeatedly and forcibly jerking, pulling, kicking, and spurring are actions sometimes made in a moment of reactive frustration or anger, and can quickly escalate to become abusive to the horse. These are reactions that are easy to fall prey to—even for compassionate riders—in an instance of disobedience or trouble from a powerful horse. It can be frightening when a horse acts up, and we react out of fear for our safety, sometimes rightly so. When you catch a horse in this kind of behavior and can respond in the moment, you do indeed

IS "BITLESS" MORE COMPASSIONATE?

Understandably, a rider wants to believe he or she is providing the most comfortable situation for his or her horse, and this is a very kind-hearted thought to have in regards to the selection of equipment. Asking this question though, I feel, furthers division within the industry over the "better choice" when weighing one type of bridle versus another. You will find many opinions based on everyone's "filters" and background experience with horses. The real question to ask is, "What is the most compassionate way to meet the needs of the horse and the capabilities of the rider?"

Bit or no bit, the rider still needs to learn to ride correctly and develop soft, quiet hands, which result from an independent seat. In correct equitation, horses are *not* "steered" by their heads. Proper riding requires the coordination of all natural aids. If a rider's hands are not fully under control, and he or she inadvertently—or need to "block" and resist the activity (see sidebar, p. 108). When it comes to resolving issues in a horse that has compromised your safety, and possibly that of his own and other horses and riders in a busy arena, show, or trail ride, we would just like to see the *intent of punishment* removed from a rider's mindset, and for *reactive* corrections to become *responsive*, nonviolent actions.

I know all too well what it feels like to have a horse misbehave. As a veteran rider of off-the-track Thoroughbreds, young, powerful Warmbloods, half-wild ponies, and spoiled and burned-out show horses, my job was to identify and solve issues. What caused them to buck, bolt, rear, spin around, refuse jumps, run backward, pull like a freight train, and any number of other vices? After many years of riding all kinds of horses, it is possible to become so sensitive to the feeling transmitted through a horse's back that you can tell how that horse has been ridden *before* even asking him to take a step. The signals conveyed through the horse's musculoskeletal system into your own body actually contain a lot of information. The key is to have the patience to sit there and listen to your horse for a minute or two before starting your ride. Here again is another good opportunity to take a few deep breaths, center, focus your mind, and get ready to pay full attention to your horse. We repeatedly mention taking this action for good reason.

purposely—pulls on a horse, *any type* of headstall can be abusive to the horse. The rider's seat and leg aids, when uneducated, can cause spinal damage, muscular imbalance, and pain throughout the horse's body.

Also, many competitive disciplines require a bit so it can be in the horse's interest over the long term to teach him to accept and yield to one. In all cases, adjust the noseband loosely enough and have it properly placed so the horse can move his jaw and breathe freely. Riders and trainers who abide by the 25 Principles of Compassionate Equitation will select the most comfortable bridle for the horse and ensure it is used with finesse and never with the kind of action intended to cause pain.

Observe your horse, evaluate his expression, or have an expert on the ground help you decide if your choices of equipment and your ability to use it with skill and care are, in fact, the most compassionate options you have offered him.

The array of punishment and abuse horses put up with still amazes me. Some eventually lose tolerance and do not have much of a life unless someone literally rescues and rehabilitates them. The question I always ask is, "How did they get that way?" Most of the time, when a horse came to me for training, his full background was rarely disclosed. It involved a lot of detective work to figure some horses out. Unless acute pain is involved, extreme issues do not develop overnight. Most likely, the subtle clues indicating something was going wrong with training were missed or ignored all along.

When communicating with your horse becomes difficult, slow it down. Walk. Breathe. Dismount if it will help both of you calm down—you will accomplish more with a productive, short session than working beyond the horse's zone of attention and comfort. Leave the arena relaxed and happy.

Returning horses to a level of trust with consistent, short, productive training sessions often proves to be a successful formula. Horses that longe quietly in halt, walk, trot, and canter, and do so via voice commands, are generally pleasant and responsive under saddle, too. Proper longeing is a terrific problem-solver, and when done well, provides a safe, bonding exercise for both horse and rider. Longeing can help maintain impulsion and build hindquarter strength without having the added pressure of a rider on the horse's back. Whatever you want the horse to do under saddle, he will be more adept if he is first able to perform most of the required movements and gaits from the ground. When choosing longeing equipment, make sure it is never intended to pull your horse into a "frame." Remember, the tools that are used are only as compassionate as the person attached to them. Protect yourself, too, by always longeing with gloves and boots. There is no need for frantic chasing, nor do I recommend encouraging horses to "play up" when they are fresh, as you don't want them to associate being at the end of a longe line with being allowed to scoot off, rear, buck, or turn around without warning. Erratic behavior while on the longe can become a real problem if you need a method of quiet exercise, to warm up at a busy show, or give a lesson.

With proper training the contact between the horse's mouth and the rider's hands is light and the pressure is mild at best. Optimally, it is so light you could visualize the reins being replaced with silk threads. Such visualizing techniques can be helpful when estimating the amount of pressure you are putting on the horse. Combine imagery with regulated, deep breathing, and the horse will actually match your breathing patterns, and the two of you can work in exquisite harmony as a result. When you get your breathing right, rhythm occurs naturally, and the horse will respond by releasing tension throughout his body. Allowing this release to occur improves proprioception and is dependent on the rider's seat remaining perfectly balanced while the horse warms up and is encouraged to establish regularity in his steps. This is quite the opposite effect of that caused by "overflexing," also known as "hyperflexion," to force a frame, which is seen too often these days.[1]

Uta Ulrike von Borstel, et al, describe the 2006 FEI review of "hyper-flexion" in the Applied Animal Behaviour Science *article "Impact of Riding in a Coercively Obtained Rollkur Posture on Welfare and Fear of Performance Horses." Much has now been written about the controversial "hyperflexed" or "Rollkur" posture, involving the positioning of the horse's head and neck in a deep and round position with the horse's muzzle (almost) touching his chest, which is thought to have detrimental effects on the horse's physical and/or psychological state (http://www.equitationscience.com/documents/Conferences/Consensus%20workshop/UtaVonBorstel_Rollkur2009.pdf).*

The positioning of the horse's neck arises from activity in the hindquarters, subsequent to rhythm, tempo, and suppleness being created by the rider. A horse correctly warmed up for his training session or competitive event moves freely forward with a swinging back and a soft, relaxed expression. He is not rushing, or falling on his forehand. His tail swings rhythmically from side to side, not swishing in irritation. The horse's back raises and sometimes the gaits will change dramatically from "flat" (no suspension) to "elevated" (more suspension) as a result. It is an extraordinary feeling when this occurs, like at lift-off when the nose of a plane elevates above its tail. Again, the rider's seat is imperative to helping the horse maintain freedom of his movement, otherwise he will flatten and the gaits will diminish in quality, subject to the way he is being ridden. When cooling down, always allow the horse a free-walk on a loose rein before leaving the arena. Find relaxation before increasing the intensity of the workout, and come back to relaxation at the end of your session.

This is a relatively brief explanation of a complex set of events that are critical to your horse's performance. For more information, I recommend perusing the outstanding selection of books and DVDs available on classical training.

Patience and consistency in training is compassionate training. Pulling the horse into a frame never allows the rider to listen for the horse's request for relief from the pressure. The horse that is ridden forward, moving freely from back to front in a relaxed position, will clearly let the rider know when he is ready for something more.

Patience is a quality most of us find difficult to sustain, whether in our homes and business lives, or when working with animals. I learned a long time ago as a teenager with young, green horses, that a loss of patience can have upsetting consequences. Everything moves so fast in our modern world and our expectation is to get instant results. Creatures of low technology, such as our animals, suffer the most for our desire to have everything happen in a virtual instant. On one hand, you need a quick, flexible mind to respond to a horse's instinctive prey-animal tendencies during training, but it is also important to understand the value of repeating those responses over and over and over again with a lot of patience and consistency.

Make sure you have a fundamental understanding of what constitutes an advanced level of training in your particular discipline, as it helps clarify the step-by-step process and reasons behind one exercise progressing into the next. Even basic interactions with horses require extensive study of the processes necessary to get the horse to the point of being started under saddle. When your goal is not competition-related or discipline-specific and you only wish to ride for recreation purposes, happily and safely, you still need a sound, responsive horse that can traverse the terrain, remain calm in traffic, is not herd-bound, and so forth. Sadly, many riders do not have the patience to learn the horsemanship necessary to either train a horse or preserve the training he's had.

Cultivating patience and eliminating the ego's need for rapid accomplishment, instantaneous fun, and accolades are qualities we encourage. It is easy to get attached to the ego. It is our identity—our "self"—and we like to protect that identity. For most of us, "letting go" of that ego requires a long process of self-reflection and becoming highly aware of thoughts, speech, and actions toward other humans, as well as horses. We cannot be perfect, but we can certainly get better at noticing how we affect others.

THE "OVERFLEXING" PHENOMENON

"Overflexing" is a modern tendency used by many riders and trainers, often to position a horse's head and neck or to increase control. In the rush to put a horse in the desired "frame" or to obtain a certain "look," or in some cases to give a rider or trainer more control of a strong or nervous mount, artificial devices, overuse of hands, and other methods are used to pull or compel the horse into position. It has been found that "overflexing" or "hyperflexing the neck," either longitudinally or laterally, may produce stress responses in the horse, such as:

- Changes in pace
- Backing up
- Bucking
- Stumbling
- Tail-swishing
- Head-tossing
- Nose-tilting
- Abnormal oral behavior

- Snorting
- Groaning
- Visibility of eye-white
- Ears fixed backward
- Stress on intervertebral discs
- Micro-tears in muscle fibers
- Inconsistent contact and/or a tendency to be behind the bit

I started running competitively at the age of 48 and learned a very important thing that certainly applies to training horses: It takes a long time—years, in fact—to build the necessary strength in muscles, tendons, and ligaments for high-performance sport. It is just a part of athletic development.

If you are patient for the best results, and you know how and when to rest, recover, and increase or decrease intensity and variety of activity, you will givie your horse the best chance to progress in your chosen area of activity. Our horses' bodies are the same as ours in this regard.[2]

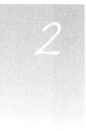

In a 2013 article in Preventive Veterinary Medicine, *Agneta Egenvall, et al, explained research examining orthopedic or other injuries in sports medicine and how they can be quantified using the "days-lost to training" concept. "Both the training regimen and the surface used in training and racing can affect the health of racehorses," they write. "Our aim was to associate 'days-lost to training' in elite-level show-jumpers to horse characteristics, training and management strategies, and the time spent working on various training and competition surfaces" (http://pub.epsilon.slu.se/11660/).*

Be patient and understanding in regards to your horse's athletic development.

Oftentimes, a horse will be trying so hard to please the rider, but the rider ignores his noble attempts and forgets to give him praise. I've watched horses enough from the ground that I'm quite certain they enjoy being told when they've done well. Be very quick to praise the horse when he has pleased you or performed a movement that you know is new or difficult for him. Understand how a loose rein allows the horse to stretch and relax, how a scratch on the neck or shoulder feels good to him, and how he responds favorably to a kind tone of voice. Horses are creatures who appreciate comfort, much like we do, and being rewarded for a job well done in relation to a particular session is going to help ensure they will be ready and willing to come back into the arena with confidence and a good attitude next day.

There are basics of general, good horsemanship—such as hand-picking a tail—that are frequently forgotten in the rush to get a ride underway. These could also include certain details, such as leaving the girth a bit loose for the walk from barn to arena, then only tightening it when you're about to mount. When you have finished a ride, if you don't already do this, consider dismounting in the arena, loosening the girth, and just allowing the horse a quiet moment to look around before hand-walking back to the grooming area, or perhaps you can strip the tack and turn your horse loose for a roll. This gives him a chance to settle and exercise his natural curiosity about his surroundings. Horses seem to appreciate a little massage on the neck and poll after a ride, and it is an opportunity for you both to take a few deep breaths at the same time, then walk quietly back to the barn. Small details of mindfulness are very important when dealing with such sensitive beings as horses. They are like young children, paying attention to every little mood change, nuance, and shift in our focus and energy. *Everything* we do has an effect on them, one way or the other. Why *not* make the experience as restorative, productive, and joyful as possible?

If we can work on ourselves to where we can ride and handle horses with patience, compassion, and consistency, leaving aggression, anger, and the ego behind, just imagine how fellow humans will react to us, as well. Whether it is meditation, breathing exercises, yoga, intense spiritual study, or simply changing your focus, whatever method you choose to reach your most Compassionate Self, you may find yourself transformed and more at peace than you ever thought possible.

Dr. Allen Schoen:

I have been very fortunate to have many compassionate horse trainers and owners as clients. They may have been a self-selective group because of my approach to compassionate veterinary medical care, integrating acupuncture, chiropractic, and natural supplements. Yet as my practice expanded, I have also had plenty of opportunity to observe the contrast between compassionate and less-than-compassionate training methods. I have seen the consequences as changes in the behavior, contentment, and well-being of the horses as well as in the frequency and number of pain and lameness issues.

Over the years I found myself inadvertently not looking forward to visiting the horse barns with less compassionate training methods. The horses in these facilities appeared angry and were more defensive and protective of their bodies. They were also more suspicious of human interaction. The entire environment in the barn ends up being a manifestation of a fundamental lack of kindness, tolerance, and forgiveness. The barn staff did not seem happy. The riders did not seem happy. The trainers were not happy. And the horses were not happy.

Focusing intention on proper riding and training with respect for the animal's welfare reflects throughout the barn.

I have seen riders who desire to reach a higher level of performance inadvertently become attracted to certain trainers with a less-than-transparent training process. Transparency or lack of may not be apparent at first—unfortunately, there are plenty of trainers who say the right things and appear to have the horse's welfare in mind, but when you look a little deeper, below the surface, the methods are not what we would consider compassionate. It is not uncommon for a naive rider with competitive aspirations to be unaware of what it took "behind the scenes" to get him or her to a particular level, show, or goal.

As a rider looking to improve and succeed with a trainer's help, you must look at the broader picture when considering a barn. How does the place feel? Are the horses happy? Are the grooms happy? Are the other riders happy? Is the trainer happy? Actions speak louder than words. Watch how people and horses move and stand. Conduct a *sensory scan* of everything and everyone at the barn. Do you sense tension? Or peace and easy camaraderie? If you do not ask the right questions you might not get the right answers. Talk to everyone there, including the attending veterinarians if you have the opportunity to do so. You seek patience, kindness, and consistency, as these qualities are of benefit to all.

"A good example is far better than a good precept."

Dwight Moody, American Preacher and Publisher

Questions to Consider
BASED ON PRINCIPLE 9

1   Are the training methods I am or another trainer is using with my horse compassionate, patient, and consistent?

2   Do I consider myself a patient person? If not, how can I become more so?

3   In what ways can I become more patient with my horse?

4   Do I feel that I have a secure, independent seat and apply my aids consistently? Or am I unbalanced, emotional, and reactive at times, perhaps causing me to apply aids suddenly or more aggressively? In what ways can I improve my riding skills to identify more with the former and less with the latter?

5   If my horse spooks or misbehaves, what tools can I employ ensuring that I react quickly with a clear correction but *without* aggression or other emotion? Can I ride with focus? Am I able to repeat my clear, corrective actions in the same way each time my horse requires?

CHAPTER TEN

A Compassionate Approach to Training and Showing

We allow for the creation of new, more respectful, humane and considerate approaches to horsemanship and all training methods.

Susan Gordon:

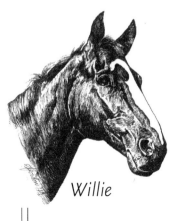

Willie

Willie frequently prompted the question, "What in the world is going through this horse's mind?" For a while I remained in denial about his obvious hostility toward dressage, which I mentioned at the beginning of chapter 6 (p. 120).

The 360-degree handstand at "P" near the beginning of a First Level test was one of his more spectacular moves. The required 10-meter circle was actually much easier than the effort he put into his acrobatics. He planted his front feet, flipped his haunches vertically, and spun 180 degrees at the same time. Then he did it again. He landed precisely on the track of the circle and carried on as though nothing had happened. I did not even know a horse was physically capable of such a movement! I could tell from the saddle how smug he was. Mortified, I was unsure of how much I dared ask him to lengthen, following the circle, as Willie may have considered it an invitation for another surprise.

Willie was schooled to Fourth Level in dressage and had also been an upper-level eventing horse. As people materialized who were able to help me piece together more of his history, it became apparent that he had a bit of a reputation. That is, a reputation for bucking people off in the show ring. Even taking steps back down to lower levels and schooling shows did not appease Willie's disdain for the dressage arena.

Eventually I realized the most sensible thing for both of us was to not show him. As I've relayed throughout his story, at some point in his life he must have found that bucking his rider off was an effective way to relieve his discomfort or get out of work. The snippets of information from various sources kept confirming that assessment to be correct. Willie's very good equine memory, combined with his now reasonable level of soundness, made for some very entertaining moments— for the judge and audience anyway—in our brief competitive career together.

For those of you interested in dressage scores, we were given a "4" for the anomalous 10-meter circle...due to "disobedience."

In these pages, we have purposefully made an effort to avoid discussing at length any particular training method, use of specific tack, or the process of starting or finishing a horse. Part of the reasoning here is that we intend to use current scientific studies and evolving research to continuously support the 25 Principles of Compassionate Equitation so far as determining what *does* and *does not* constitute putting undue pressure and stress on a horse, *no matter which training method or style of tack is used or wherever in the training process you may be*. These studies are contributing greatly to more humane methods of training, clarifying the benefit of certain techniques, and will continue to provide new insights on methods new and old in the years ahead. And of course, even those techniques we do touch upon briefly in this book are subject to reassessment as time goes on. We believe that technology and sophisticated data-sets may prove the need for adjustments in methodology and philosophy for as long as humans and horses are bound together.

The entire equine industry has undergone considerable shifting in recent years. Riding and horse ownership has become too costly for many. Those who do continue to ride often do not invest in regular lessons, and some may simply think they do not need consistent instruction. It seems as though patient training over years and long-term goals have given way to short workshops and clinics, online seminars, and video instruction. This conveniently allows online marketing and potentially lucrative opportunities for building a fan-base well beyond the local area instructors and trainers usually tap. High-tech tools for equestrian education are indeed marvelous, but they are meant to be *in support of* and *not a replacement for* the amount of time it takes to learn how to ride and train horses well.

This new economy has also given rise to opinions and methods that often pit one person's version of training against another. Well-known methods are copied, then individualized and branded with a new twist. While not all of these techniques are necessarily *bad*, it is possible that some have contributed to a contentious and divisive atmosphere for both competitive and recreational riders.

One of our goals for Compassionate Equestrians is to have riders learn to look carefully at their chosen disciplines and training methods. Decide *for yourself* if what you are doing to and with your horse is really in his best interest. Be discerning and cautious when exploring trainers and trends that deviate from common sense and classical training and handling. Claims of humane treatment may be made but not necessarily practiced. Some individuals may have little, if any, actual training experience, or training experiences that are not applicable to horses and disciplines outside of their scope of knowledge and ability.

We tend to gravitate to an "image" and respond to likeable personalities. This does not mean that training methods or products are as good as might be claimed.

I believe it is the human *ego* that is the root cause of much suffering, in the case of both horses *and* humans. We all have an ego, whether we are competitive or not. It is how we identify ourselves and how we adapt that persona to the outside world. Sometimes it can lead us to being overly confident or toward an unhealthy level of narcissism. Or, the ego can be better understood and used to help retain the desire to reach a certain goal. Perhaps the ego combined with our emotional attachment to horses is what produces a tendency for equestrians to be defensive. When we feel our horses or our riding are unfairly judged, the ego wants to step in and tell the individual making that judgment exactly how we feel. When we work very hard to accomplish a riding or horsemanship goal, the sting of criticism bites even harder. That said, we also want to develop resilience in the face of bullying or mental abuse by others. As already mentioned, I feel levying criticism of another's horse or another's riding, is *also* an ego-based inclination. It is neither compassionate nor productive. And then what we have are two ego-oriented horsepeople debating who is right and who is wrong, somebody's feelings get hurt, and the horses ultimately suffer from the resulting anger, frustration, or sadness felt by the riders involved.

Everybody has his or her own story. We may not be aware of how much fear or pain is actually behind comments or criticism coming from another person.

The best riders are often the most humble. They are frequently the most highly successful athletes or trainers who also understand how easy it is to be the gold medalist one day and sitting out of competition the next. This is particularly the case when horses are involved as injury, sponsorship, and ownership can change in the blink of an eye. It is more satisfying in the long run when personal accomplishment results from *task-* or *goal-orientation* rather than *ego-orientation* (see sidebar, p. 180). And more than anything else, having a high regard for the horse's welfare that we hold *above* our own desire to reach a goal or compete and win, is the compassionate choice. In fact, the FEI states just that in their code of ethics: "the welfare of the horse shall be regarded above all else." It is also up to

WHAT IS *EGO*?

The medical definition of *ego*, according to Merriam-Webster, is *the self especially as contrasted with another self or the world*. Ego is also one of the three divisions of the psyche in psychoanalytic theory that serves as the organized conscious mediator between the person and reality—it is the part that remembers, evaluates, plans, and in other ways is responsive to and acts in the surrounding physical and social world.

individuals to be self-affirming, however. If you can sense your horse is having a problem and your ego says, "Show him anyway," practice looking within and saying instead, "No, help him heal and save the ribbons for another day." This is the difference between a well-managed ego and one that is overly self-centered.

"Our attitude towards suffering becomes very important because it can affect how we cope with suffering when it arises."

Dalai Lama XIV, *The Art of Happiness* (Riverhead Books, 1998)

Riding in a particular discipline for competitive purposes has many positive effects on both horses and riders when high standards of training and deportment are upheld. It teaches discipline, focus, responsibility, and potentially good sportsmanship, which means controlling the ego and any tendency toward "one-upmanship." Those who are driven by their ego tend to have increased levels of anxiety and stress, and as we have already learned, this can have a negative effect on the rider, the horse, and others around them.

Is it contradictory to be both competitive *and* compassionate? Some may think so. As a competitive athlete in both equestrian events and running, I admit it is a challenge to learn how to be compassionate at all times, under all circumstances. As we know, horses may or may not agree with our desires to be the best on any given day. The most seasoned competitor has learned that the quickest way to become humbled is to trot into the show ring thinking you are going to win the class!

TASK-ORIENTATION VS. EGO-ORIENTATION

In *task-* or *goal-orientation*, we learn and/or develop based on what we perceive we are capable of with an understanding and willingness to commit maximum effort to the achievement. When motivated by a goal, we will often persevere in the face of failure, choose challenging tasks, and experience greater natural interest in the activities at hand.

In *ego-orientation*, our perception of our own abilities gains importance and we strive to demonstrate superiority in comparison with others. We are less inclined, perhaps, to choose challenging tasks or those we intrinsically love because it is more important to succeed.

What is your motivation to compete in equestrian sports?

The key is in your *intention*. When you *intend to beat your fellow competitors at all times*, you may find yourself disappointed when that simply does not happen. If you fail to see a loss as an opportunity for personal growth, you will possibly cause yourself even more mental anguish and frustration before the next event comes around. Worse, you might take your frustrations out on your horse. My students, like all students, sometimes won, but would also sometimes lose a class and then be very down or self-critical about it. At these moments, I chose to say that nobody could win every class, all the time. If one person was guaranteed to win, no one would want to compete against him or her, and what fun would that be for anyone? When you realize it is in human nature to want "to do well," you can view competitiveness from a different angle. Excelling can be a tremendous confidence boost, but we must balance this by having compassion and being capable of letting other people have their turn in the spotlight, and be happy knowing how good it makes *them* feel. For every ribbon or medal we win, there is somebody else working just as hard and hoping to win just as much as we are. Everybody is on common ground when it comes to competing.

In competition, as well as everyday interactions with other beings, try your best to remain considerate, open-minded, and view everyone as equal. Then when you do well, even *exceptionally* well, the most important opportunity you are afforded is that of inspiring and teaching the aspiring riders around you. In the process of learning how to *compete well*, comes the bigger challenge of learning to *win well* and wanting the best for others. In the running and triathlon community, I have always been moved by the spectators who cheer for everybody, especially the youngest, oldest, and last-place finishers. At horse shows, who *doesn't* feel empathy for the rider who perseveres through nerves or struggles with an anxious horse?

When it comes to trainers, leaving the ego out of our tendency to want to tout the better training method, the better breed, or the better equipment is difficult. There is often a compulsion to be defensive when we feel our preferred methods or breeds of horse or style of riding have been unjustly criticized and it is hard to let that go—I know from experience. It is human nature to judge and compare others according to the view we have of ourselves, and yet many of us recognize how much we end up suffering for our attitudes. In cultivating compassion, we can release that defensiveness and ego-driven competitiveness.

PUTTING THE HORSE FIRST

Even aged show horses that are semi-retired and relatively pain-free seem to enjoy continuing to show if they have always thrived amidst crowds and excitement. If you have ever felt a jumper "pump up" at the in-gate and surge into a gallop at the sound of the starting buzzer you know what I mean. If you have a horse that sulks when he's left at home, he might actually stay in better health if taken to a few shows a season and only shown within the limits of his physical capabilities. Each horse is an individual, as we've mentioned repeatedly, and the compassionate approach is to recognize places and situations that help your horse feel *wanted* and *needed*. He might not be your superstar any longer, but he may be thrilled to pack a young rider around his or her first competition.

Whatever his age, be mindful of your horse at all times when attending a horse show or clinic. Riders like to sit on their horses and chat between rounds, classes, or lessons, and the horse's expression or behavior will begin to indicate signs of distress or boredom. If you had to carry a weight on your back and shoulders all day long, and never set it down, how would you feel?

Some of the most meaningful moments I have experienced at horse shows did not involve winning ribbons but displays of good sportsmanship and friendship. Supporting other competitors and thanking judges, trainers, and show support staff, uplifts everyone and reflects well on you.

You're always either training or un-training the horse you're mounted on. Riding and training horses are activities based in the fundamental knowledge of sports physiology.

Compassionate training methods translate to *respectful* and *humane* in that our techniques do not come from the ego—we are willing to quell our instinctive competitiveness and feelings of "us versus them" in the name of equine welfare, above all else. Be aware of how a particular training technique may push a horse more quickly than he can comprehend, or ask more of him physically than his body can handle. Some training practices can set a young horse up for a short career and early onset lameness due to asking for too much, too soon. The same holds true in human sports training and physiology where excessive overtraining and improper muscular development can lead to early breakdown in muscles, tendons, and ligaments, and produce lingering fatigue that removes all enjoyment from an activity if the activity is possible at all.[1,2]

1,2

In the October 2011 article "Regenerative Medicine for the Treatment of Mulsculoskeletal Overuse Injuries in Competition Horses," Paola Torricelli, et al, explain a study likening equine and human athletes: "Competition horses are involved in highly demanding activities, thus being a similar model for the high mechanical overload typical of human athletes (http://pubmedcentralcanada.ca/pmcc/articles/PMC3174295/).

Dr. Liz Walmsley, BVSc, Resident in Equine Surgery at the University of Melbourne Equine Centre in Australia, writes in "Diagnosing and Managing Muscle Tears in Horses" that "Muscle strains account for more than 50% of musculoskeletal injuries in human athletes. However, the frequency with which they are definitively diagnosed (with proof they are the cause of lameness) in horses, is far lower. This is likely due to a number of reasons including difficulty in accurately palpating the deep muscle of horses, low levels of lameness caused by mild injuries, and the inability of horses to 'tell us where it hurts'" (http://www.racingvictoria.net.au/asset/cms/Vet%20Services%20PDF/MuscleTears-LWalmsley.pdf).

HORSE SHOPPING: A TRAINER'S OPPORTUNITY FOR COMPASSION AND CONSCIOUSNESS

As head instructor and barn owner of Inner Circle Farm in Patterson, New York, Laura Parker has 38 years of serious and professional experience in loving and learning with horses. She is the former Assistant Director of Riding at Pace University in New York and acquired her Master's Degree from NYU in motor learning and kinesiology, which has greatly benefited her students because of her understanding of the human body in motion. She studies and teaches classical dressage, and is one of Dr. Schoen's clients. Here she shares one story of a trainer's responsibility when helping match human and horse.

"In the course of a career, trainers have a unique opportunity to assist their clients in the purchase of a horse," says Parker. "The honor and responsibility of this position I do not take lightly. I recently was blessed to be a part of the joy once again of uniting two souls, human and equine.

"In this case, my new student had sadly experienced a true lack of compassion and consciousness on the part of her first dressage trainer. This lovely and sincere young woman had waited a very long time but had finally the means to purchase a quality, well-trained horse. Her former trainer quickly guided her to the purchase of a horse that although beautiful was riddled with physical problems that made riding him extremely difficult. Even though she questioned whether it was appropriate to ride him due to his physical issues, she was made to feel that her novice riding skills were at fault.

"The opportunity to field such a request by a student is always a dream come true for me: Someone really interested in learning with the financial means to support and care for a horse, who at the same time is giving a horse a chance at a loving supportive partnership.

"As dreams do come true, my student's first horse is here with us, feeling and looking like a different being, muscled, relaxed and appreciating the original intention this wonderful woman had for him. He is now being worked only within

Continued →

(Cont.)

his comfort zone and is treated with the healing modalities necessary. Meanwhile, my student's new tall, dark, and handsome riding partner—physically capable of teaching her and developing continuously himself—is a daily reminder of how compassion and consciousness is a choice in every crevice of the horse world."

Even horses used in recreational activities such as trail riding are susceptible to injury if worked especially hard on weekends then left standing around during the week with no additional exercise. As we touched upon in the previous chapter, compassionate training and riding encompasses a fundamental understanding of the biomechanics of the horse's musculoskeletal system. There are limits to the duration and intensity of workouts given the horse's stage of development. And as we've also discussed previously, it has been confirmed that horses have a weight-bearing load tolerance (see p. 83). Riders are cautioned to be aware of exceeding the horse's comfort zone and ability to carry their weight plus tack without doing spinal damage. It is up to each individual to be truthful regarding his or her own level of competence in approaching any method of riding as it relates to equine development so as to do no harm to the horse.

It is in the best interest of the horse if we place compassion at the base for our training, whether for competition or recreational purposes, and remain open to new ways this objective might be met. When we take our ego out of the equation, at least to the degree that it is not the dominating reason behind our equestrian activity, we expand our field of vision to that of observing—not judging—the industry at large and the welfare of *all* equines. To refer to "all training methods" as Principle 10 suggests, is quite encompassing, and the view can be disturbing in some cases. For our own well-being, we are positively affected by establishing a calm, clear state of mind with which to approach and interact with horses and other horsepeople. If we strive to maintain that state, we will inevitably inspire and educate others to do so, as well.

Dr. Allen Schoen:

Some trainers purposely apply painful methods to horses in order to control their behavior. As a Compassionate Equestrian it is not possible to support such a method, as the horse's behavior may be related to pain in the first place.

With regards to my perspective on various training approaches, I do not feel like I am an expert by any means on the advantages and disadvantages of particular training programs. In an attempt to look at various approaches from a more expansive viewpoint, I am sharing my thoughts as an integrative veterinarian who witnesses the *results* of how horses have been handled and trained.

I recently read an online discussion regarding a device designed to stop horses from bucking. The device puts pressure on a sensitive part of the horse's head, and is only activated when the horse bucks. The overriding discomfort from the device shuts down the horse's tendency to buck, and the individual promoting the device claims the horse can then be safely ridden again.

We all know how pain can be used to affect control—in horses and humans— but my real concern in scenarios such as this one is that *there may still be an issue with the horse's back or body*, the cause of the buck in the first place, and the device that trains the horse it is not comfortable to buck is *not* getting to that root cause. First and foremost, you must try to find and resolve the root of the problem, rather than continuously using tricks and devices to control undesirable behaviors. It seems the behaviors are a physical expression—the horse's communication of pain and discomfort. He may not speak English, but in "Equish" (my humorous term for equine language) he may say things quite clearly in his own way. Sometimes, if we do not listen, that communication can become more and more violent until we finally hear what he is saying. The result when it gets to this point could be harmful to both rider and horse. It seems wiser to try to listen to the horse from the get-go and be sensitive to his behavioral communication continuously, adapting to and resolving issues earlier rather than later.

I used to get caught up in long-winded debates over the "best approaches" to various horse-and-rider issues. When I was pioneering my complementary veterinary approaches, many skeptics and cynics would verbally attack new ideas and then wonder why I was not responding to their accusations or engaging in their arguments.

You can spend your whole life responding to these kinds of discussions.

It seemed to me, at some level, these cynics were not open to hearing another perspective, but rather wanted to cement *their* positions as the only ones. Science is always evolving and changing. As a first-year veterinary student it was often heard that, by the time you graduate, a significant amount of what you learned would later be disproven, changed, or evolved. An idea that was thought to be real one year is later left by the graveyard of disproved facts. Ideally, science is an open-minded, respectful field, exploring the universe and all that exists. But as with much of the modern media, it seems rudeness and ruthless attacks have become the accepted means of communication in "scientism," and science has become a dogma. A comparison can be made here to the equestrian industry.

EXERCISE IN COMPASSION

Be The Change You Wish To Be

1   Create more quiet time for yourself in nature.

2   Take your horse on quiet, relaxed trail rides and enjoy peaceful, calm moments together, in the stall or pasture or ring.

3   Evaluate how you can quiet your heart and mind throughout the day.

4   Ask yourself: How else can I be the change I wish to be?

At one point in my life I realized that I needed to be even more of the change I wanted to see.

As the world seemed to be spinning faster and faster, increased traffic and road rage felt like it was everywhere, improved technology allowed us to be more efficient, yet also somehow created busier, more distracted lives, I realized I needed to experience more time being quiet in *nature's resonance*. I sense one of the big issues with the horse world in general is, in fact, *nature deficit disorder*: We bring all the stress from our modern-day life into the barn with us, and at some subconscious level, we think being with our horses will connect us to nature. The reality is that, instead, we can bring busyness and "mind traffic" to the horse, and envelope him in a *neural-net web*, covering him like an umbrella with our own beliefs, programming, and imprinting. The horse becomes a prisoner of this *neural net* of ours, and *instead of the horse transforming us* through his peace of mind, *we disturb the horse's sense of being* until he is in the same state of imbalance we are.

I notice, actually, how happy horses and riders seem after relaxing trail rides through the woods or quiet moments hand-grazing in a natural setting. I sense that it may be beneficial to increase the call for these relaxing, non-goal-oriented moments into many of our interactions with horses, whether just training at home or seriously competing.

What is going on in the industry right now that makes people respond to horses and training the way they do?

If we do not ask the right questions, we will not get the correct answers. In terms of the issues with horses that we see throughout the industry, across disciplines and borders, first we must clarify, "What is pain and what is discomfort?" To do so, we must look at the horse, study him closely, and understand him better.

The Dalai Lama was once shown an experiment meant to measure and compare "liking expressions" in rats and human babies: each tasted both sugar water and bitter water. Upon tasting the two waters, the expressions between the rats and human babies were very similar (rhythmic licking for the sweet and mouth-gaping for the bitter). The Dalai Lama, however, was most concerned when he discovered that the rats were tested with a photonic line (a wire emitting light) inserted in their heads. The researchers insisted the rats were not in pain or discomfort. The Dalai Lama's response was, "I am not sure they're *not* in pain."

Two questions arise in my thoughts based on this story. First, what constitutes pain and discomfort and how is that determined by our mental "filters"—that is, what we *want* to see based on our training and programming? Here, the researchers were looking at the rat behavior through the filter of scientific training, and they did not think to consider whether the line was causing pain in the rats.

Second, the researchers were comparing the expressions of rats to those of babies, and thus finding a way to "decode" what a rat might be "saying" in terms of "like" and "dislike." I do not think it is unreasonable to assume we can learn to read the facial expressions of horses. You must learn to really *look* at your horse and be intimately familiar with his individual stances and expressions: what he does when something hurts or is annoying, and how he acts when he's contented or comfortable. It is commonly thought that when a horse's ears are back and he looks tense, he is probably in some sort of discomfort. In contrast, when his facial expressions are relaxed and interested, they are less indicative of pain. Continuously reevaluate your riding and training techniques based on your horse's responses and expressions.

When I have to repeat the same adjustment on a horse, time after time, I have to ask, "What is going on with this horse's riding and training that's making the repeated adjustments necessary?"

Say your horse requires repeated chiropractic adjustments of a similar nature. Ask yourself: Is it a biomechanical problem due to a chronic issue the horse has? Or is there something that can be changed in the riding, training, equipment, or shoeing that can provide long-term resolution of the issue? Seek advice from your veterinarian, trainer, or other equine professional, but whenever there are recurring problems, be willing to explore whether there is something *you* could be doing differently to help improve the situation.

Besides offering hands-on treatment, part of my protocol is teaching clients what they can do to prevent physical issues—for example, tightness—from becoming chronic. Various stretching techniques, acupressure, and other natural therapeutic approaches can be applied before and after riding to prevent tightness issues. Yet sometimes, the tricky part is in getting the rider or trainer to correct *riding habits* that are causing the horse's problems.

The issues I'm typically called to address are not necessarily related to which type of bit or saddle or other equipment is used. Sometimes it is not the "tool." Sometimes it is the person behind it. When seeking the cause of a horse's discomfort, if you keep going back further and further, and digging deeper and deeper, the key is often the *mind* and *heart* of the person who has worked with or is working with the horse. As we said in the sidebar on p. 166, bit or bitless, either can be beneficial or harmful, painful or not painful. It all depends on the rider.

When training is too intense and pressure is never relieved, the horses seem miserable. It breaks my heart.

The rider's hands hold more than just the reins...they hold a metaphor for life. Perhaps softening the grip or relaxing the connection between hand and halter, or hand and bridle, is the same *softening* and *letting go* we need to offer ourselves as we ride through life. This is not meant to be a judgment; just a thought you might be interested in exploring. The whole concept of *letting go* is a dance. Like playing a violin, you do not want the strings too loose or too tight.

Our unique filters tell us what *letting go* means. Some people have tremendous fears and want to be in control of everything in their life. So *letting go* of the reins, on the horse, is something they really struggle with. They might manage it for a brief moment that is too late or not enough. Whereas others who are perhaps a bit careless and detached in life might drop the reins entirely, and so the horse scoots off. It is all about being *mindful*—attentive to the moment-to-moment interactions with your horse. But find a happy balance—not to an extreme—where you support the horse and the horse supports you.

From my perspective as veterinarian and animal behaviorist, *letting go* is a very personal thing. We bring all our own baggage, "mind traffic," patterning, and imprinting to the very concept of *letting go*...but then *can we let go* of all that? To be *present*, to be with the horse in the moment, to not overreact by throwing away the reins or suddenly tossing a training method or piece of equipment out the window, but to approach riding questions in a moment of mindfulness, so we can decide if we are *reacting* or *responding*—this is our aim. Remember, the key is for our movements on horseback to come from *conscious response* rather than *reaction* (see p. 130).

When we let go of everything all at once, it is usually a reaction rather than a response.

Our goal with the concept of *letting go* is the *release of all preconceptions* so you can be present in the moment with your horse and attentive to the horse in that moment of response. It's like the song, *The Gambler*, made famous by singer Kenny Rogers—you have to "Know when to hold 'em, know when to fold 'em." It is very subtle. It is also a message that you are giving to the horse. Sometimes the hardest thing is to go forward when the horse (or the human) is "stuck."

When leading, riding, or driving a horse, we are physically connected to another creature's head, and *that* is a huge responsibility. We put ourselves in control of his body *and* mind. If the horse is in discomfort or pain, ensuring that *we* have a clear-thinking, beautiful mind means we will be sensitive to and aware of reactions and resistances indicative of a need for treatment.

I recently treated a horse for a client who was aware of the symptoms of Lyme disease from previous horses I had diagnosed and treated for her: chronic aggravation and hypersensitivity to grooming; irritation with tack and

The Mindful Art of Letting Go

You can find a balance when *letting go* by keeping the following in mind:

- Do not get attached to words or concepts.
- Clear your mind and let go of previous imprints.
- Quiet your mind, and quiet your heart.
- Practice "wiring what you fire" (see p. 47). The more we "fire" *open* heart, *open* mind, and refuse to be mired in old imprints, the clearer we can be, and we can bring that awareness to our interactions with the horse.

rider, recurring lameness, and so on. She also had contracted and experienced the discomfort and pain of Lyme disease herself, so she knew how it felt and had empathy for the horse.

Animals with Lyme disease act really painful and stiff and commonly are very sensitive to touch. They may react with discomfort and pain to even the slightest amount of pressure.

Just to be safe, the horse was put on a course of antibiotics, pending the results of the Lyme titer (the test for Lyme based on dilution negative/positive antibody response), and there was some improvement. My client's attending veterinarian did not feel the horse had Lyme when the titer came back negative, so the treatment was stopped. Then the symptoms returned within days and were worse than before. Based on the information the client presented, I suspected that *it was* in fact Lyme disease causing the horse's behavioral (and other) issues.

My experience with active pathologic Lyme disease and neurologic Lyme disease is that if it isn't treated appropriately at the beginning it can cross the blood-brain-barrier, go into the brain and spinal cord, and cause many behavioral issues. I recommended minocycline (an antibiotic) to my client and communicated my findings to the other veterinarian. After a month on the antibiotic, he was no longer lame, and his poor behavior and other issues were resolved.

A skeptic might say his recovery was due to the anti-inflammatory effects of the minocycline, but the horse had been on phenylbutazone ("bute") and other non-steroidal anti-inflammatory medication (NSAIDs) without a change in his noticeable level of discomfort. It was obvious that the anti-infectious effect of the minocycline was working in this case. This story illustrates how when approaching a horse with benevolent mindfulness, part of that mindfulness is about being aware of his possible discomfort and then taking all necessary steps to find out exactly why the horse is in distress and alleviating it if possible.

When you've done "everything right" so far in terms of a horse's training but his response is regressive rather than progressive, waste no time in discovering what the source of the problem could be.

Acknowledging the potential source of a horse's physical or behavioral problems, then taking immediate action, is the mark of a good trainer and rider. That is *the* key for those who work with horses. Because we bring our own imprinting, "programming," and personal issues (such as abuse, addictions or negative patterning—see p. 12) to everything we do with horses, we suggest exploring personal growth programs as part of your journey as a Compassionate Equestrian. When we deal with our own "stuff" *outside* the barn, we can find a clear vision of how to be with the horses *inside*, as well as how to help others be with horses in a mindful way.

In Principle 1 (see p. 21) we acknowledge the horse's ability to feel pain and our awareness that we are sitting on the bones, nerves, muscles, and soft tissues of another living being. We owe it to that living being to find and alleviate a source of pain when one is present *before* causing further mental and physical damage by making the horse continue to work under such circumstances.

By addressing the physical and emotional challenges with ourselves and our horses, plus keeping up with current research insofar as an awareness of the need to be flexible in regards to acceptance of a particular training method or device, we will be able to look forward to the creation of new, more respectful, humane, and considerate approaches to horsemanship and all training methods.

"THE GREAT IMITATOR": IMPORTANT INFORMATION REGARDING TICK-BORNE DISEASE

In this book, I refer to equine Lyme disease and other tick-borne diseases in several chapters. I bring it up a number of times because all too often I have seen a horse in pain, and because of a questionable or low Lyme titer (a measurement of the amount or concentration of a substance in a solution—in this case, antibodies) other veterinarians have felt that Lyme or tick-borne disease was *not* the cause. It is stated in *most* Lyme disease titers that the titer may not accurately reflect the presence of the disease in the animal and should be considered *along with* clinical signs in the animal. Lyme disease is a diagnostic dilemma: it is both under-diagnosed and over-diagnosed.

When "everything else" may have been taken into consideration and treated, and the titer is low, a horse might then be simply labeled a "bad horse" due to his problem behavior (clinical signs of tick-borne disease). This, as we've discussed, can lead to him being treated harshly or punished, and so he experiences more pain because he's reacting to his pain.

I also use the term *tick-borne disease* as well as *Lyme disease* (an infectious disease caused by the spirochete *Borrelia burgdorferi*) because there is a new spirochete called *Borrelia miyamotoi* that shows all the same signs as Lyme disease, but there is no test for it. There may also be other infectious tick-borne diseases that we do not have tests for.

In March 2013, Dr. Richard Ostfeld, Disease Ecologist at the Cary Institute of Ecosystem Studies, was reported to warn against the potential for emergence and spread of disease caused by *Borrelia miyamotoi*. "A January 2013 study from the *New England Journal of Medicine* provides evidence of *miyamotoi* infection among people in the United States for the first time," states the press release on the Tick-Borne Disease Alliance website. "In addition, new research from the Yale School of Public Health shows that adult female ticks can transmit *miyamotoi* directly to their larvae, which is not the case for other tick-borne pathogens."

Questions to Consider
BASED ON PRINCIPLE 10

1 Are there any training techniques or riding styles that I use that may unintentionally cause discomfort or pain in my horse?

2 What can I do to determine if my horse is in pain? What can I do to determine whether my training or riding is the cause?

3 When looking back in my riding and horse-owning history, are there times that Principle 10 could have been beneficial in dealing with a horse's behavior or training problems?

4 What might I do differently now, based on Principle 10?

5 What kind of industry-wide changes related to Principle 10 would I like to see occur?

CHAPTER ELEVEN

Training with Common Sense

We acknowledge that common sense is a component of compassion. We agree that our hearts be open to the bigger picture of how the horse industry has evolved, and how it will evolve into the future, as kindness, tolerance, and forgiveness are restored to all aspects of the equestrian world.

Susan Gordon:

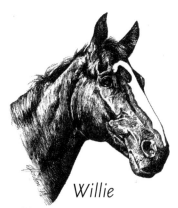

Willie

When a train is coming down the tracks, and you are walking on the tracks, common sense would dictate to most people that the best move would be to get off the tracks. This applies to all life's lessons, including those horses teach us.

Common sense where horses are concerned may not be quite as obvious as getting off the tracks as a train approaches. Of course, an angry horse charging could be likened to a train. Your immediate sense of danger tells you, "Get out of the way...angry horse coming through!" But then, stepping aside only reinforces the horse's aggressive, dominant behavior. Common sense also dictates that if you do get run over by a thousand-pound animal, the likelihood of serious injury is high. And so you see part of our quandary when it comes to deciphering exactly what might be termed "common-sense horse training."

Does applying the brakes and gas in your car at the same time make sense? No. I have never actually tried it, but common sense says it isn't good for either the engine or the brakes. How about kicking a horse and jerking on his mouth at the same time? Willie was a prime example of the results of these conflicting aids. As soon as you put leg on and touched the reins, he figured a battle was coming. He would immediately assume a defensive posture. When a rider is scared or angry, common sense is often overridden, and he or she enters defensive mode, too. When both horse and rider are defending themselves from one another, the end result is ultimately a horse that is very difficult to motivate, much less enjoyable or pleasant to ride, and an exhausted, frustrated rider.

Modifying Willie's behavior, especially his charging on the ground, to get him to a point where he was not so dangerous to handle took a lot of thinking. It was important to have him not feel as though he was being punished, as that is what I believe led to his aggressive behavior in the first place. Since there was the potential for him to run right over top of me, common sense dictated a method that would place him on a longe circle but protect me from harm when he turned in and charged. I utilized an unusual training aid: a 55-gallon plastic barrel. I set it in the middle of the round pen and free-longed Willie around the perimeter. My plan was to stay behind the barrel, then kick it over and roll it at him when he took a run at me. Sure enough, unorthodox *as it was, it worked, and rather quickly, too. He only had to experience "roll the barrel" a couple of times. He would stop in his tracks and cock his head, looking at the barrel sideways like a curious puppy. It completely took him out of the moment and he forgot why he was charging at me in the first place. Nobody got punished, nobody got hurt.*

According to Wikipedia:

"Common sense" has at least two specifically philosophical meanings. One is a capability of the animal soul (Greek psukhē) proposed by Aristotle, which enables different individual senses to collectively perceive character- istics, such as movement and size, which are common to all things, and which help people and other animals to distinguish and identify things. It is distinct from basic sensory perception and from human rational thinking, but works with both. The second special use of the term is Roman-influ- enced and is used for the natural human sensitivity for other humans and the community. Just like the everyday meaning, both of these refer to a type of basic awareness and ability to judge, which most people are expected to share naturally, even if they cannot explain why.

Common sense really is a complex system of thought and philosophy. No wonder it can be so elusive and confusing sometimes! Combine it with the training of horses and questions abound. Horse training is covered in an endless number of books, videos, and workshops, but how many people are really clear as to what it means, what it all entails, and what the goals are? Do you know what constitutes a "finished" horse in your chosen method or discipline? If you ride, you need a horse that is trained to some degree, even if it isn't to the extent of an advanced level—but you also want to know where your horse's performance is situated in relation to the standards of your discipline. When that horse receives his training from a compassionate horseperson who will help prevent the onset of vices through kind, yet correct training, he will have a good chance at relative soundness and be rideable for a long time to come.

Yes, common sense dictates that horses be trained to respond to humans in the safest manner possible while evolving into a good pleasure or performance horse. The person gauging and evaluating a horse in that regard, however, is always coming from his or her own perceptions of what "common sense," "safe," and "good" mean.

There are many different systems for training horses, depending on the horse's intended use. Fundamentally, the methods are most conducive to incremental progress when executed in a series of steps designed to produce a safe, content, sound, and well-mannered saddle or driving horse. Basic school figures that improve the horse's balance, quality of gaits, and muscular development are ideally part of the program. It is easy for a newcomer to be misled into techniques that may appear kind and humane, yet inadvertently produce horses that are poorly mannered, stiff, and hard to control when mounted. If the method does not appear to be derived from a foundation of good sports physiology, and the exercises involved do not have an athletic explanation or reasoning behind them, the novice equestrian is advised to use caution and perhaps consult other sources of education and training.

Developing a deep bond and authentic relationship with the horse is extremely important, but common sense would dictate that groundwork, including the use of a round pen, contributes to the athletic development of the horse, as well as helping you connect with your horse. While you can love horses dearly and feel tremendous compassion for them, once you are on their backs, no matter how lightly they are worked, they are being asked for an athletic performance, as are you, the rider, and they need to be prepared accordingly.

Without concern for a correctly developed musculoskeletal system, the horse will sooner or later suffer from the effects of asymmetry and gait irregularities.

A systematic training method was introduced in the *Art of Horsemanship* written by the Greek horseman Xenophon over 2,000 years ago. This is the foundation of authentic classical horsemanship and is still valid to this day. It was the most humane method developed for training horses used in wars. The horses had to be maneuverable and respond on loose reins as they carried soldiers wielding

LISTEN...AND BE VERY FAIR

One of Dr. Schoen's clients, Mikki Kuchta of Aiken Bach Farm in North Salem, New York, has ridden her whole life, and has been eventing for 30 years, competing up to the highest levels of the sport. She started her competitive career on the hunter/jumper circuit and has served as a Pony Club examiner and instructor for the Metropolitan Region of the United States Pony Club. Kuchta was one of the first trainers to become certified with the ICP (the United States Eventing Association's Instructor Certification Program). When asked if she could pass on one concept to other horsepeople, what would it be, she replied:

"First, understanding the natural instincts of the horse enables one to remain calm around them, which allows for harmonious training. They are prey animals and in some fashion or another they will act like prey animals, and this cannot be changed. Many riders perceive the flight instinct as a threat to the rider, and this creates fear and tension and decreases the opportunity for clear communication.

"Listen to the horses. They communicate with actions and reactions; and much information can be gleaned from these...which also helps a trainer to alter methods to facilitate progressing a horse in training.

"Be very fair! The line between acceptable behavior and unacceptable behavior cannot vacillate. It must be black and white consistently, so that the animal knows what to expect from the human."

weapons, and they had to be desensitized to the sights and sounds of combat. Modern-day dressage has evolved from the exercises and school figures that were developed by cavalries to create bold, responsive horses that conformed to the needs of their various regiments. Hence the precision of quadrilles and airs-above-the-ground, such as those performed by the Lipizzaner horses of the Spanish Riding School of Vienna.

Xenophon emphasized lightness, kindness, and benevolent techniques without force.

Throughout history there has been very little deviation as to what the basic requirements are. Horses had to go forward and be extremely responsive to their riders or drivers. From the viewpoint of being reliant on a horse for your very survival, it would have made the most sense to have an excellent relationship and understanding of your horse to go along with his careful training. Due to the need to quickly mount new recruits, however, cavalry riders were trained as quickly as possible. Without the benefit of years of training, the tendency for any rider is to follow his instincts to "clutch, grab, and go." As a result, the finesse of the horse's true abilities as made apparent through Xenophon's training methods was soon relegated to the domain of only a handful of influential equitation masters, and his techniques were abandoned by many.

"Anything forced, cannot be beautiful."

Xenophon

Having horses for transportation and agriculture was still a necessity, even in the lifetime of my grandparents. It has been a very recent evolution for horses to go from being relied on for food and livelihood to having no particular purpose other than sport and pleasurable recreation. When horses were necessary en masse for military, farm work, and transportation, harsh equipment and techniques were commonly used to dominate and control them to ensure a quick transition from "unbroke" to "useful."

As there was no research supporting the intelligence or emotional life of animals, horses were generally thought of in the same context as machines. My grandmother always enjoyed telling me stories about one of her family's buggy horses that reared a lot. She had no explanation as to why to the horse might have been rearing, and gave no indication that anyone thought the horse might have been in pain or frightened by harsh training. There were so many horses available at that time that when a horse did not perform as required, another quickly replaced it. In big, busy cities, you can only imagine the conditions on streets crowded with horses. Beside the extraordinary amount of manure,[1] there were frequent accidents due to horses spooking, kicking, biting, or trampling bystanders. *Compassion* was not a concern when it came to horses, as their primary reason for existing was to service a growing human population.

When that era was over, it was also over quickly for thousands of horses. It took less than 20 years to go from an equine-based society to a motor-vehicle-based society. "In 1900, 4,192 cars were sold in the US; by 1912 that number had risen to 356,000," wrote Eric Morris in a 2007 issue of *Access*. "In 1912, traffic counts in New York showed more cars than horses for the first time. The equine was not replaced all at once, but function by function. Freight haulage was the last bastion of horse-drawn transportation; the motorized truck finally supplanted the horse cart in the 1920s."

In his article "From Horse Power to Horsepower" (Access, 2007), Eric Morris stated: "In 1898, delegates from around the globe gathered in New York City for the world's first international urban planning conference. One topic dominated the discussion. It was not housing, land use, economic development, or infrastructure. The delegates were driven to desperation by horse manure" (http://www.uctc.net/access/30/ Access%2030%20-%2002%20-%20Horse%20Power.pdf).

Less than a century into the world of motor vehicles, dressage—the horsemanship of Xenophon— converted from a test of classical riding standards to a display of costly, highly-bred horses. And they, like many other sport horses, are at risk of being pushed too quickly into upper levels, not allowing their bodies the time they need to develop as athletes. This trend in all disciplines appears to be due to unrealistic expectations and an unwillingness to spend enough time building slowly toward an end result. I can understand the thrill and glamour of riding and showing advanced-level horses in any sport, but *all* horses and riders have to start with a strong foundation of basics. Sometimes they need to stay there for a long time, or be willing to move on only to return to basics again if that is in the horse's best interest.

I have heard people say they do not want to show at a lower level, as though it is embarrassing or beneath them to be there. This is the ego speaking, much to the detriment of the horse, and the equine industry as a whole. For example, consider an average horse in terms of build and bloodlines executing a beautiful, relaxed Training Level dressage test versus a finely bred Grand Prix horse with diminished movement that is ridden with a tight curb rein and false break behind the poll.

As mentioned earlier, when proper muscular development does not occur early on in the horse's training, the horse is set up for a limited career, no matter how wonderful his gaits are or how well bred the horse is. It does not make sense to rush a horse through training knowing the potential for damage.

You can't be a jazz virtuoso without first learning the musical scales.

Years ago, compassionate training methods may not have been on the mind of a cowboy breaking a colt destined for driving and roping cattle, or at the forefront of a general's mind as he rode off with his unit to the front lines. When people in this day and age say they do not want to use force or severe methods on horses, part of that means understanding the origins of some of those harsher methods. As we've already discussed, in the past, working horses were the majority of the equine population. Outside the schools of equitation, forceful methods became the norm due to the high demand for "useful" animals. If a cowboy needed a new horse, he threw the saddle and bridle on a youngster, jumped on, and rode the horse until he quit bucking. It was "common sense" to people at the time to "break" a horse as quickly as possible.

Some techniques used today to rush horses into a frame, show ring, or race-track do not fall into the realm of common sense for *our* time. Asking for too much, too soon, or pushing a horse that is not suitable for the demands being made of him, are training errors we see all too often. Nor is it necessarily appropriate to *only* ride a horse in his *natural* frame if his way of going includes being high-headed, hollow-backed, and crooked—as those tendencies could be exacerbated and eventually lead to lameness. Horses are designed to move freely forward and prefer to do so, but when carrying a rider they also must be balanced. Thought must be given as to how their musculature will be slowly built over time to carry a rider and prevent unsoundness. This is still the base of classical, correct equitation, as we learned from Xenophon. With the addition of *compassion* to classical training ideas, we can merge new and old paradigms in the pursuit of a benevolent method of consistently producing well-schooled, happy, healthy, horses—whose happiness and health then positively affects all those around them.

All horse people—regardless of discipline—benefit from knowing the fundamentals of classical horsemanship. It is like learning the musical scales before deciding on which style of music you prefer to pursue. You cannot be a jazz virtuoso or rock superstar without first learning C, D, E, F, G, A, B, C, then their majors, minors, 7ths, and so forth. It makes sense to understand the goals of a well-trained horse and how to accomplish those goals before pursuing a specialty discipline or sport.

We believe the majority of horse owners want what's best for their horses. It is the process of determining what actually is best for the horse that can become confusing in our modern world of information overload and instant access.

Many people in today's horse world are eager and willing to absorb new information. "Horses" are a lifestyle choice that have given rise to a slew of products and trends, especially those that make life with horses more personal, simpler, and easy to manage in this busy, highly technical modern world. There is a great *love* for the horse amongst the current demographic of owners, and most want the absolute best for their horses. But it can be very hard to determine what actually *is* best for the horse when trying to decipher the enormous amount of information available online and with the rise of branded equipment and clinicians. While we want everything faster, better, bigger, and more productive, as we've said in this book, horses themselves have not changed much beyond their original, herd-binding, free-ranging natural tendencies and psychologies.

Unfortunately, many issues in the equine industry have arisen as a result of *our* changing when the horse has not, and deviations from classical concepts of horse training. Today there is often an emphasis put on fragmented aspects of horsemanship rather than the whole. We have to recognize there are no short-cuts or substitutes for the years of study and practice necessary to becoming a masterful rider and trainer. Having an understanding of equine behavior and a wonderful relationship with your horse is one thing, but getting on a horse and acquiring competent riding skills is yet another. Good riding requires a whole other level of instruction and practice. There is no point establishing a respectful relationship on the ground, then getting on your horse and causing him pain or distress because of your unbalanced seat, incorrect application of the aids, or problems with the tack. We need to have respect for the horse *when we ride him*, too, and that means common sense training for ourselves as riders.

A conscientious horseperson—from the very beginnings of benevolent horsemanship as first written by Xenophon—*always* puts the comfort and welfare of the horse *first*. As mentioned, circumstances of the times have given rise to more forceful methods over the years, but they are once again, thankfully, falling out of favor. If you study the masters of equitation—such as one of my favorites, Colonel Alois Podhajsky (author of the revered *My Horses, My Teachers*)—you will find the compassionate base from which the kinder techniques originated.

A FEW BASIC CHARACTERISTICS OF A MODERN, WELL-TRAINED HORSE

- Leads correctly (that is, he respects your personal space, does not pull, hang back, or push on you).

- Ties.

- Loads in a trailer easily.

- Has good ground manners (for example, allows all body parts to be touched, lets you pick up his feet, is easily caught, and stands quietly for grooming, veterinarian, and farrier).

- Longes or free longes correctly.

- Stands still for mounting.

- Responds to light aids (that is, understands a squeeze of the fingers, subtle shifts in the seat, and touch of the legs, rather than requiring heavier application of aids to generate a proper response).

- Forward, supple, and rhythmic with three good quality gaits (or well-confirmed breed-specific gaits) with clean footfalls, free movement, a good attitude, and an appropriate level of soundness.

Common-sense methods begin with concern for the horse's conformation as a basis for determining if he will likely be able to carry a rider comfortably. Ideally, this is still the case today as we want a horse that will stay sound in the feet and legs, show the kind of movement that can be enhanced with correct training, and maintain an excellent disposition (more likely if he stays sound).

Good breeding is essential to producing the kind of horses people want to work with, however, breeding too many horses of *any* quality is *not* in line with the 25 Principles of Compassionate Equitation. "Overbreeding" has resulted in the suffering of too many horses that end up abused, abandoned or at slaughterhouses due to not being able to find long-term homes.[2] Even today, some large operations breed a lot of working horses, and in some cases the mindset is that the good ones are kept, whereas the culls are looked upon as "salvage livestock." This is highly contentious given the extreme range of opinions as to what the best answers are in matters concerning excessive numbers of horses.

> *According to a 2013 post by The Humane Society of the United States, they recommend the following when it comes to addressing the over-population of horses: "We can limit overbreeding, provide shelter, and expand adoption work. More than 160,000 horses were sent to slaughter last year [2012] alone, and a vast majority of them would have been good candidates for new homes. The USDA documented that 92.3 percent of horses sent to slaughter are in good condition and are able to live out a productive life" (http://www.humanesociety.org/issues/horse_slaughter/facts/facts_horse_slaughter.html).*

Common sense dictates that *all* of these aspects be taken into consideration when thinking about what contributes to compassionate training methods. It is plain old common sense to develop correctly educated riders, well-trained horses, and restricted breeding programs. These seem to be necessary and not unreasonable steps toward a sustainable future for the equine industry. It does not serve the horse industry well to support methods that, whether they appear to be humane or not, produce poorly trained or unsound horses. Putting compassion and common sense at the base of all training methods, combined with a clear understanding of optimal training goals, creates healthy, happy horses with potentially long and useful lives— whether they're used for Western sports, English disciplines, driving, racing, or not ridden at all.

Dr. Allen Schoen:

We must be sure we do not mistake compassion for being overly naive about a horse and allowing dangerous behavior, or putting ourselves or the horse in jeopardy.

Discipline—distinguished from *punishment*—is common sense. An animal (or human) that doesn't known appropriate boundaries can be dangerous. As the behaviors of a spoiled horse can often mimic behaviors of a horse responding to pain, it is important to be as clear as possible in determining the difference.

Spoiled *or* in pain, the horse's size and quick reactions can lead to injuries for a human handler.

By using common sense and having respect for yourself and your horse, you are being compassionate because you are not increasing risks for the animal. If the horse is spoiled and allowed to continue to be, somebody else will have to discipline him. The horse may also inadvertently harm another being.

It is compassionate for all involved to have a well-trained, well-behaved horse that won't be in the position of having bitten, kicked, pushed, or run away with someone. Practical horsemanship is based in common sense and designed for the safety and welfare of both horses and their human handlers and riders. As the UK organization Blue Cross for Pets says, safety around horses "requires both common sense and an understanding of horses. Horse riding is a high-risk activity, but handling horses from the ground can be just as dangerous for the unwary. Whether a beginner or an experienced horse keeper, safety awareness is vital both on the ground and in the saddle."

We do not want to see compassion mistaken as a lack of common sense regarding the training and handling of horses. With this in mind, when compassionately applying common sense to horsemanship, follow these basic guidelines:

- Be nice to your horse, but teach boundaries.

- When something appears to be causing your horse pain and discomfort, acknowledge it.

- Trust your instincts if you feel a training method is detrimental to your horse's progress, or mental or physical well-being.

- Listen to your veterinarian, farrier, and other knowledgeable individuals if they question your horse's behavior.

- Be humble enough to ask for help when you are unable to correct your horse's behavior by yourself.

- Do not breed poor-quality horses with conformation faults and genetic predisposition to disease.

Questions to Consider

BASED ON PRINCIPLE 11

1   Do I understand how and why ensuring my horse is well-mannered and correctly trained is being compassionate to him?

2   Can I see how producing a good quality horse with solid training basics might be conducive to the long-term soundness, longevity, and general happiness of that horse?

3   Do I and others I ride with or others in my barn abide by guidelines that exemplify common-sense horsemanship?

CHAPTER TWELVE

Learning to Recognize Pain and Discomfort

We are committed to educating everyone involved with horses in the understanding of how pain and discomfort are expressed by a horse.

Susan Gordon:

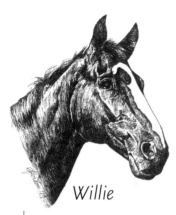

Willie

If only they could talk. If only we would listen when they do.

My blog "Ask Willie: The Thinking Horse" features Willie's point of view, conveying messages "straight from the horse's mouth." He was always quite expressive, as many horses are. Many mothers would have been covering their children's ears around him had Willie been able to speak our human language!

One night I had a dream about Willie in which he escaped from his stall, smoked a pipe, and taught philosophy to the other horses in the barn. It would have been just like him! If he did not have a "voice" in my waking life, he certainly did in my dream state. The dream is what ignited the idea to write from his viewpoint about his history, beginning from a high point as a winning show jumper to a low as a broken-down gelding nobody wanted.

I often tell people to trust their "gut instincts" when it comes to horses (see p. 229). If you are listening to what horses are "saying," that is generally how you will sense their messages to you first. Or, in some cases, a "picture" will pop into your head. A message can be less than a whisper. I had that feeling when Willie jumped his last oxer-to-oxer, in-and-out combination. His arthritic joints could not make the distances between jumps, even though he tried, and he barely cleared the final rail. In another instance with a different horse, I sat at the in-gate, waiting for my jumper class, and scratched the horse right then and there because something did not "feel" right. This was a powerful, but nervous big bay that had stopped at a large oxer with me the day before in schooling. We had jumped several rounds clean, with no problems. But all of a sudden, while waiting for that class, I felt a shift in his energy. I sensed that he had reached his limit, and I felt we needed to be done for the day.

If Willie had lessons in philosophy to teach other horses, he certainly had a few he felt people needed to learn, too. Couldn't sit straight in the saddle? Willie would curl his body up like a cat's, track awkwardly as he reflected the rider's crooked seat, and "scowl." You could almost see the cartoon "thought-balloon" over his head, explaining to the frustrated student that if he or she would just sit correctly, he would also move correctly. He could out-stubborn anyone until the rider got it right.

Had someone tried to put Willie on a lesson string when his tendency was to buck on a daily basis, his teaching career obviously would not have turned out so well! But eventually he learned to tolerate a beginner rider. A schoolmaster is genuinely worth his weight in gold. Unfortunately, a lifetime of uneducated seats will ultimately affect a horse's back, and so our most valuable four-legged souls are to be commended for their contribution to the education of up and coming equestrians. We therefore owe it to them to keep them as comfortable as possible.

There are tremendous learning opportunities worldwide for equestrians to seek out further education and training at every level. As examples: In Canada, most instructors are certified by Equine Canada's stellar coaching program.[1] Such a system standardizes rider education and ties in to the National Canadian Coaches Program, which is a blanket organization for many other sports. Certification in the United States is not required for instructors, but there are excellent programs such as the Certified Horsemanship Association and American Riding Instructor's Association.[2,3] The FN system in Germany teaches riding and licenses trainers, and the British Horse Society in the United Kingdom offers professional qualifications.

Equine Canada describes its coaching program in the following way: "As in any sport, athletic accomplishment, and teaching or coaching are separate skillsets. In equestrianism, horsemanship (ability to work with/train the horse) is a third area of competency. Being a good athlete or accomplished trainer does not necessarily give a coach/instructor the skills for being an effective teacher and coach. Equine Canada certification recognizes the coach/instructors' teaching and coaching skills as meeting professional, and internationally recognized standards for coaching practice" (http://www.equinecanada.ca/index.php?option=com_content&view=section&id=126&Itemid=743&lang=en).

The Certified Horsemanship Association (CHA) strives "To promote excellence in safety and education for the benefit of the entire horse industry... by certifying instructors, accrediting equine facilities and publishing educational resources (http://cha-ahse.org/).

The American Riding Instructors Association (ARIA) Certification Program assesses "all aspects of each candidate's demonstrated knowledge of the discipline he/she wishes to teach, attention to professionalism and safety, and business and personal integrity. Even at Level 1, ARIA certification is hard-earned, which makes it respected and important. Major insurance companies recognize ARIA Certification, and offer those instructors a substantial discount on their insurance needs" (www.riding-instructor.com).

A good horsemanship education is vital to our discussion of riding and training, and also invaluable to being a competent "ground person" or observer of horses.

There are, of course, other established rider/trainer certification programs and respected schools of classical equitation where horses and riders are taught time-tested methods. *The Compassionate Equestrian* supports those schools that have traditionally put the welfare of the horse first. There is a need to clarify this aspect of horsemanship, as there has been considerable debate, online and elsewhere, concerning some traditional techniques and their potential harm to the horse.

Unfortunately too many high-profile instances of glaring abuse have surfaced in show arenas or on racetracks in recent years. I feel that in some cases the evidence of what's "bad" within the horse world has caused some to associate aspects of classical training with non-compassionate methods. Therefore, when discussing Principle 12, I'd like to reaffirm that the true foundations of classical training were designed to keep horses sound and happy throughout a working lifetime, with the intention of allowing them to perform as freely under saddle as they do when turned out and playing with other horses. The mere act of placing a bit in the horse's mouth, or a saddle on his back, or requesting movements that he has been bred, trained, and well prepared for, does not mean that the horse is experiencing pain or unhappiness as a result.

The current trend of using the term "natural" to describe the most desirable way to keep and train horses (generally in reference to an array of training techniques based on research derived from studying equine herd dynamics, ethology, and behavior) has helped disseminate knowledge of horse psychology, body language, and instinct, and has been extremely enlightening for many people. *But* the moment we engage a horse and ask that he respond to our human language, we are experiencing something contrary to what is *natural* in the horse's mind. After all, horses are *prey* and we are *predators*. The best we can do is to understand *how we affect* their ability to "just be horses" in the requests that we make. And yes, we want to be aware of how the horse conveys pain and discomfort to us. Even better, we would like to prevent the horse from being uncomfortable in the first place.

DEVELOP A GREAT SEAT (THAT DOESN'T CAUSE YOUR HORSE PAIN OR DISCOMFORT!)

Before riding, make sure you are physically balanced and in alignment, as well as calm and centered in your heart and mind. The following situations are the most ideal ways to develop a balanced, independent seat, but they may not be available to everyone. Choose the opportunity or opportunities that are best applied to your situation.

- Practice on a seasoned, schoolmaster lesson horse.
- Spend countless hours on the longe line with a patient, highly qualified instructor.
- Ride without stirrups.
- Ride without reins.
- Watch other riders with excellent seats and hands.
- Cross-train for cardio, core strength, and flexibility.

In traditional schools of equitation such as the famed Spanish Riding School of Vienna, Austria, a strict adherence to age-old methods has produced consistent results, decade after decade. Horses and riders are set on a standardized course of education with results generally predictable, as they have been for over 400 years. Most riders learning in the fast pace of our modernized world do not have the patience required in such a system where new riders, known as *cadets,* are put on the longe line without stirrups and reins for the first years of their education. It is only after four to six years of intensive education on a fully trained Lipizzaner stallion that the cadet is evaluated for progress and allowed to participate in the school's quadrilles under the supervision of the head rider. It takes eight to twelve years to become a fully qualified rider at the school, and only *then* is a student allowed a young stallion to train.

The wheel, so to speak, has not been "reinvented" when it comes to training horses. We just have more tools available now to be able to tell what does and does not cause distress to horses. Researchers in the science of equitation continue to update this information.

Impatience is one reason for the mistakes made with horses today, especially as newer horse owners may be influenced by a confusing array of information targeted at inexperienced owners, expecting a rapid and special connection with horses. However, modern human expectations of instant gratification aren't always in the best interest of a horse. Reading and studying in depth while off the horse is imperative to attaining a thorough grasp on your chosen discipline. The problem nowadays is sometimes caused by our tendency to receive, and in fact prefer information in short sentences and brief video segments. We simply cannot abbreviate the *correct* training of a horse and rider.

The fascinating part about a seasoned, well-trained horse is the ability with which he's able to become the teacher, as Colonel Podhajsky so eloquently states in *My Horses, My Teachers* (Trafalgar Square Books, 1997). Given the opportunity, a schoolmaster is a genius in action, and from an instructor's viewpoint, a highly valued assistant when working with the human student. Learning to ride means learning to *feel*, and much of that *feel* cannot necessarily be taught through verbiage. It is done by sitting in the saddle, hour after hour, transition after transition, until progress is made toward an independent seat, legs, and hands.

What the instructor sees from the ground is meant to be of tremendous assistance in translating to the rider what he or she feels when in the saddle. The *eyes on the ground* may catch signs in the horse that indicate distress and discomfort, and this information is relayed to the rider so he or she begins to learn to feel the correlation between "ears pinned" and "heel accidentally digging into the ribs," for example. Besides just teaching the student how to apply the aids to tell the horse which gait or movement to perform, a good instructor helps the rider develop a sensitive feel, to be ever mindful of the horse's subtle (or perhaps not-so-subtle) reactions to pain and discomfort, and also to take note when the horse is moving correctly with freedom and comfort. Eventually, we get better and better at reading the information silently conveyed to us by the horse as to how he might be feeling, whether we are on the ground *or* in the saddle.

If you want to be good at something, spend a lot of time doing it.

During my career as a professional rider I was frequently tasked with determining the reasons a horse would buck, bolt, or stop at jumps. I was often told, "He gives no warning." Usually, I found that was not true. There was always some kind of "alert message" that I could feel come up through the horse's back or shoulders, perhaps as little as a split second before the reactive behavior would start. Riders *can* learn how to be mindful of the subtle signals given by the horse, often by simply paying more attention to what they are feeling in the horse's body language. Almost every major reaction is due to something hurting in the horse's body. And the only reason I became sensitive enough to "hear" what the horse's body was saying was by riding many horses, day in, day out, over a lot of years. I realize this kind of experience is not available to the average rider, but you can certainly spend time understanding the depths of your own horse's behavior, and through the bonding process, you will become attuned to his subtle signals, as he will become more in tune to your body and emotions as well. You can also learn a lot by attending horse shows and observing many different horse-and-rider combinations. Practice evaluating your observations, and see if you can identify various issues in horses that might make you sensitive enough to even predict how a particular horse might perform in the competition arena, or perhaps see if your opinion of how a class should place agrees with that of the judge.

As we've learned, riders need to be compassionate with themselves, too, and realize it is easy to miss signs of pain or discomfort in the horse. In becoming a Compassionate Equestrian we always allow that we do *the best we can, to the best of our abilities*. This is also true when learning to recognize how horses indicate how they feel and what they may need. It takes a lot of careful observation and qualified evaluation by an equine professional to be clear when the horse's behavior is *not* pain-related.

If you have a sore rib, and somebody pokes you in that rib, your reaction will be swift and probably not too congenial toward the person who provoked the pain. While it is believed horses have a much thicker skin than we do, they can still bruise, break, and be strained due to the athletic activities we impose on them. If we accidentally poke, kick, or pull on a sore part, we are likely to be met with a less-than-favorable reaction. It could be anything from ears suddenly pinned, to an attempt at biting you, or kicking at your leg pressure when mounted. As we've said already in this book, relegating such responses to "behavioral issues" is doing a tremendous disservice to the horse and reacting by punishing him only serves to make the horse equate pain with more pain. How would *you* respond if you were "attacked" by the person who poked you in the sore rib just because you reacted to the poke?

HOW HORSES SAY "OUCH"

- Sudden changes in expression or personality, especially from bright/interested to dull
- Bucking
- Rearing
- Agitated tail swishing
- Sinking the back when mounted
- Moving away from the rider during mounting
- Pinning ears when the saddle is placed on the back
- Biting or restless when being groomed
- Resisting backing up
- Out-of-context sweating
- Unusual stance: for example, pointing one foot forward or rocking back on haunches

- Difficulty negotiating hills
- Teeth grinding
- Looking at the belly, trying to roll, and pawing (common colic symptoms)
- Reluctance to move
- Muscle tremors
- Abnormal gait
- Anxious appearance
- Increased respiration or heart rate (other than related to exercise)
- Dilated pupils
- Flared nostrils

Do you or trainers you know or work with require a recent veterinarian's exam before working with a new horse?

Before beginning a reschooling project on your own or sending your horse to a professional trainer, especially for issues that you feel may be behavior-related, try to have the horse be free of all pain and discomfort issues to the best of your ability and knowledge. While you or a professional trainer may be able to observe whether or not a horse is likely in pain, and while you might even be able to determine where the soreness originates, it may take a veterinary exam to pinpoint the primary cause. It's possible this practice, if more widespread, would result in fewer problems and better safety for both horses and humans. For example, I know a rider who was hospitalized after a violent bucking episode, and her horse was sent to another trainer for correction of the behavior *without* having a veterinary evaluation for possible pain. He was eventually found to have *osteochondritis dissecans* (OCD—a developmental disease that affects the cartilage and bone in joints), and the veterinarian confirmed that his extreme bucking was most likely related to severe joint pain.

This is a common scenario, perhaps more so than many horsepeople realize. It is up to the individual to decide if he or she will require a veterinary "soundness exam" prior to beginning training with a new horse or accepting a new equine client. As Compassionate Equestrians, owners or sellers of horses can also choose to be responsible and fully disclose any information that may have led to a horse experiencing traumatic or chronic pain, to the best of their knowledge and understanding. I realize this is an ideal that might be difficult to conceive in the traditional world of "horse trading" where honesty is not presumed, but I do believe it is a goal to which we should aspire.

Learning to recognize pain and discomfort in the horse begins with an open-minded and considerate evaluation of him. There may also be personal issues the rider or owner is experiencing in his or her own life that could relate to the horse's problems. This is how we can begin to create a holistic system of education for all horsepeople. We observe the horse first of all, as he cannot verbally express what makes him hurt, and thoroughly examine and decipher what he might be feeling due to the equipment and pressures we are putting on him.

Dr. Allen Schoen:

Evaluating a horse that has been beaten while in pain can be a very challenging experience for a veterinarian, as it produces a very defensive, reactive animal.

"Watch out! Be careful!"

These were the first words I heard as I was asked to evaluate an eight-year-old chestnut mare.

"This horse hates people, especially men, and she may kick you or bite you without any warning," cautioned the trainer as I gently approached "Witch," a mare with a clearly defensive attitude. I listened as the trainer revealed her history: whenever she was being difficult, previous handlers had beat her, claiming she was stubborn, obnoxious, angry, and other negative adjectives.

I observed her behaviors, used nonverbal communication, and gently approached her, calmly putting my hand on her neck and stroking her. I assessed her through the Diagnostic Acupuncture Point Palpation Exam (DAPE) and musculoskeletal alignment evaluation, which I do on all horses I see. I could feel tremendous resistance as I tried to palpate in the area of her atlas and upper neck. She raised her head higher and higher as my hands approached her poll. When I palpated an acupuncture point behind the saddle that can be sensitive when a mare is in heat or has ovarian issues, her ears went back, her back stiffened up, and she almost made to kick out at me. I asked the trainer if Witch was "marish" at times. The trainer rolled her eyes and laughed.

"Are you kidding!" she said. "She will try to kill you when she is in heat and even when she is not."

I suggested that some of the mare's attitude might be due to ovarian pain. The trainer chuckled and said that I was the first man she knew who acknowledged that ovarian pain could cause back problems.

I suggested possible treatments for the mare, including conventional medications for ovarian issues, acupuncture, Western herbal supplements, or some Traditional herbal formulas that I have found to be clinically beneficial in some cases. We began with a conservative approach at first: acupuncture and herbal formulas. Once I performed acupuncture on the acupoints for the ovaries, the mare immediately relaxed, her head dropped down, she began to yawn, her back muscles loosened, and her entire demeanor changed. The trainer was amazed to see such an instantaneous response to the acupuncture therapy. I explained that I felt that many of the behaviors the mare had long demonstrated were defensive responses to discomfort, and she actually was quite a nice horse if not punished for being in pain.

DO YOUR HOMEWORK

When considering the lease or purchase of a new horse, follow your horse's history back as far as you can to find out what his early training was like. Watch for subtle cues as to whether he was handled compassionately or not. Look at his ears. Look at his eyes. Look at how he interacts with people and other horses. If there are issues from the horse's past, determine if they are resolvable using compassionate training methods *before* taking on the horse. If you determine the horse is going to be too much of a challenge for you or your trainer to handle in a tolerant and forgiving manner, perhaps this is not the right horse for you.

Horses can experience muscle spasms in the area right behind the saddle that can set off episodes of bucking or bolting. A veterinarian trained in acupuncture or acupressure points can help determine why that particular part of the body is so sensitive. This is helpful when determining whether a problem is a training, tack, rider, or lameness issue due to a primary back problem or an internal medicine cause (such as an ovarian cyst in a mare).

When addressing possible causes of pain in the horse, it is important to come from an integrative medicine perspective. For example, as I deduced in the case of the chestnut mare, certain acupuncture points on the back can be very sensitive when a mare has significant ovarian issues due to being in heat or the existence of ovarian cysts. She may exhibit severe bucking and behavioral reactions, or experience muscle spasms right behind the saddle. A veterinarian who is also trained in acupuncture, as I am, can identify a specific sore point, suggest the possible reasons why it is so sensitive, and decide if other parameters are also related to the sensitivity of the pressure point. It helps to narrow the focus of the diagnosis when a broader scope of modalities can be applied in the diagnostic process.

Before proceeding with any kind of training, before taking your horse out on the trail or into the show ring, ensure you are coming from a compassionate mind and heart that has acknowledged and resolved any potential discomfort your horse may be experiencing. In some cases, you might have to *let go* of preconceived notions regarding the horse's ability to respond comfortably and progressively to the plans you initially had for him. When your horse's training is set back due to injuries or illness, be patient in the rehabilitation and recovery process, allowing time and treatment necessary before returning to an intense training protocol or showing schedule. This goes back to always asking yourself the same kind of question: "What would be the most compassionate approach for this horse, at this time?"

In the case of the chestnut mare, the problem was, no one recognized she was in pain. I see this far too frequently, and this really saddens me.

I feel that ideally, education regarding the recognition of pain in horses should be encouraged for *all* horsepeople. This includes explaining equine behaviors that are related to pain and discomfort and various options for alleviating them. This is the essence of Principle 12 of Compassionate Equitation. The latest research in this area is actually available online and on your smartphone via an application known as the Horse Side Vet Guide® (horsesidevetguide.com). Dr. Douglas O. Thal, the creator of HSVG, makes essential equine healthcare information available at your fingertips in order to increase the quality of communication between owners, riders, and equine caregivers and their veterinarians—for the benefit of the horse.

Scientists have also developed a new standardized "pain scale" that helps equestrians determine when a horse might be experiencing discomfort by observing changes in facial expression—what is known as the *Horse Grimace Scale (HGS)*. "The assessment of pain is critical for the welfare of horses," write Emanuela Dalla Costa, et al, in their article on PLOS.org "Existing pain assessment methods have several limitations, which reduce the applicability in everyday life. Assessment of facial expression changes, as a novel means of pain scoring, may offer numerous advantages and overcome some of these limitations."[4] There is now an HGS app available from Animal Welfare Science Hub (animalwelfarehub.com).

4   *In "Development of the Horse Grimace Scale (HGS) as a Pain Assessment Tool in Horses Undergoing Routine Castration" (PLOS/One, March 2014), Emanuela Dalla Costa, et al, describe their study wherein "Forty stallions were assigned to one of two treatments and all animals underwent routine surgical castration under general anaesthesia. Group A (n = 19) received a single injection of Flunixin immediately before anaesthesia. Group B (n = 21) received Flunixin immediately before anaesthesia and then again,*

OTHER SYSTEMS FOR DETERMINING PAIN IN HORSES

The following methods of determining the existence of pain or discomfort in horses are used primarily in the veterinary care field. As we have acknowledged, pain in horses is difficult to assess because of their inability to communicate with humans through verbal language. This could be further compounded by horses potentially suppressing the exhibition of obvious signs of pain in the presence of possible predators (that is, humans) as is suggested with other prey species.

- *The Post Abdominal Surgery Pain Assessment Scale (PASPAS)* is a multidimensional scale that can be used to quantify pain after laparotomy (a surgical procedure involving a large incision to gain access into the abdominal cavity).

- *The Composite Pain Scale (CPS)* focuses on the presence of pain-related behaviors and the change in the frequency of normal behavior patterns and physiological parameters. It has been successfully applied following surgery (for example, castration, as in the HGS study—see p. 220), injury, and disease.

Researchers do note, however, that behavior-based assessments of pain are not without limitations. These include the need for trained and experienced observers, prolonged observation periods (particularly in conditions inducing only mild pain), and the palpation of the painful area, in some cases.

as an oral administration, six hours after the surgery. In addition, six horses were used as anaesthesia controls (C). These animals underwent non-invasive, indolent procedures, received the same treatment as group A, but did not undergo surgical procedures that could be accompanied with surgical pain. Changes in behaviour, composite pain scale (CPS) scores and horse grimace scale (HGS) scores were assessed before and 8-hours post-procedure. Only horses undergoing castration (Groups A and B) showed significantly greater HGS and CPS scores at 8-hours post compared to preoperatively. Further, maintenance behaviours such as explorative behaviour and alertness were also reduced. No difference was observed between the two analgesic treatment groups" (http://journals.plos.org/plosone/article?id=10.1371/journal.pone.0092281).

Increase your own awareness of what kind of signs indicate pain in horses. Study various pain-assessment programs. Study equine behavior. These steps will be beneficial in improving the health, happiness, and safety of both horse and rider. When you are tuned in to early signs of discomfort, you can resolve issues more quickly and thereby prevent future behavioral issues.

Questions to Consider
BASED ON PRINCIPLE 12

1   Are there behavioral issues my horse exhibits *now* that might be due to pain?

2   What can I do to determine if my horse's behavior issues are due to discomfort? What can I do to help find the root cause of the discomfort?

3   What can I do to resolve any issues that may be causing pain in my horse?

CHAPTER THIRTEEN

Recognizing Subtle Signs of Resistance

We recognize that horses may exhibit subtle signs of discomfort and pain. These signs could indicate the early onset of potential lameness and lead to more serious, chronic problems. We agree to increase our mindfulness, awareness, and understanding of the subtle signals conveyed to us by the horse's silent language.

Susan Gordon:

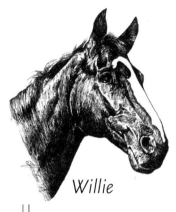

Willie

It was very disconcerting to have Willie "lose" his canter altogether. At the time, I was preparing to show him at Second Level when his canter all but vanished. I chalked it up to hot weather, laziness, and the fact that he really did not like dressage anyhow. The only way he was inspired to school a few dressage movements was with a brisk gallop across the field, a leap through the water jump, and about 10 minutes in the ring, at most. Second Level required the beginnings of collected canter though, and it simply was not happening. His gaits were still regular, so I suspected something internal.

After scratching from a couple of shows, I requested the veterinarian evaluate him, and in particular, check his bloodwork. Willie was found to be severely anemic. The veterinarian, who always had great advice, told me it was common amongst Warmbloods in hot climates.

Oops. I missed that one. Poor Willie. He was back to normal in due time after being put on a good blood-building supplement. He would have received the necessary supplement sooner had I been far more attentive and responded when I sensed that something had gone awry as soon as his training began to backslide. It is a good example of how our desire to have a horse perform at a certain level can delay a proper response to the horse's actual needs. Even though Willie was giving me signs he was struggling with something, I was initially in denial of the messages he was trying to convey because I wanted to go to those shows. You can be sensitive to horses and still end up allowing human desires and ego to interfere with that connection. It's kind of like static in the "energy field." This is where what we've learned about self-compassion so far, and what we will learn about forgiveness (in chapter 25, p. 391), is so important.

There are many clues horses can give us when something is "not right," and it is up to us to pay attention and investigate what might be causing a change in behavior, or a stall or backslide in progress.

Watch the breathing patterns of the horses you work with; pay attention to their responses to everything in their environment. Their sensory reactions say a lot about how to determine the best way to proceed with a workout. It is important to be familiar with your horse's normal baseline of behavior so you can recognize changes that may be of concern. For instance, if a horse is uncharacteristically spooking at things, one possibility (of many) is he is having eye problems. If he is sweating out of context, he may be experiencing severe pain.

In order to gain the ability to recognize pain and discomfort in a horse, it is imperative to have a very good understanding of what the normal expression is for a working, athletic horse and one that is at rest.

Developing a consistent routine with your horse helps determine what is "normal" for him. Let the horse tell you where he is most comfortable during pre-ride preparations: The aisle? The wash area? If it means grooming him in his stall, then that works, too. Look for big sighs, slow breathing, and signs of relaxation *before* heading to the arena or trail. Any lingering signs of tension by the time you are tacked up and ready to go may mean a change in plans or the workout. This is especially true when working with a youngster or riding a new horse. Sometimes, it's true, you just do not know what might be triggering a horse's stress, but it is still important to decide how you will calm him before proceeding with the pending session. The best policy for recognizing subtle clues of distress in the horse is to know and understand the horse's personality and what may bother him under "normal" circumstances.

We learn to interpret the horse's body language and that helps inform our decisions as regards training and workouts when we witness a new or different response. This is one reason why thorough grooming is so critical. When anything physical is sore, stiff, or just sensitive, we not only notice, but we may also be able to treat a minor problem before it becomes a serious one.

Groom your horse thoroughly and pay special attention to his feet, joints, and legs every time. It is good to be a little fanatical about keeping feet and legs scrupulously clean—if nothing else, it tunes you in to the physical changes in these areas.

I learned late in my career that you can never say, "I've seen everything!" when it comes to horses. I was caring for a buckskin mare while her owner was away. One day, I led her into the barn and placed her in the cross-ties, and the horses in all the nearby stalls immediately stuck their heads out and began licking—at nothing in particular. I had never seen that kind of group behavior before and thought it was odd, but since the mare seemed normal, I carried on grooming as planned. The next day I brought her into the barn and the same thing happened. This time even more horses in the 20-stall barn stuck out their heads started "air-licking"! Some licked so much they had foam around their mouths. I felt it had to have *something* to do with the buckskin mare. I went over her closely and noticed a bit of swelling over her right eye. It looked like she had bumped her head on something, but there wasn't any hair missing and no obvious wound. I placed my hand over the swelling and it was hot, and heat plus swelling is a sign of serious trouble. Usually this means an infection, but I still could not find a wound anywhere. Meanwhile, the other horses were licking furiously, reaching over their doors, trying to reach the buckskin. Her behavior was still normal, and she ignored the strange interest of the other horses. Now I was not just curious, I was a bit alarmed.

I followed the swelling and heat to a spot at the base of her forelock. There, hidden under her thick, black, wiry hair was a minuscule hole. I gently pressed around the tiny opening, and it became immediately obvious that this was indeed a badly infected puncture wound.[1] The horses in the barn were responding to the smell of the infection, long before I was able to detect it. A quick call to the veterinarian prevented things from getting any worse. I have seen horses "air-licking" since then, and now I am quite aware of what it means. If the buckskin mare was sending subtle clues to me about her injury, I was not picking up on them. The other horses sure knew what was going on, though!

1

Puncture wounds in horses can become serious very quickly. Take action right away if your horse has sustained such an injury, especially when a joint is involved. In the January 2004 EQUUS magazine article "Pasture Puncture Wounds," Joanne Meszoly writes that punctures near joints or tendons are most urgently in need of medical care because the by-products of infection can irreversibly damage cartilage and tendon sheaths.

"If the wound penetrates the joint, assume you've got a joint infection and call your veterinarian," says Jerry Black, DVM, in the article. "The knee and fetlock in particular have no significant soft-tissue cover, so it doesn't take a lot of penetration. Even a quarter-inch puncture in the fetlock is serious. It needs to be tended to within a matter of hours" (http://equusmagazine.com/article/puncture010804).

One of the huge benefits to slowing down a bit, breathing deeply, and clearing your emotions prior to being around horses is the fact that you can focus on your horse in more specific detail. Horses are big animals, but they are not indestructible by any means, and there are some that *always* seem to find different ways of getting hurt or into trouble. I am a bit obsessive when it comes to inspecting legs and feet before and after rides. It takes extra time to check tendons and joints for heat and swelling, and inspect shoes and nails for problems, but it could make the difference between a very lame horse and one that just needs a break. A bad injury can be expensive and long-term, so it pays to look for the signs a minor issue may need attending to.

Since beginning my own running program, including high-mileage with speed intervals, I have had the opportunity to learn what a minor injury probably feels like to a horse. Some days it is just a matter of being stiff and not feeling like exercising. Other days there might be a knot in a calf muscle that says, "Be careful." but you can still run. Slowly. Ask for speed and you may end up with a higher grade of injury, even a tear. Foot problems? Those hurt. Have you ever stubbed your toe or bruised a toenail? Do you ever wonder why horses limp so dramatically when they have a stone bruise or get trimmed too short? It does not take much of sore spot in the foot to produce an "off" gait in a runner either. Sometimes what seems like a minor incident can trigger an injury days later, or when you can still run just fine, a compensatory injury develops on the side that *was* sound. As humans, we can decide for ourselves whether or not we hurt too much to risk further injury with a workout, or talk ourselves into running when we are merely stiff and sore, but horses do not get to make such choices. Because we make these decisions for them, we have to watch closely and read their signals carefully.

As I mentioned in chapter 12, a valuable lesson I learned over the years is to pay attention to my "gut instincts" when it comes to horses. After all, the gut is like a second brain.[2] Once again, a very quiet, focused state of mind (see QFI on p. 8) is helpful in learning to discern where those "gut feelings" are coming from. For example, when you have "butterflies" because you are nervous about a class at a show or riding a new horse, you can self-talk your way into a more confident state and "trot on." But when your stomach is in knots because you feel your horse is telling you something is amiss, you may want to, scratch, dismount, and explore the issue further before requesting the horse perform in any way. With practice, you will find your instincts to be quite trustworthy once you learn to separate out your emotions and be objective. A quiet mind is also a more perceptive mind, and you may begin to notice things about your horse that you had not before.

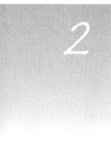

In his September 2012 cover story "That Gut Feeling" in the American Psychological Association Monitor on Psychology, *Dr. Siri Carpenter writes, "Gut bacteria also produce hundreds of neurochemicals that the brain uses to regulate basic physiological processes as well as mental processes such as learning, memory and mood. For example, gut bacteria manufacture about 95 percent of the body's supply of serotonin, which influences both mood and GI activity. When you consider the gut's multifaceted ability to communicate with the brain, along with its crucial role in defending the body against the perils of the outside world, 'it's almost unthinkable that the gut is not playing a critical role in mind states,' says gastroenterologist Emeran Mayer, MD, director of the Center for Neurobiology of Stress at the University of California, Los Angeles" (http://www.apa.org/monitor/2012/09/gut-feeling.aspx).*

What if *you* were hurting and unable to explain to anybody that you were experiencing pain, where it was, and what it felt like? Imagine being a horse in that situation that might like to say, "Help me!" if he could, but can only try to tell you through his body language.[3] The exercises in breathing, slowing down, and centering that we have suggested in previous chapters will help you become more aware of the subtle clues your horse sends you when he needs to "talk."

C. Lesimple and M. Hausberger ask, "How accurate are we at assessing other's well-being?" using horses in their Frontiers in Psychology *article (January 2014). "Here we show that caretakers strongly underestimate horses' expressions of well-being impairment," the authors state (http://www.ncbi.nlm.nih.gov/pubmed/24478748).*

Dr. Allen Schoen:

When speaking about lameness, some of my professors in equine medicine when I was in veterinary school would say, "Don't listen to a horse's trainer or rider because it can mislead you."

My professors' message was that "insight" from a trainer or rider could guide a veterinarian in the wrong direction because the trainer or rider's perception altered the information he or she provided. There is, of course, some truth to this because, as we've already discussed in this book, everyone sees things differently. As veterinary students, to avoid this issue, we were trained to watch the horse for ourselves and complete a conventional lameness exam.

HAVE A "GUT FEELING" SOMETHING'S "NOT RIGHT"?

Here are some behavioral signs that something might be wrong with your horse and warrant further investigation:

- A horse that's normally fine about walking into the arena hesitates, maybe even stops at the gate and takes a step or two backward.

- He doesn't want to be caught, even in his stall.

- His ears lay back when he is saddled or his girth is tightened.

- He tilts his head or spooks at objects that he usually ignores.

- His ears lay back or he tries to bite when you look at or gently touch an area of his body.

- Movements under saddle begin to deteriorate instead of continuing to improve.

- He has trouble getting up after rolling.

- He is reluctant to go up or down a hill.

- There are distinct changes in energy levels.

- His posture changes—for example he points one foot or "bunches" his legs up underneath his body.

- He takes longer to warm up than usual.

- If he jumps, he has trouble making the distances between fences.

Compare this with the list "How Horses Say 'Ouch'" on p. 216. Do you see the crossover between pain and behavior and understand how subtle the clues can be?

A few years later, as I was integrating acupuncture, chiropractic, and other methodologies into my practice, I noticed how different acupuncture point patterns related to different kinds of lameness and to pain in different areas of the body that may not have caused lameness *yet*. Then I became aware that a pattern of *trigger points* and *muscles spasms* sometimes showed up *before* the lameness was apparent. So, while as veterinary students we were trained to say to owners, "Your horse is not lame enough for *me* to see the problem. Ride him until he's obviously lame and I'll come back," you can see how this seems ill-advised in terms of trying to treat or prevent soundness issues! Being able to sense trigger points *before* the horse was lame seemed a profoundly better solution.

One of the first racehorses I had worked on with acupuncture in the early 1980s was a wonderful teacher in this regard. This mare showed me how acupuncture could improve my ability to diagnose and treat subtle lameness *prior* to becoming clinical. The chestnut Thoroughbred had to be rested for a while because of an undiagnosed intermittent lameness. The trainer asked me to look at her, because even after being rested, she still was "not quite right." Upon evaluation of her acupuncture points (also called *acupoints*), I found her hocks and back were quite sore. I did acupuncture for her back and acupoints at that first visit, and I suggested the trainer inject her hocks. The trainer decided to race her a few days after my acupuncture treatment, prior to the hocks being injected. The mare won her first race in over a year. The trainer was so thrilled that not only did I begin to treat all his horses, but he then based a large part of his training program on what I was finding on his horses *before* they became lame. This transformed the string's success rate, other racehorse trainers began to notice, and then began a period when I saw many horses at the racetracks in New York.

When I was first learning about diagnostic acupuncture points,
I quickly realized that acupuncture enabled me to discover
underlying causes of many of these subtle lameness issues
before they became clinically evident.

Based on my background in neurophysiology, my mind felt more comfortable choosing acupoints based more on a neurophysiologic and somatovisceral perspective, as well as a biomechanical perspective. Interestingly enough, they normally coincided quite closely with points based on Traditional Chinese Medicine.

The fact that it was possible to detect "pre-clinical" lameness issues, *prior to a horse becoming lame*, was one of the great benefits of interpreting diagnostic

AN ACUPRESSURE PRIMER

Acupressure and *acupuncture points* (also called *acupoints*) on the body are the same, usually small depressions between muscles or between muscles and bones. Acupressure uses pressure versus acupuncture's needles. Acupressure on specific acupoints can be beneficial: You apply steady, rotating pressure with a fingertip.

1   If you want to *relax* the point, gently massage *counterclockwise* over it. If your horse tends to be nervous or hyperactive or sore in an area, counterclockwise movement usually calms and relaxes the sore muscles.

2   If you want to *stimulate* and give it more energy, rub *clockwise*. This is appropriate when your horse is generally lethargic and weak—it often perks him up. (Note that this has not been "proven" by double-blind studies by any means, but in Chinese acupressure, this is what is recommended.)

When applying acupressure to your horse, breathe deeply, slowly, and regularly. Your breath will relax both of you and create your rhythm. If you are hyper and irritable and try to apply acupressure to your horse, he will sense your energy! The wrong energy can make him anxious or cranky and not want to be around you. This is a good practice to help you slow yourself down and relax. Offer massage of the acupoints daily or as often as possible. (See my full article on this topic on my website www.drschoen.com.)

acupuncture points. Based on the level of sensitivity of the specific points, I could pick up many different issues, treat them, and resolve them *before* they got any worse.

Then, when studying veterinary chiropractic care I began to appreciate how even some of the slightest misalignments or fixations could cause some very subtle pre-clinical lameness issues as well. For instance, one client told me how short-strided her horse was up front. Her attending veterinarian was unable to detect any significant lameness. She then had me evaluate her horse's diagnostic acupuncture points and palpate for various misalignments, asymmetries, and musculoskeletal fixations. In my examination, I found that there was decreased flexibility in the horse's shoulders, the sternum was slightly off to the right, a few thoracic vertebrae were displaced slightly to the left, and two ribs were compressed more tightly than the others. Based on my findings, I then evaluated her saddle fit. I found that the saddle was pinching the horse's withers, tight behind the shoulders, and impinging on the shoulders. I corrected the misalignments and fixations with adjustments and acupuncture, and her horse was able to flow freely with her front legs again—and there was no evidence of lameness. The client's saddle fit had to be corrected to prevent the issues from recurring.

VET TALK: COMPASSION Q & A

My good friend and colleague Steve Engle, DVM, graduated from Texas A&M University School of Veterinary Medicine & Biomedical Sciences in 1978. He is certified in equine acupuncture and chiropractic and has developed his own specialized, integrative approach. Dr. Engle has treated some of the top show jumpers and dressage horses in the United States and around the world. I asked him to share his perspective on a number of equine industry issues.

AS: What are the biggest issues regarding incorporating compassion in the horse world?

SE: The biggest barrier to compassion is money. It is the double-edged sword: much needed to provide facilities and care for those that are desperately in need, but it is often the desire for money that puts the well-being of a lot of these horses in jeopardy.

AS: What do you see that is needed? Lacking?

SE: Education and awareness. Compassion comes from awareness. Unfortunately the younger generation in the United States seems to be steeped in self-indulgence and instant gratification. There does seem to be an effort by our educational system to incentivize students to perform community service, which is a great start. I would like to see the various equestrian organizations create more awareness programs targeting young riders.

AS: How do you integrate compassion in your work with the horses and everyone involved, each day?

As I go over an acupoint, I feel different levels of sensitivity. The more super-ficially I palpate the point and get a reaction, the more likely it is indicative of more acute, more serious, or more evident lameness. If I palpate the points and only get subtle reactions, that can indicate subtle pain. Or, it might be a secondary compensatory issue. The level of pain, or the level of reaction at the acupoints, also assists me in figuring out what is a *primary* issue and what's *secondary*. Usually the more *acute* the problem is, the more *reactive* the point

SE: I am in the business of pain relief and so am uniquely aware of how pain affects the horse's demeanor, his weight, his hair coat, even his digestive system, let alone soundness. By becoming engaged in this area of medicine this has afforded me the realization of how grateful these animals can be. Much like people, there *is* a certain percentage of horses that would rather "hold on" to their body of pain than have it addressed; these are the animals that I can't help much. Fortunately, the vast majority of horses want to be free of pain, and it is with those that I am rewarded by their response to what I do.

AS: What would you like to see change in the horse world to make it more com-passionate in the future?

SE: The trend is a little disheartening at this time. But there are those that are trying to do good for animals that have been discarded once they have exceeded their usefulness. Increased tax incentives to draw more money into the facilities that help support retired and unwanted horses would be of value. I'd also like to see a way to get youth volunteers to help in rescues through the community service programs in our schools.

AS: Do you have compassionate tips that you use that you would like to see other horsepeople incorporate in their work with horses?

SE: Spend more time touching your horse or horses. A horse is uniquely bonded to the one who rides him. Spending more time on the ground touching, grooming, connecting just might enhance that bond, as well as awareness. More often than not I see these animals treated more like they are tools than living, feeling beings.

is upon superficial palpation, and the more indicative that is of that being your *primary* or *more significant* issue.

It is *quite common* for me to see horses where the acupoints may be reactive prior to a lameness becoming more evident. For example, I might say, "These points are reactive, suggesting a possible front foot issue." Then the horse's trainer might counter with, "No, the horse is fine in the front feet, no problems." But a few minutes later, he or she will remember, "Well, actually, the other day, when going over a jump he hesitated at takeoff and the landing wasn't quite right." Or, a day or two later, he or she might call and say, "Oh my gosh, the horse just went lame from an abscess in the foot!"

In spite of my early instruction to the contrary (see p. 228) I feel that by working in conjunction with a good trainer or a good rider, and the synergy of us putting our heads together, assists with the detective work often necessary to track down the source of pain in the horse. Then we can collectively say, "Ah-ha, maybe *that's* why the horse is doing this!"

There is an art in seeing lameness in the horse.

I am aware of certain Olympic-level veterinarians who are exceptionally good at noticing the subtle clues that indicate lameness in horses. A few have outstanding skill in combining integrative and complementary medicine with conventional medicine, and also have great empathy for the horse. This is why an integrative approach is best when there is a possibility that something might be developing "under the surface" concerning your horse's soundness. A veterinarian skilled in spotting the early signs of lameness is invaluable in the process, and one open to combining complementary and conventional modalities may offer further insights and options for treatment. This kind of compassionate, capable individual cannot only help your horse recover as quickly as possible, he or she can also prevent minor issues from turning into more serious ones.

As with the other Principles, we always conclude by asking, "What is the most compassionate thing to do for this horse?" When your horse is exhibiting subtle signs of pain or lameness or requiring progressive desensitization due to his experiences and history, the Compassionate Equestrian strives to be aware enough to enlist the most beneficial professional help while remaining open to new and innovative approaches. The Compassionate Approach is to create a team that works well together to help evaluate your horse when he experiences physical or behavioral issues, and then to welcome the team's insights as to how you can resolve them.

Questions to Consider
BASED ON PRINCIPLE 13

1   Have I recently noticed any subtle symptoms of lameness or atypical behavior in my horse?

2   How can I become more aware and mindful of subtle issues?

3   Is there a considerate, capable, and open-minded professional who can help me decide if my horse is experiencing minor discomfort that could become serious?

4   Can I learn from previous experiences when horses perhaps *did* show subtle signs of stress or pain that I may have missed?

5   What can I do and who can I work with to resolve lameness or behavioral issues?

CHAPTER FOURTEEN

Healthy Environments and Preventive Care: Incorporating the Precautionary Principle

We acknowledge that all beings deserve to live in a holistic, balanced, healthy environment. This is imperative to preventive health care, both physically and mentally, in humans and horses, and includes the creation of barns and other environments free of toxic compounds.

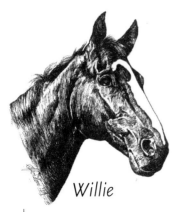

Willie

Susan Gordon:

Willie had some opinions about his environment. He pretty much had clear opinions on everything, but I was surprised at how specific his preferences were when it came to dealing with his basic needs and wants. When he first moved in with me, my backyard was only an acre, but it was sufficient for one horse. There was a lot of cacti: big prickly pears, cholla, barrel, and other succulents. The feeding shelter was shaded and there were several citrus trees close to the fence.

A low-hanging clothesline was cemented into the ground, close to and on the inside of the fence. I was concerned about its location because if a sizeable horse like Willie was to wedge himself between the clothesline and the fence, he could feel trapped, panic, and get hurt in the process. It was a rented property, though, so I left the clothesline as it was, although most would warn that taking such chances when it comes to horses is putting the horse at risk of injury. If I could do it again, I would most certainly take my own best advice and "err on the side of caution."

Sure enough, the morning after Willie arrived, I found him exactly where I thought would be the worst possible place. I froze upon entering the paddock, staring at the huge horse jammed in between the fence and the clothesline. He had even ducked under the line to wedge himself in there. Anticipating trouble as he tried to extract himself, I stood quietly and waited for him to make the first move. He pricked his ears in anticipation of breakfast, and then carefully backed himself out of the tight spot, lowering his head under the clothesline, then turning and walked calmly toward the barn. I breathed a sigh of relief and realized this wise old horse knew what he was doing and was very aware of his body. I was lucky this time, as not every horse is so savvy in this kind of situation.

Over time, I came to learn that Willie loved to cram himself into tight spaces. For a large horse, I thought it an odd behavior. He also favored lolling about in the shade of a big orange tree. When we moved and I had to search for a boarding barn for Willie, I found a peaceful facility surrounded by citrus groves with pipe-rail stalls, two arenas, and a 25-acre pasture. There were two pens available, and I was asked to choose one for him. Knowing Willie, I wanted him to make the choice. One of the pens was quite accommodating, but it did not have a tree of its own. It was exposed to the hot sun and only partially shaded by the tree in *the pen next to it. The other pen had its own wonderful, large, shade tree, but it was considerably smaller, and the roots of the tree made the ground uneven.*

I informed the owner that Willie liked both trees and small spaces, even though the logical choice for most owners would have been the larger pen. I'm sure she thought I was a little strange, but she agreed to let me turn Willie loose so he could to "pick one."

He did.

With both gates open, he checked out each pen and "chose" the small one. He was so happy with his new space that on more than one occasion I would go out to the big pasture to catch him, only to find that he had wandered back into his pen and was happily relaxing under his coveted tree.

Not too many horses are given the opportunity to have a say about the kind of environment in which they live. It would certainly be interesting to be able to record their personal preferences and the kind of environment most conducive to maintaining their physical and mental health and well-being. I believe their input would be as fascinating as it would be valuable.

Today, with the constant stream of news from around the world, it is hard to escape the incomprehensible degree of suffering humans inflict upon one another. When you factor in how climate change and mounting costs from catastrophic weather events are ruining so many lives and properties, sometimes it seems like the endless wheel of events sends us from one emotional extreme to the other and just won't let up.

The more we pay attention to all the bad news the more we are likely to succumb to emotional swings that mirror the outside events. Suddenly, we are instinctively always on the lookout for things that might cause us harm. Watching and listening to the media seems to provide us with a perpetual list of subjects to be wary of, keeping our stress hormones on high alert. This makes us more like horses than ever before.

It seems unfair to be taken on such a rollercoaster ride of highs and lows when staying in emotional balance is far more conducive to our good health and well-being, as well as that of our horses. There are so many occurrences that can take us from happy to sad to everything in between. All living beings exist in the same program—a cycle of birth to completion, form to formless, existence to nonexistence. A myriad of opportunities arise along the way to help us understand how to conduct ourselves so as to get the most out of life that we can.

We are stewards of the environment. This means from the micro to the macro, or from our internal environment to that of the Earth's. Our well-being is the planet's well-being.

Inevitably, we are stewards of our own environment, whether that means our internal selves or our immediate surroundings. Every place and every moment allows us the chance to be mindful and create the kind of space where joy and peace can flourish and expand. Everything you do in this effort has meaning, no matter how insignificant it may seem. Even tasks as simple as cleaning the bit when you finish a ride, wiping the mud off your boots before putting them away, or cleaning your horse's stall *just so*, your thoughts and actions are responsible for providing yourself and others a clean, pleasant, safe space in which to be. There are many small details that may initially seem mundane but are very important to the creation of a holistic, balanced environment.

As we have tried to emphasize throughout this book, when you give of yourself in a kind, compassionate way, the ripple effect is palpable, whether you are aware of it in the moment or not. Similarly, when you leave a barn angry, or have said unkind words to someone, then everyone leaves the barn upset, and everyone in their immediate path suffers, as well. Even if you are the only person hanging out in your backyard with a horse or two, you go from your home and your family or personal and business relationships to the barn, and then back again, and your anger or unkind thoughts travel with you—unless you consciously release them. The living body holds both *positive* and *negative* energy, and it has to dissipate somewhere. *We can choose to become a conduit for the more positive energy.*

In seeking *balance* for ourselves, we begin to look for stability in the environment around us and the elements that allow us to live free from fear and illness.[1] In the most natural state, our minds and the minds of our horses are primarily concerned with survival. Without actual predators, we conceive of them anyway—in the form of other people who may not like us, stress at work, or hazards on the streets and in crowded places. Sometimes we are not even aware when we are adversely reacting to a toxic environment; we become so accustomed to it. How many people would love to escape the city every now and then and just be in nature? To just be with horses? Quite a few, I am sure. The challenge is leaving the stress and toxicity behind.

Rick Hanson, PhD, writes in "Relaxed and Contented" on WiseBrain.org: "It's remarkable but true: part of your nervous system exists to make you feel peaceful and all right. Its formal title is: 'the parasympathetic wing of the autonomic nervous system' or PNS, for short. You can trigger the PNS at will, which immediately lowers your sense of stress, brings health benefits like reducing blood pressure and strengthening the immune system, and lifts your mood. This gives you more control over your inner landscape—a nice thing at times when the outer world seems driven by forces that are beyond your influence, from local traffic jams to global warming" (http://www.wisebrain.org/ParasympatheticNS.pdf).

Balance *in this case refers to achieving equilibrium in the* autonomic nervous system, *made up of the* sympathetic, *or "fight/flight" response, and the* parasympathetic, *or "rest/digest" response.*

When driven by concerns of survival, humans are affected in the same way herd animals are when all their focus is on the very basic needs required to sustain life. The sheer "will to live" can create a considerable amount of stress as our sympathetic nervous system remains overactivated. Stress leaves us compromised in areas that need the most attention when we are striving to bring everything back into balance.

At the primary, physical level, humans, horses and all living beings are made up of complex chemical interactions that work in harmony with each other and require nutrients to maintain the best quality of health. The food and water that provides us with nutrients varies dramatically in quality throughout the world and can be both the cause and cure for disease.

Understanding how the biochemistry of nutrition affects general health is of great benefit to all of us—for the sake of ourselves, our families and our horses.

The number of chemicals that have entered food sources since World War II is extraordinary. Many are not well researched or even approved for consumption. This includes additives and persistent organic pollutants in both human and pet foods.[2]

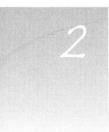

In "Persistent Toxic Chemicals in the US Food Supply" (Journal of Epidemiology and Community Health, 2002), K.S. Schafer, S.E. Kegley explain how "persistent organic pollutants (POPs) have spread throughout the global environment to threaten human health and damage ecosystems, with evidence of POPs contamination in wildlife, human blood, and breast milk documented worldwide" (http://jech.bmj.com/content/56/11/813.full).

Dr. Schoen and I are concerned that there has been virtually no research done on the potential harmful interactions of different chemicals that are now commonly found in human and pet foods. There have been very few studies done on the long-term detrimental effects of chronic exposure to many of these chemicals. This includes pesticide-based fly-drips and sprays used in barns, food containing genetically modified organisms (GMOs), and possible electromagnetic pollution and WiFi radiation, all of which we are exposed to but do not even see.

The presence of toxins in the environment can be overwhelming when you start looking around. Damaging, eco-disruptive products seem to be everywhere—from paints and glues with toxic compounds, to pesticides used around the barn and on horses, to contaminated groundwater, petroleum-based products, artificial supplements, and airborne particulates. It can be a daunting task to "clean up" the places our horses and we call home. However, living spaces for *all beings* may be created in such a way they are considered *sacred spaces*, as are our own bodies. When we view living species as part of a whole, interconnected system, it is possible to understand the importance of keeping them *balanced* for total well-being. Everything is connected to everything else.

Besides manmade chemicals that have been introduced to the environment, there are naturally occurring toxins that can make their way into horse feed.[3,4] This includes poisonous plants particular to your region. Some hazards are harder to identify, however, such as *mycotoxins* produced by mold. Mycotoxins can be present in feed or bedding, or in plants when the right conditions occur. Most horses instinctively avoid toxins when they are given a choice of good, clean food. It is difficult for them to avoid contaminated bedding though, and sometimes mold or weeds in the hay are palatable enough to horses for them to ingest enough to be problematic. Those responsible for feeding horses are best equipped to do so if they know to keep an eye out for mold and spoilage in hay and grain, as well as having knowledge of which plants and weeds are toxic in their area.

Christine Skelly, PhD, of Michigan State University writes on My Horse University that "Equine feedstuffs can be exposed to toxins during growth, harvest and storage. Plant disease, environmental conditions and insect infestation can all increase the likelihood of toxins being present in grains and hays" (http://www.myhorseuniversity.com/resources/eTips/November_2010/Didyouknow).

And in her May 2014 article, "The Danger of Mycotoxins," on TheHorse.com, Janice Holland, PhD, says: "Specific molds and fungi produce mycotoxins in soils, grains, and forages when environmental conditions are favorable. Once produced, they are generally very stable and will persist for a long time during storage. Horses that consume grains and forages contaminated by mycotoxins can suffer from a variety of health issues" (http://www.thehorse.com/articles/33898/the-danger-of-mycotoxins?utm_source=Newsletter&utm_medium=nutrition&utm_campaign=05-19-2014).

The ideal for both humans and horses is to follow a real-food, organic diet whenever possible. We are not synthetic beings, and neither are our horses. This alone is a good reason to look carefully at what we put in our bodies, and theirs, and what we surround ourselves with in terms of what we eat, drink, and breathe on a daily basis.

TREAT YOUR BODY WITH COMPASSION

As a successful, competitive athlete, I need *high-density nutrition* that helps me perform at my best and provides enough energy and anti-inflammatory qualities to do so. As author Matt Frazier espouses in his book *No Meat Athlete* (Fair Winds Press, 2013), whole, plant-based foods are a great source for the amount of calories and nutrients I need. I have also discovered through study, trial, and error, that holistic and alternative medicine works best to help *prevent* illness and keep me free of health complaints, even well into my fifties. This is not a replacement for professional nutrition or medical advice, but just a suggestion to be open-minded and receptive to possible ways you can treat *your body* with compassion, too.

Being a good steward of the equine environment includes the barns and arenas, plus the property itself and its relationship to the surrounding geographical area. Nutrient management strategies,[5] pasture and paddock rotation, recycling, energy efficiency, noxious plant control, and proper management of streams, wetlands, and throughways for wildlife are all areas of concern for a healthy environment.

5 *According to Ontario Ministry of Agriculture, Food and Rural Affairs environmental specialist P. Doris, in Canada, "Under the regulations of the Nutrient Management Act, 2002, farmers must have an approved nutrient management strategy (NMS) before applying for a building permit for facilities for housing horses or for manure storage on farms with greater than 5 nutrient units...The NMS sets out the environmentally acceptable methods for managing manure and runoff generated on the farm" (http://www.omafra.gov.on.ca/english/engineer/facts/10-057.htm).*

EXERCISE IN COMPASSION

Form a Nutrient Management Strategy for Your Barn

Whether you keep your horses at home or board them at a nearby facility, take the time to consider the following questions with your local environment in mind:

- How much manure is produced and stored on the property?

- Have you planned (or has barn management planned) appropriately for the siting of new barns and manure storage facilities in relation to sensitive features on your own and neighboring property, such as wells and surface water?

- How is runoff managed?

- Do you or does barn management have knowledge of the landbase that manure is applied to or other locations where it is stored?

- Do you or does barn management have a contingency plan for unforeseen circumstances or emergencies regarding waste disposal on your property?

When assessing your barn and property for toxicity, seek guidance from environmental and agricultural offices in your area in identifying plants and materials of concern, as well as making recommendations for removal and remediation as necessary.

If you are boarding at a barn and you do not feel proper management of the property is practiced, it's best for both you and your horse to move to a cleaner, safer location. When this is not possible, research how your horse's home could possibly be made safer, cleaner, and less toxic, and bring a list of reasonable steps to the barn's manager. Offer to help. Many equestrian operations tend to run at low to no profit, so issues of finances are often the first to be considered when changes are suggested. Even when those changes would lead to a much better environment for both horses and humans, the costs may seem prohibitive. Encourage small, affordable steps, as little changes can ultimately make a significant difference in the horse's well-being.

If you are on your own property with just your own horses, you can make a personal project out of determining what will help make your barn and property less toxic and more environmentally friendly. Put together a step-by-step plan, and, then start with the simplest thing. Do what you can under the circumstances and always remember you are benefiting all beings just by becoming conscious and aware of environmental concerns. Horses and equestrian facilities have a significant impact on their immediate and neighboring surroundings and it literally "takes a village" of like-minded participants to *become aware* of issues with the keeping, feeding, watering, and transportation of animals, and it takes that village once again to actually improve the state of things.

There are basic standards that are fundamental to cleanliness, and promoting good equine health and safety, for every barn. In some areas, these standards are even regulated, so far as weed,- dust,- and manure-control is concerned, although they may not necessarily be enforced. For the most part, it is up to attentive owners and managers to want to set the highest standards for their horses and maintain a facility that reflects these parameters. We have taken a formerly wild species and domesticated it, creating a manmade environment around *our* convenience. The most compassionate way to manage that environment is to make sure it is free of toxins, pollution, and danger since the horses cannot escape it of their own accord.

As feed prices, land, and construction costs rise, so does the cost of building or retrofitting structures for horses. Understandably, the realization that perhaps your facility is not the best possible environment for horses or people is going to cause some stress in itself. If you are already up to a very high level of "green thinking" and have incorporated sustainability in your equine operation, then kudos for the effort you've made in getting there. You are likely reaping the rewards of a peaceful and healthy home for your horse already, and we, as cohabitants of the planet, are better off as well.

Part of a healthy environment for horses is ensuring their safety and the safety of everyone who participates in equine activities. This means maintaining fencing, minimizing hazards, and implementing helmet and footwear rules, without exception. Here are some easy steps you can take to make your barn clean, safe, and nontoxic:

- Reduce consumption of non-renewable resources and provide recycling bins where applicable.

- Address nutrient, sediment, and pathogen discharges.

- Manage commercial fertilizer and animal manure input costs.

- Improve surface water quality and ensure horses have access to clean, fresh water at all times.

- Identify and remediate toxic plants and materials in and around the facility.

- Manage nitrogen, phosphorus, and potassium and consider all sources of such nutrients.

- Establish a rule that all persons under the age of 18 must wear helmets when mounted, and state that helmets are suggested for all adults when mounted. Riding *without* a helmet puts a rider at risk for a Traumatic Brain Injury (TBI), no matter what his or her age, experience, or preferred discipline! Even *one* TBI can dramatically alter a person's quality of life.

- Require closed footwear in and around the facility and closed footwear with a heel for all mounted riders.

- Review fencing on a regular basis to ensure it is safe and well managed. Barbed wire and large-hole web or wire fencing can cause serious injuries if horses get caught or tangled in it. These are not suitable for use with horses.

- Encourage continuing education regarding sustainable practices for all those using, working at, or visiting the barn.

THE ENVIRONMENTAL IMPACT
OF THE EQUINE INDUSTRY

The following are just a few ways horses and horsepeople impact the environment at large. These are factors that require thought in order to ensure the equine industry is not negatively affecting our world but rather contributing to it in the best way possible.

- Transportation of feed.

- Maintenance of buildings and facilities to house horses.

- Consumption of water.

- Management of manure and barn waste.

- Transportation of horses to shows, clinics, training facilities.

- Creation of waste related to products and services needed to maintain domestic horses.

- Runoff from pastures and paddocks.

- Overgrazing land both domestically and in the wild.

- Ovepopulation due to overbreeding and unwanted animals.

Elevating our standards of training and equine care to holistic, humane levels are equivalent to establishing *best practices* in a sustainable environment. When we respect all life, an eco-friendly environment will be evident in the day-to-day operations of our handling and training of horses. It doesn't start and end with grooming and tacking up, but can become a permanent lifestyle shift incorporating all our other activities in and out of the barn. A Compassionate Barn supports the wellness of *all* living beings within and around the facility. In the stable, cleanliness and order are strong indicators of the mindset of those who run things. Like so many other concepts we have talked about, this has a trickle-down effect from the horses to the health professionals who help care for them to the youngest horse enthusiast who visits.

What kind of barn would you like to walk into today?

We encourage equestrian facilities to adopt the principles of a less-toxic environment and apply sustainable, green technologies to their horsekeeping in as many ways as possible, to the best of their abilities. All creatures enjoy the benefits of holistic care in a more natural setting. Your barn may already meet these high standards, and this may simply be a cheerful confirmation of what a great job you are doing being compassionate toward your horse, other beings, and the world. Or, it may take some rethinking, re-evaluating, and perhaps even major changes in your barn to attain this estimable level of care. Some changes need not cost a thing, as they mean simply taking an honest look at your own heart and mind, perhaps adjusting your perspective and determining how you might be able to be even *more* compassionate. The most important thing about embodying a peaceful nature and having respect for all life is to *just start doing it* with a nonjudgmental, happy, positive, creative attitude.

Dr. Allen Schoen:

I often joke with my clients about what I call "Mindful Mucking Therapy," and I am always impressed with how many people comment that they actually love the time they spend mucking their horses' stalls. They truly find it quite meditative and internally quieting. They find that it helps empty their mind of their endless "to-do" list. They love the smells of the horse barn, the quietness, and it allows them a time to truly be in the moment focused only on the cleaning process. I often see barn staff quietly attentive to their mucking, a gentle smile on their faces. Others actually "whistle while they work" or sing happy tunes while listening to cheerful music.

Yet, there are others who have a grumpy look, muck quickly and impatiently, are not focused on their task, and are not respectful of the horse when he is still in the stall. These are the contrasts in our facilities now. We have an opportunity to shift our view of the task and possibly that of others.

At boarding, training, and large professional facilities, grooms and barn staff are key players with an integral role in the creation of a safe and healthy environment for our horses.

One trainer lamented to me one day how she wished she could find more compassionate grooms and barn staff. I connected her with another barn, whose management had told me they were blessed with a group of happy, peaceful, competent grooms and staff who referred others of the same ilk to their barn because everyone was so happy there. I also asked her to make up a list of what she would like to see exemplified in Compassionate Grooming. She included being sensitive to the horse; learning how hard or softly to brush them, which ones liked a softer or firmer touch; being aware of skin issues or behavioral changes and reporting them; and being aware of any potential issues in the barn in terms of both the physical plant maintenance and staff and boarder morale and relations. Her list included a wish that grooms would share what *they thought* could be improved to make the barn a happier place for horses and humans.

I have seen and encourage owners, trainers, and riders to continuously thank their grooms and staff, and acknowledge them for taking good, loving care of their horses and their horses' environment. "Honey attracts bees," as they say. Every being appreciates being acknowledged for conscientious or hard work. When they are, they are happier and do an even better job, repeating the acts for which they were acknowledged in the future.

When assessing the horse's environment we want to look at everything *he is in contact with.*

When a barn is having an excessive rate of respiratory issues, for example, we want to evaluate the entire environment to determine the causes. This means looking at the food quality, the amount of time the horses are in and out, ventilation and air quality in the barn, and possible toxins in and around the products and materials used in the horse's care.

My personal preference is to be as "natural" as possible, including stall bedding, which can vary in type and quality according to region and availability, but today sourcing "natural" products is very much about "buyer beware" and trying as best as possible to do our due diligence when making selections.

For example, pyrethrin, a "natural" organic compound, could be in your "natural" anti-insect repellant. "Natural" though it may be, as a chemical it can be enhanced with various oil-based carriers that may possibly be toxic in the long-term to the horse. Such chemicals may precipitate allergic responses and respiratory issues. Toxic aerosols in barns may be precursors to Chronic Obstructive Pulmonary Disease (COPD). Simply stated, COPD is an allergic

GET HELP WITH ENVIRONMENTAL MANAGEMENT—AROUND THE WORLD

Globally, the equestrian industry is beginning to place more emphasis on protecting and preserving the environment, incorporating new initiatives for sustainability at all levels:

- Canada's University of Guelph in Ontario, for example, offers an excellent online program, which includes stewardship initiatives through outreach education and increasing the network of financial and technical assistance programs available to the equestrian community (www.equinestudiesonline.ca).

- In the United States, the Audubon Lifestyles Program has a detailed section for equestrian facilities (http://www.thesustainabilitycouncil.org/audubon-life-styles.html). A considerable amount of information and a certification program is provided to help barns meet the goals of a healthy, sustainable environment. The program works for both existing and planned facilities. What I love about this program is that it not only sets high standards for reducing the overall "footprint" of a facility, such as minimizing waste, but it also highlights the importance of equestrian safety as part of creating a healthy environment.

- The German Equestrian Federation (FN) has supported a new project aimed at preserving and promoting biological diversity within the equine environment (http://www.pferd-aktuell.de/biologischevielfalt).

- The British Equestrian Federation (BEF) has developed a facilities and sustainability strategy to improve the quality and quantity of facilities in the United Kingdom to assist in meeting the development and competition needs of the sport at all levels (www.bef.co.uk).

- The Fédération Equestre Internationale (FEI) has also introduced a "sustainability handbook" full of initiatives that are designed to help event organizers protect the environment at equestrian events (www.fei.org).

bronchitis—a reaction to products in the environment, such as moldy hay or chemicals that have not been documented to be hazardous. I have actually found I have to leave a barn occasionally if some fly spray systems come on while I am there, as I can develop acute respiratory signs such as congestion and coughing when the spray is dispensed.

I still feel bad for horses subjected to the chemical fly spray systems because I wonder what kind of reaction some of them may be having due to chronic exposure. I have seen some horses move away from the sprays and stick their heads outside their stall windows to avoid the spray while it is turned on.

A healthy environment also includes the visual environment.

I've seen horses that are only in indoor arenas or their stalls, just going around and around or standing idle, all winter long. In climates with cold or snowy winters this is a common scenario. Quite a few horses that have been indoors all winter and seem "bored" enjoy a natural, varied, visual experience beyond their controlled indoor environment. I find these horses seem to be frustrated in these very limiting, enclosed spaces for extended periods of time with little or no exposure to the outdoors or views of interest.

EXERCISE IN COMPASSION

Dream Barn

Imagine a barn that feels:

- Calming
- Friendly
- Quiet
- Happy
- Clean
- Welcoming
- Beautiful
- Inspiring

Now think of five other adjectives you'd like to be able to use to describe *your* barn. These adjectives can help you find ways to set achievable goals in making your barn all you'd like it to be for those who enter.

Engage In "Mindful Mucking Therapy"

Stall cleaning—a thankless job. Or is it? As the Buddhists say (and we extrapolate to the horse world): "Before enlightenment, muck stalls, carry water. After enlightenment, muck stalls, carry water."

The key point is, *who* is doing the mucking? Metaphorically, this can be applied to other aspects of our lives. Are you opposed to the task of lifting those heavy manure piles and wet spots into the wheelbarrow? Does the prospect of scrubbing water and feed buckets make you procrastinate and find something to distract yourself from the necessary task?

If you feel natural resistance toward mucking, or any daily chore, whether related to the barn or not, *Mindful Mucking* is an opportunity to change your struggle against a potentially negative task and turn it into a positive one. Notice what "buttons" are pushed within as the chore of stall-cleaning arises each day. Can you detach yourself from the resistance you feel and turn your "conditioned belief" that you dislike, abhor, or are "too good for" mucking into a positive, more accepting attitude?

- *Gratitude.* Think about the value of a clean stall and the gratitude of those for whom the stall was cleaned. Consider the fact that a clean stall is imperative to preventing certain health problems in horses. In fact, stall mucking is a very important part of maintaining the overall good health and wellness of horses.

- *Quiet and calm.* Mucking stalls can become an exercise in meditation and mindfulness. You, or whoever cleans the stall for your horse, will be in a good frame of mind if you first practice our suggested 10 minutes of quiet contemplation (QFI—see p. 8) and release of any negative emotions. Whether the horse is in the stall or not, entering the stall while stressed or angry can leave an "energy imprint" that will affect the whole atmosphere in the barn, not to mention the horse.

- *Emptiness.* It is ideal when your horse can be out of his stall when the cleaning takes place, but this is not always possible. If he is turned out while mucking, you literally have more "space" to work, both mentally and physically. Treat the horse with care if you have to move him from one spot to another while picking out manure and wet spots. Yelling at the horse, elbowing him, or hitting him with a fork is unacceptable and can eventually lead to him being frightened by quick movements, and aggressive when he feels trapped in a small space.

- *Equanimity.* If you are the owner, trainer, or rider of a horse and someone else is doing the stall mucking for you, thank the individual for his or her mindfulness in regards to the horse and attention to the healthy environment he or she is helping create.

- *Breathe!* When you are cleaning stalls, be kind to yourself in the process. It is physically demanding, as is most work around the barn, so keep your breathing from becoming shallow as your heart rate increases, and be mindful of your own body's needs.

- *Clearing and centering.* Organize your equipment and find a rhythm in your routine. Think of "Soiled bedding out, fresh bedding in," as a mantra. All negative thoughts and feelings go out with the manure; all new, positive thoughts replace them with the fresh bedding. You are creating a safe, healthy place for your horse, and a safe, healthy place for yourself.

Leave the stall with a smile and lightness in your heart, content with the good care and fresh, sweet-smelling environment you've provided your horse. This is a compassionate job well done by *you*!

Listen, look, smell, *really use* all your senses to evaluate the barn environment from both your perspective and your horse's. *Sound* is also part of a holistic, healthy environment, which we already discussed in chapter 8 (p. 149). By being mindful and aware of the products you purchase and use on your horses and in your barns, you lessen their chances, and your own, of having allergic or adverse reactions to toxins. If the environment is also peaceful and the energy is conducive to compassionate interactions, everyone will be able to focus more clearly on the horses' needs and on each other's. This is, in itself, conscientious, preventive health care. We are here to minimize suffering for all beings in the barn in the most holistic way possible.

I once was evaluating a horse's environment because he was developing an allergic bronchitis. I considered his history, looking for any possible environmental triggers: bad hay, mold, pesticides, sprays, and so on. Some possible causes were evident, including an overhead fly-spray system. I went into the horse's stall and breathed in, first standing up and then kneeling down. There was a noticeable difference lower to the ground in terms of lack of airflow. After adjusting the horse's environment to improve ventilation and remove the possible trigger, the horse improved significantly and was able to stop using previously prescribed medications altogether.

A healthy environment is directly related to being a Compassionate Human and a Compassionate Equestrian.

Essentially, a healthy environment is a compassionate one because we are preventing disease in both horse and human by limiting exposure to toxins. More and more toxins are being "put in the fine print" on products, and as mentioned, we also have to inspect the labels of "natural" products for hidden chemicals. The goal here is what you *don't* get—meaning, when you control the products and environment in the barn you and your horse *won't* get the contact and respiratory allergies, gastrointestinal issues, and various dermatological problems that are common reactions to toxins.

Strong precaution holds that regulation is required whenever there is a possible risk to health, safety, or the environment, even when the supporting evidence is speculative and even if the economic costs of regulation are high.

Part of *The Compassionate Equestrian* model is to recognize the *Precautionary Principle* in application to our equine environments.[6,7] The Precautionary Principle suggests that science can reliably assess and quantify potential risks to the natural environment and that measures can be taken in advance to protect both the environment and humans from *human-caused damage*.

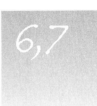

The Canadian Environmental Law Association states that "The precautionary principle denotes a duty to prevent harm, when it is within our power to do so, even when all the evidence is not in. This principle has been codified in several international treaties" (http://www.cela.ca/collections/pollution/precautionary-principle).

And in the 2005 document The Precautionary Principle from the World Commission on the Ethics of Scientific Knowledge and Technology (COMEST) and the United Nations Educational, Scientific and Cultural Organization (UNESCO) it says: "The Precautionary Principle is often seen as an integral principle of sustainable development, that is development that meets the needs of the present without compromising the abilities of future generations to meet their needs. By safeguarding against serious and, particularly, irreversible harm to the natural resource base that might jeopardize the capacity of future generations to provide for their own needs, it builds on ethical notions on intra- and inter-generational equity" (http://unesdoc.unesco.org/images/0013/001395/139578e.pdf).

EXERCISE IN COMPASSION

Assess Your Horse's Environment

- What's in his bedding?

- What are the stalls painted or stained with?

- Is the air laden with dust, fly sprays, and drips?

- What is the ventilation like?

- Which potentially harmful chemicals are in the products used in your barn? Read the labels!

- What qualifies as "natural"? Consider carefully such claims on all products, supplements, and feedstuffs.

- There may be hidden chemicals in *your* products, too. What's on *your* skin when you reach out and touch your horse? Read more labels!

The Environmental Sense Scan

In this exercise, strive to consciously sense every aspect of your horse's surroundings and identify any possible environmental exposures that can be harmful. Is there anything you:

- *Smell* that is potentially noxious or irritating?

- *Hear* that is disruptive to your peace and that of your horse?

- *See* that may be dangerous to you or your horse? Or do you see very little in terms of variety and interest, which can also be harmful?

- If you were your horse, how would your food and water *taste?* Fresh and clean? Stale? Metallic?

- *Touch* the shavings, the edges of the stall doors, the footing in the arena.

- *Sixth sense:* Is there a "feeling" or "energy" or "aura" that is cause for concern? Electromagnetic pollution? Possible carcinogens? A general sense of unhappiness and ill health in the barn?

Applying the Precautionary Principle to the equine industry means we decide, in advance, what the implications are for the future of horses that may be exposed to the products that are still in development and may not be properly researched or regulated. This requires examining the *risks versus benefits* of product use, and the many other considerations involved with our ethical responsibility to the environment. If there is an opportunity to prevent irreversible damage to the world at large and avoid dangers to our own health and that of our horses, then that is the most compassionate choice for all of us.

As says Sakyong Mipham Rinpoche, head of Shambhala International (Shambhala.org), "At this crossroads for our planet, how humanity views itself at some deep level is going to make or break the situation."

Questions to Consider
BASED ON PRINCIPLE 14

1   Am I committed to undertaking the task of removing toxic substances from my barn?

2   Do my horses receive adequate stimulation from a natural, varied environment?

3   Am I able to make the connection between a barn that is kept to a high environmental standard and the emotional and physical well-being of its occupants and visitors?

CHAPTER FIFTEEN

Integrating Conventional and Complementary Approaches to Health

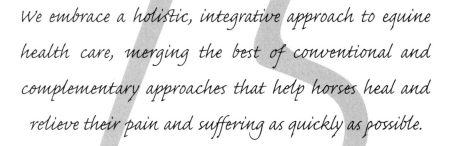

We embrace a holistic, integrative approach to equine health care, merging the best of conventional and complementary approaches that help horses heal and relieve their pain and suffering as quickly as possible.

Susan Gordon:

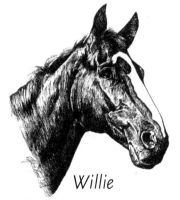

Willie

Willie was given all of the normally recommended vaccinations and standard veterinary care to keep him as sound as possible. The facility I moved Willie to "post-backyard" used a veterinarian who was a certified acupuncturist as well as a conventional DVM. While I did not request acupuncture treatments for Willie, she was still always helpful in explaining how the acupoints related to the conditions he was being treated for—for example, in one case it was the anemia, and in another situation I discovered he was very allergic to red ant bites (he broke out in hives during a ride, and his respiratory system almost shut down).

"It matters not whether theories are Eastern or Western, so long as they prove to be true."

Dr. Jen-Hsou Lin

Even in the 1990s, holistic veterinary medicine was still just emerging, and it was fascinating to me, as an enthusiast of alternative medicine for humans, to see how it could work for horses, too. Willie had already experienced a "tapping" technique I had been using for a decade or so at the time, which involves an approach derived from Shiatsu massage—three fingers "tap" the acupoints in a rhythmic, steady pressure. I benefited from the experience of another trainer who had also been treating her horses with this kind of "tapping massage"—which is very similar to the popular method for humans known as Emotional Freedom Techniques (EFT)— and found her horses seemed to enjoy it immensely. She taught me how to apply the technique to my own horses.

Because I was not "trained" in acupressure, and also due in part to the general attitudes toward alternative and natural medicine, I pretty much kept the technique to myself. I quietly used my tapping technique on all the horses I rode, even while mounted, to help relax and relieve any tension in their upper body. The method usually worked, sometimes in very beneficial ways.

Willie loved to be tapped, like all the other horses I had worked on before him. It relaxed him and always produced the breathing and head-lowering effects I was *looking for, both from the ground and the saddle. The contented expression and bodily responses I got from Willie when I used a three-finger tap on his poll, neck, and back were enough of a positive response to make me continue the practice.*

Willie was also the beneficiary of my training with the continuing education program of The College of Syntonic Optometry in Boston, Massachusetts (collegeofsyntonicoptometry.com). Syntonics, or optometric phototherapy, is the branch of ocular science dealing with the application of selected light frequencies through the eyes. I had read the book, Light: Medicine of the Future *by Dr. Jacob Liberman (Bear & Company, 1990), and became enamored with the study and application of colored light and its health benefits for humans. Around that time, several companies were making devices that used monochromatic red light in the visible and near-infrared range, and there were some that were made especially for use on horses. In what is called photonic therapy, the light frequencies are applied directly to the acupoints on the body (not through the eyes as with syntonics) via cluster-heads or a pad containing light emitting diodes (LEDs).*

I made a series of appointments for Willie with a practitioner trained in the application of the photonic therapy, as he had become quite body-sore when his school horse duties increased over time. The results were very satisfying, as his pain and stiffness appeared to decrease immensely, his energy returned, and his range-of-motion (ROM) increased exponentially. (Note: For current more advanced technology recommended by Dr. Schoen, consider low-level laser therapy such as Multi Radiance Veterinary Laser Therapy (www.multiradiance.com/Compassionate).

I could have had more extensive workups and multiple X-rays done on the big guy, but most of the information in regards to his condition would have come as no surprise, and I was on a limited budget. I made the presumption that the very obvious lumps, bumps, and stiff joints were indicative of what was going on below the surface. The old scar tissue from past accidents could not be helped much with conventional medicine, so noninvasive approaches—like my tapping and photonic therapy—were a reasonable alternative to consider, and seemed to help in very positive ways. To keep an old horse comfortable, my thought was always, "Why not try gentle, natural, inexpensive methods that may help relieve his pain and mobility issues?"

I was introduced to holistic medicine for humans shortly after I began working with horses full time around 1981. I began to increase my own use of natural remedies for maintaining good health, based on the advice of professional practitioners, and found them to be very effective. In the 1970s, when I first started riding, conventional veterinary medicine was the primary method by which most horses were cared for. Veterinarians usually did not suggest anything that approached herbal remedies or holistic, natural treatments, as those modalities were not being taught in standard veterinary medicine at the time. The old standby methods we used in the barn for treating injuries *were* simple and natural, however: cold-hosing, ice packs, leg wraps, mud poultices, and the occasional application of a well-known veterinary liniment made of oils and herbs. Medications such as phenylbutazone ("bute") were sparingly given for pain relief. At the time, there just weren't veterinary acupuncturists, chiropractors, or equine massage therapists to help with a horse's healing process. Holistic veterinary medicine was still a very young field, and not generally available to horse owners.

In the decades past, as participation in equestrian sports increased, whenever complex lameness arose the normal diagnostic protocol was based on observations of movement, nerve blocks, X-rays, and clinical experience. Modern advanced diagnostic imaging—such as digital X-rays, ultrasound, MRI, and nuclear scintigraphy—were not available until more recently. Over the years I had several horses with "mystery lamenesses" and spinal deformities that conventional medicine could not resolve at the time. The show jumpers and off-the-track Thoroughbreds, in particular, were subject to many injuries given the intensity of training, showing or other post-racing careers.

As any high-performance athlete is aware, increasing
endurance and speed also increases the odds of injury, and
sometimes tracing back to the source of injury can be difficult.

I have observed the rising popularity of various methods of alternative practices that seem to be producing some promising and beneficial results. Of course, sports medicine and new technologies have also advanced considerably in the past few decades. They now offer many new options for diagnosing and treating lameness. Still, I find the effectiveness of simple, noninvasive techniques convincing and the evolution of integrative approaches both fascinating and worth exploring.

Ideally, the goal of holistic medicine is to find the root cause of a particular condition through the history, physical examination, observation, and diagnostic tests. It is not uncommon that the cause may be multifactorial. Once a proper diagnosis has been made, then one can look at which approach or combination of approaches is most appropriate to help the horse heal as quickly and as well as possible.

Practitioners of holistic veterinary medicine are graduates of an accredited veterinary college or university.

Nowadays there are various schools for pursuing the alternative methods that were only just emerging in 1980s and 90s. In addition, there are post-graduate integrative veterinary training courses for certifying licensed DVMs all over the world. I am extremely grateful to pioneers such as Dr. Schoen, for developing unique, effective, holistic, complementary approaches from modalities that were previously made available exclusively to human medical practitioners. He helped pave the way for integrative options when considering the evaluation and treatment for sick and injured horses.

Experience and observation changed me from a "believer" in holistic medicine to knowing without a doubt that it has its place in the evaluation and treatment of pain and disease. In appropriate cases, when applied correctly and professionally and in conjunction with conventional practice as necessary, the results can be impressive. We owe it to our horses as Compassionate Equestrians to investigate and consider holistic, complementary approaches to their care and well-being. Such approaches may not only relieve their discomfort but perhaps aid in a much faster healing process.

Dr. Allen Schoen:

No one form of medicine has all the answers or cures all problems.

The vision of holistic, integrative animal health care is to take the best of natural approaches and combine them with the best of conventional veterinary medicine. Each therapy has its indications and its limitations. It just seems prudent to take what works in all fields and integrate them into a comprehensive form of animal health care.

What this means in practice and to horse owners or caregivers is that we do everything as naturally and health-consciously as possible to *prevent* disease and injury in the first place. If this is not enough and a horse becomes ill or hurt, then we look at all the best approaches to both diagnose and treat the problem. This may include conventional medical examinations, blood tests, and X-rays, to name just a few common diagnostic practices. In addition, a holistically-oriented veterinarian may look at other possible causes of disease and injury such as environmental conditions, nutritional deficiencies, saddle fit, shoeing, rider issues, training methods, dental problems, traumatic incident, and more. Treatment might consist of conventional medications *as well as* holistic approaches to help the animal heal more quickly. While practicing, teaching, and writing about this field, I have come to appreciate that there is a balance between exploring the benefits of natural health care and acknowledging the benefits of conventional Western medicine.

I have been pleased to see that the concepts of holistic, integrative care that I have been sharing for the last 30 years are being incorporated into equine practices in many unique ways.

There are veterinarians who limit their practice to just integrative approaches—such as acupuncture, chiropractic care, nutrition, and herbal medicine—and there are other practitioners who have integrated all of these into their conventional, all-around veterinary approach. By integrating holistic methods into a complete equine practice, practitioners are able to add, say, acupuncture, as an adjunct to their conventional treatment, as well as in different emergency situations. In addition, they may be aware that in addition to conventional lameness evaluation and treatments, complementary therapies may help with a more comprehensive approach to lameness by treating secondary compensatory problems. I have also seen some veterinarians take basic training in complementary therapies simply so they could be aware of their indications and then refer their clients to those veterinarians who have chosen to specialize. Since "practice makes perfect," this way, they can focus on the areas of medicine they are best trained for, while allowing that other practitioners can support the horse's health in additional ways. This, too, is the advantage of the veterinarian who specializes in complementary therapies—he or she develops a more focused technique, which sometimes a general practitioner may not have time for.

When I began pioneering this specialized approach over 30 years ago, I chose to focus on it because very few veterinarians were, and I wanted to see how far it could be developed and advanced. I am grateful that over three decades, I have worked with most of the veterinarians in my practice area in a respectful and appreciative manner, and after they have seen the benefits of acupuncture and chiropractic care, many of them have either gone for training or are simply open to suggesting them as therapies to their clients.

GUIDELINES WHEN CONSIDERING COMPLEMENTARY THERAPIES

1   It is important to begin with an appropriate diagnosis or differential diagnosis (a way of distinguishing a condition or disease from those that present similar symptoms) from a licensed veterinarian.

2   Discuss the therapeutic options with your veterinarian and/or a veterinarian trained in complementary therapies.

3   If considering approaches that are allowed to be administered by individuals without veterinary training, make sure the complementary treatments do not delay or interfere with appropriate veterinary care and attention.

4   When a non-veterinarian recommends an approach and says not to listen to your licensed veterinarian, consider that a "red flag." Therapies should be complementary, *not* adversarial.

5   Beware of conflicts of interest when someone is marketing his or her products or methods as the *only* ones that can help.

6   Be aware that non-veterinarians are not legally permitted to diagnose diseases or conditions. Check if a lay practitioner is allowed to do what they are claiming to do and if they have the appropriate training.

7   Know which therapies you can be trained to administer to your own horse and which therapies should be only applied by veterinary or other certified professionals.

8   Develop an integrative program in conjunction with your veterinarian if he or she is open to such options, or with a veterinarian who is knowledgeable in both conventional and complementary approaches and works with others who have the appropriate training in complementary therapies.

As I've said, there is an advantage to having someone who does *just* the complementary therapies because that is his or her particular, unique area of expertise. In general, I think it is best when your conventional veterinarian is open to an integrative approach. In this way, he or she can work together with someone who specializes, like me, to offer both conventional and complementary therapies to help your horse heal. For instance, it is not uncommon for the conventional veterinarians in my area to have their clients ask me to evaluate their horses from an acupuncture and chiropractic/musculoskeletal alignment perspective, *in addition* to their own work on localizing a primary lower leg lameness.

This is a pretty common example. In a primary lameness, the *reductionist approach* (gaining an understanding of the nature of the lameness by *reducing* it to more fundamental aspects or to one specific anatomical location) of isolating that lameness is crucial. What has been lacking in equine medicine for so long is a commitment to addressing all the secondary, compensatory responses for primary lameness. On numerous occasions, an owner or rider has told me that a horse's hock or ankle had been injected because issues were found there based on a lameness evaluation and radiographic images, but the horse was *still* "not right." It is not uncommon in these scenarios that once you take care of all the *secondary compensatory problems*, the horse then improves.

The benefit of integrative, complementary approaches is that they may be able to resolve the secondary, compensatory issues, allowing the horse to improve overall. You are also often able to pick up subtle soft-tissue issues before the horse actually goes lame, and by treating them, you prevent lameness.

Many of my clients will actually have me see their horses *before* they go to their regular veterinarian because of the ability to pick up subtle issues. When a client feels the horse is not lame, but "not quite right," what we will often find are issues such as improper saddle fit, or the shoeing angle is off, or there is an asymmetry in the musculoskeletal system that is not creating actual joint or tendon lameness but the horse is not performing as well as he could be.

So as you can see, there is validity and good reasons for both approaches: for taking a conventional approach first or for seeking the complementary, integrative approach initially. When the horse is not obviously lame, it is not unreasonable to go with an integrative approach first. If your horse is distinctly lame, you definitely want to go the conventional route to isolate and treat the lameness, and *then* have someone rebalance the horse through the various complementary therapies. It is also not unreasonable to have your primary care veterinarian evaluate your horse first anyway to make sure he or she is not seeing any other issues from his or her perspective.

LEARN MORE

If you would like to read more about complementary and alternative approaches to veterinary medicine and animal health care, Dr. Susan Wynn and I co-edited the classic textbook *Complementary and Alternative Veterinary Medicine* (Mosby, 1998). The book reviewed all the scientific evidence available at the time, as well as the practical applications of the various complementary therapies, including:

- Nutrition-based complementary therapies
- Physical medicine approaches, such as acupuncture, chiropractic and osteopathic care, physical therapy, and various massage approaches
- Energetic medicine, including low-level laser therapy, low-level photon therapy, and magnetic field therapy
- Botanical medicine such as Western herbal medicine, Traditional Chinese Herbal Medicine, and Ayurvedic (Indian) herbal medicine
- Homeopathy
- Miscellaneous therapies such as environmental medicine, aromatherapy, and Bach Flower remedies

There is also a section on how to integrate these approaches into conventional equine veterinary practices, as well as discussions of veterinary bioethics, the human-animal bond, vaccine-related issues, and ethnoveterinary medicine.

Did the horse create a biomechanical problem in the person or did the person create the problem in the horse?

It so often comes to the big question of, "Which comes first, the chicken or the egg?" That is part of the diagnostic challenge and puzzle when working with horses and their riders. In some cases, a client's biomechanical challenges and asymmetry clearly creates similar issues in the horse. In other cases, a chronic lameness in the horse can cause him to be asymmetrical and compensating, which leads to lower back and sacroiliac issues in the horse, which in turn causes problems in the rider.

This last hypothetical begs the question (a common point of discussion): "Which comes first, lower leg lameness or back issues?" Again, I have seen it go both ways. Some are primary lower leg issues with secondary compensation in the back and sacroiliac region as I just described, and others are primarily back issues that can cause the horse to favor a particular leg, which leads toward lower leg lameness.

These are all diagnostic challenges: evaluating what part of the issue is caused by the rider, what part by the horse, what part is lower leg lameness, what part is the back, what component is due to saddle fit, shoeing, training, or riding. *That* is why we need to look at the *whole* picture when it comes to Ultimate Healing.

Compassion is not about labels.

I never say it is one or the other when it comes to what is best for the horse. That is why I call my approach "integrative." I also try not to get attached to labels because what I have found occasionally, and unfortunately, is that there are veterinarians and owners, riders, and trainers who are adversarial, antagonistic, or dismissive toward anything titled "alternative" or "complementary." If we *let go of the labels* and just ask our favorite question, "What is best for the horse?" then we can embrace all of these modalities, which ultimately leads to a better outcome. And *that* is why we are here.

The adversarial aspect became apparent to me earlier in my career when I started getting more involved with chiropractic study, and I lectured a number of times in a certification course. I could see the schism: some chiropractors worked with veterinarians and vice versa, but there was also often a lack of open-mindedness on both sides, as well as competitiveness. The more I looked at these relationships, and at chiropractic with my background and master's degree in neurophysiology (which has always been the foundation for my whole approach), I began to question the wisdom of applying some of the "human" chiropractic terminology to veterinary medicine.

What can at times make veterinary and human medicine and chiropractic adversarial are some of the terms, such as "subluxation."

In human medicine *subluxation* is diagnosed based upon an X-ray as an actual anatomic issue that can be measured. Human chiropractors view it also as a functional and dynamic issue—a movement in and out of alignment. They then sometimes speak loosely about "putting things back into place." But skeptical equine veterinarians would say, "There's *no way* you can move an equine bone with your hands on big horses." When lecturing on the subject, I try to clarify this misunderstanding by explaining that you are not actually "moving bones" per se, but actually releasing trigger points, knots, and spasms in various ligamentous, tendinous, and muscular attachments *between* bones, and thereby the tensions on the vertebrae are released, and there is a realignment of structures back to a more normal symmetry.

I realized that part of the skepticism was based on miscommunication and misunderstanding due to the actual terminology and labeling. I do not think using human chiropractic terms in veterinary medicine is appropriate or works well. My preference is to use terminology that I feel is more appropriate for what I see, such as "misalignment" and "fixations." On my medical forms, you don't see the word "chiropractic," rather, "musculoskeletal alignment." My practice title reads "Veterinary Acupuncture and Complementary Therapies," and I have been exploring different terminology to help ease our industry's difficulty with other labels, as well.

At this time, I presently prefer using the term Veterinary Physiatry© *for the approach that I have developed, integrating scientific acupuncture with various approaches to musculoskeletal alignment, including chiropractic care, osteopathy, trigger-point therapy, acupuncture, and physiatry.*

There is a field in human medicine called *physiatry*, but very few people have ever heard of it, and very few doctors refer to themselves as physiatrists or physiatric medicine practitioners. Wikipedia defines physiatry as "physical medicine and rehabilitation (PM&R), or rehabilitation medicine—a branch of medicine that aims to enhance and restore functional ability and quality of life to those with physical impairments or disabilities, specifically with injuries to the muscles, bones, tissues, and nervous system." And there is now a field of veterinary medicine called *Physical Rehabilitation Medicine*, which incorporates various physical therapy modalities.[1]

> *The International Association for Veterinary Rehabilitation and Physical Therapy (IAVRPT) is dedicated to the practice, teaching, and research of veterinary rehabilitation and physical therapy, furthering scientific investigation, and providing better patient care based on sound scientific study (www.iavrpt.org).*

Over the years I realized there is a place for all approaches. My broader goal was to get acupuncture and complementary medicine accepted and integrated into the conventional veterinary establishment. I realized that for these approaches to gain acceptance I needed to teach and practice it based on neurophysiology wherever possible. By doing so holistic, integrative animal care was indeed accepted more broadly and was eventually integrated into veterinary conferences, continuing education programs, and many veterinary schools throughout the world. I eventually became an assistant clinical professor, teaching these approaches at Colorado State University College of Veterinary Medicine and Tufts University School of Veterinary Medicine in Massachusetts, as well as part of an elective program at Cornell University in New York State.

The challenge is—as with "natural" products—"buyer beware."

There are so many more resources readily available to horse owners now, through both growing awareness and online outreach. While this means there are many more ways we can be of benefit to horses, there are also *many* questionable therapies offered by less-than-scrupulous individuals, and these can potentially prevent your horse from getting the care he needs as soon as possible, possibly causing more harm than good.

In addition, while, as we mentioned earlier, complementary medicine does sometimes open the door so that a layperson can study and apply a therapy to his or her own horse, the key is understanding when this is acceptable, and when it should be handled by a veterinarian trained and licensed or certified in that area. You must check your state or country's regulating bodies to know what is allowed. For instance, veterinary acupuncture should only be practiced by a veterinarian trained in that modality, although a limited number of states in the United States allow a human acupuncturist to practice on animals *in conjunction with* a veterinarian. This applies to veterinary chiropractic care, as well. Laser therapy, on the other hand, can be used by veterinarians, as well as appropriately trained technicians and assistants. This is also the case for magnetic therapies, pulsed electromagnetic field therapy, red-light therapy, and other energetic modalities. Equine massage, "tapping," and many other alternative therapies can be practiced by individuals who have received appropriate training, whether they have veterinary experience or not. In these scenarios, a basic understanding of equine anatomy and biomechanics is to be recommended.

There is a broad spectrum of viewpoints related to complementary approaches, with advocates and skeptics and cynics at each end of the spectrum. There are still some disbelieving veterinarians who require a double-blind, placebo-controlled study before they will consider an alternative therapy. There are some questionable individuals selling a particular approach with only a few testimonials to back it. And there are also some very gifted healers out there as well, who may defy our current knowledge base. The Compassionate Equestrian needs to be open-minded, yet also ready to use his or her own discernment and wisdom when it comes to the well-being of his or her horse.

Rest is an essential component to healing.

It is amazing how we never give enough credit to *rest* and the healing power of time. In this day and age, the last thing anyone wants to hear about their horse is, "Give him some time off." Yet how many horses do you see that, given a year "sabbatical," will come back and everything will be healed? Of course, this depends on the injury, but there are so many little things that will heal when the horse is just given *time off*.

I do not see many polo ponies in my practice, but I spoke with one veterinarian who said that this is an area of care where polo players and trainers are often compassionate: when a horse is injured, they just turn him out for a year. They have so many ponies on a string, they can give a horse the time he needs to heal, and it is *amazing* how much of a difference time makes. In an ideal world, *time off* is very healing for both horses *and* for us. But today it seems there is no space for rest for anyone. And when you ask yourself, "Who is making me do all this stuff?" Well, it is *you*.

This is where *The Compassionate Equestrian* asks some deeper questions. Whether it is politics, business, environmental action, or veterinary research, oftentimes it is simply and sadly said, "Follow the money." When it comes to human-horse interactions, perhaps we can change the aphorism to, "Follow the mind." Perhaps we can even go one step further to, "Follow the heart." Maybe then, we can get in touch with our feelings, thoughts, and emotions, and come from a more compassionate place within when making choices for our horses and for ourselves.

When consciousness focuses it can excel, and it is actually an important survival mechanism.

The best hunters in prehistoric times were the ones who studied their prey, understood how the animals communicated, and were able to focus when the moment was right and hit their mark. The challenge with that focus is that sometimes, when you get *too* focused, you do not see the forest for the trees. With the neuroplasticity of the brain, the real "dance" is between excelling at whatever you focus on, but then having enough awareness and consciousness to look at the bigger picture and see how it is all integrated together.

What it comes down to is that every horse needs a *team* of compassionate, aware, specialized people committed to his well-being for his optimal health and performance. There are many conventional and complementary approaches to help horses. We can all benefit by balancing an open mind with knowledge and discernment when exploring various therapeutic options. We need to respect one another's abilities, talents, and areas of focus, and work together for the best outcome for our horses.

EXERCISE IN COMPASSION

Identify Your Filters

When the human brain focuses on a particular viewpoint—and as we've discussed, we *wire what we fire* in the brain—we tend to see lameness from our own perspectives. I own that for myself, too.

There is the old cliché when you are looking at a house, "If you are a carpenter, everything you see is a nail," or "If you are a plumber, everything you see is a pipe." Well, when it comes to evaluating a horse for a possible issue, if you are a lameness/lower leg veterinarian, you likely look at those factors. If you are a trainer, you analyze his training program. If you are a saddle-fit specialist, examine his back and his tack.

Ask yourself: Which filters color *your* vision when evaluating your horse? Do you focus on what you know best to the exclusion of other possible answers?

This is part of the mind-body medicine approach...consciousness has a natural tendency to focus. We should note here that there is a great benefit to filters and focus, too. If I am having brain surgery, for example, I would want the consciousness and focus of the best brain surgeon available!

Questions to Consider
BASED ON PRINCIPLE 15

1   Do I have a good, comprehensive, cooperative team of properly trained practitioners to offer the best diagnostic and therapeutic approaches for my horse? If not, how can I improve my team approach?

2   Do I have an open-minded, yet wise and discerning approach, and people I can turn to for advice?

3   Are there any areas of conventional or complementary medicine that I would like to learn more about?

Optimal Foods and Supplements

16

We offer the most natural food sources and supplements available.

Susan Gordon:

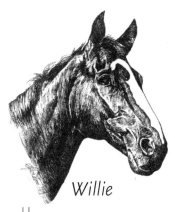

Willie

The free-choice hay-feeding method I tried with Willie was something I had never done before with another horse. When I first got him, he was so thin he required a strategy that would bring his BCS (body condition score) up to a normal standard in a safe way. The most natural way for a horse to eat is by grazing about 18 hours a day. Our artificial feeding schedules, based on convenience and economics, tend to cause problems in an animal that is inherently designed to eat almost continuously.

A hungry horse, much like a hungry person, is not in the best of moods. Hunger was not helping Willie, so riding him was out of the question until he had put on more weight. Fortunately, one of my local feed suppliers had gotten a load of clean, broad-bladed Timothy that was perfect for feeding on a free-choice basis (alfalfa hay is too rich in protein and calories to use in this way). I had a load of Timothy delivered and started the process of bulking up my scrawny new horse.

Rather than providing him an entire bale of hay at once and exposing it to the elements, Willie received a few flakes at a time on the concrete pad of the barn, and I noted the length of time it took him to finish it. As soon as he was done, he was fed a few more flakes, and his water supply was topped-up. It is critical to make sure your horse has a continual supply of fresh, clean water when offering free-choice hay, as the dry roughage has considerably less water than naturally growing grass.

Willie ate non-stop for about a week. He looked like a different horse by then, too. He finally walked away from a pile of sweet-smelling Timothy, satiated at last. I began offering him small quantities of a senior-horse grain mix, and he continued to blossom. His copper-colored coat began to shine, and his entire expression seemed to convey a satisfied horse. I had to look beyond how much it was costing to feed so much hay to one horse and be content and kind toward my choice to rescue this special old gelding. There is "dollar value" and then there is "worth." Willie was worth whatever it took to restore his faith in humanity. Simply feeding him well was the most compassionate thing I could do for him in those early days of our relationship.

Feeding horses used to be relatively straightforward, with limited selections of locally produced hay and available grains or pre-mixed sweet feeds. Early in my career, we would give horses basic vitamin, mineral, and coat supplements, but decades ago there was nothing like the array of choices we have today, ranging from natural herbs to synthesized vitamins, and from hoof growth to ulcer prevention. Besides lack of choices, we also did not have the present degree of scientific research pertaining to the feeding of horses. Given the extent of the current information available, making the right choice for each individual horse can be somewhat confusing.

At boarding barns, horses are often fed according the knowledge and expertise of management and staff, as well as economically based on the boarding fee. This may or may not work out for the individual horse or horse owner, as specific nutrient requirements are obviously different for horses working hard versus horses that are more sedentary. Feeding each horse appropriately is, in fact, an intricate part of running a barn. The larger a facility is, the more complicated it could get, and therefore the more generalized the feeding program might be.

Consider studying some of the excellent courses available in equine nutrition to understand what an optimal feeding program would be for your particular horse and discipline of choice.

As with human athletes, nutrition is fuel for the horse's activity and provides for proper recovery after exercise. We all require a perpetual intake of nutrients to stay alive and possibly a very specific diet for optimal performance in high-intensity athletic events. With humans, the person preparing to run a fast marathon will have very different nutritional needs than someone in training for their first 5-kilometer race. Marathoners need nutrient-dense diets high in complex carbohydrates (such as cereals, pasta, and grains) to produce the optimal fuel for their finely tuned muscles. A newcomer to running might have to structure his or her diet around losing weight while at the same time gaining strength and endurance for even the shortest of runs. This runner would want a reduced caloric intake, perhaps a lower percentage of and change in the sources of fat, and a different carbohydrate-to-protein ratio than the high-mileage endurance athlete, depending on his or her baseline physical condition. Comparatively, the upper-level eventing horse (for example), requires a different kind of feeding schedule than an easy-keeping trail horse who only sees a saddle on the weekends.

FACTORS TO CONSIDER FOR OPTIMAL PERFORMANCE

According to "Lessons from Human Sports Nutrition" on the *Pegasus Health* blog (www.pegasushealth.com), despite the differences in physiology between horses and humans, there is much to be learned from the feeding of human athletes, especially when it comes to muscle function. Therefore, consider these factors when feeding for optimal performance:

- Regulating amount of calories, protein, and carbohydrates required for each individual based on physiology, training load, and goals.

- Timing protein intake.

- Maximizing carbohydrate use.

- Managing hydration and electrolyte intake.

- Ensuring supplements are from reputable sources, are not contaminated, and do not contain banned substances.

- Limiting fat intake to 10 percent of total dietary energy intake.

Do you know what your horse needs to perform what you ask of him? Do you know what you need? Riders are athletes too!

Randomly supplementing a horse's diet does not always result in good health and well-being if the most basic requirements of a natural equine diet are not being met. Sometimes people spend a fortune on supplements, yet their horses still do not appear "bloomy" or in excellent health, as the hay might not be good quality or the water supply is inadequate or unclean. The best diet for a horse begins with high quality hay and feeding it in the correct amounts, according to the weight of the horse.[1]

If we do not feed horses in the most natural way possible, their health and welfare tends to suffer in a variety of ways. Think about how you feel when stressed and hungry or undernourished. It is only fair to the horse to understand how he feels when his natural grazing instincts are interrupted and replaced by a manmade feeding schedule. Human lifestyles are so disrupted by rushing around that one of the top-selling, over-the-counter drug categories is related to issues caused by diet and eating habits.[2] Be aware that what *we* may have become accustomed to is not the healthiest way to consume food, and we don't want to allow *our* unhealthy habits to impact how we expect our horses to eat.

> *The International Alliance for Animal Therapy and Healing (IAATH) says, "There's more to feeding a horse than offering free-choice hay, as not all hay is created equal when it comes to equine health. Different types of grass hay, such as Bermuda, Timothy, Orchard, Brome and Rye, along with small amounts of alfalfa or grain hay, give your horse a variety of textures, tastes and nutrients" (http://www.iaath.com/feedingnaturally.htm).*

> *Kathlyn Stone lists the United States' over-the-counter drug industry sales in "Top-Selling OTC Drugs by Category, 2012" on Pharma.about.com. That year, sales of heartburn and anti-gas medications were $2.3 billion, and laxatives sales reached $1.4 billion (http://pharma.about.com/od/Over-the-Counter-Medicine/a/Top-selling-Otc-Drugs-By-Category-2012.htm).*

1,2

Are you "bolting" your food because you are in too much of a hurry all the time? Stress causes stomach problems for both humans and horses. Be compassionate and feed yourself responsibly with whole (as in the "Real Food Movement"), natural foods, too.

As you learned in chapter 6 (p. 122), horses can get ulcers, just like humans. They cannot tell us outright when they have minor stomach pain, though. You might just note it as a "bad attitude" when it comes to being groomed, being tacked up, or mounted. While human ulcers are equated with a particular bacterium, Equine Gastric Ulcer Syndrome (EGUS) appears to be a manmade problem—removing horses from their natural environment, putting them on regulated feeding schedules, and adding intense training and showing programs.[3] Specific factors that could lead to EGUS include:

- Infrequent feeding

- Feeding too much high-soluble carbohydrates (grain and sweet feed)

- Not enough turnout

- High-intensity training

- Increased stress

- Overuse of anti-inflammatory drugs

3

In "Fix It with Feed Part 4: Prevent Ulcers by Mimicking Nature" (Chronofhorse.com, February 2011), Coree Reuter writes, "While there are no particular breeds that are more susceptible to ulcers than others, any horse that has a nervous disposition or operates in a high-stress environment is prone to EGUS. Some researchers estimate that 93 percent of racehorses have ulcers, and 63 percent of non-racing performance horses develop ulcers during their careers." (http://www.chronofhorse. com/article/fix-it-feed-part-4-prevent-ulcers-mimicking-nature)

Your horse may not have ulcers yet, but there are a few common behavioral signs that can clue you in when and if they develop: Your horse tightens or tenses up when he's girthed; he loses weight; or he seems more anxious and nervous than usual.

Climate change, transportation costs, loss of grazing land, and other factors are contributing to a "brave new world" of horsekeeping.

We have come a long way with both human and equine nutritional science in only a few years. We are going even further with new breakthroughs, such as the field of *nutrigenomics*, (the scientific study of the interaction of nutrition and genes, especially with regard to the prevention or treatment of disease—see more about this on p. 282) based on state-of-the-art genetic tools. It may help take more of the guesswork out of feeding horses appropriately, based on their genetic expression. A principal factor in nutrigenomic science is based upon the knowledge that everything we eat has an effect on our DNA, and therefore this new research has implications for the horse breeding industry, too. Or, it may determine alternatives to the feeding of hay and grain, which is becoming less available and far more expensive than it was in the past.

It does not seem like it has taken very long to go from simple, natural feeding programs, to an extremely complex, new-economy, genetically modified food chain. Natural is best, but if nature keeps changing, and human technology insists on changing nature, then our perspectives on what is most natural, and therefore best for our horses, may have to change, too. The compassionate response is to stay aware and informed and plan to have our horses cared for in the way that best supports their instinctive grazing needs while integrating that need with our own environmental challenges.

TEST YOUR HAY AND PASTURE

In the United States, the National Forage Testing Association (NFTA) was founded in 1984 as a joint effort of the American Forage and Grassland Council, the National Hay Association, and forage testing laboratories to improve the accuracy of forage testing and build grower confidence in testing animal feeds. NFTA laboratories are certified and provide an accurate diagnosis of the quality of hay or pasture your horse is receiving. For further information, visit www.foragetesting.org.

If you live outside of the United States, look for local authorities in your area that will test your hay and pasture quality to obtain a clear analysis of nutrient quality in your horse's feed.

Dr. Allen Schoen:

Genetically modified hay and beet pulp has already entered the food chain and is fed to livestock. Genetically modified organisms (GMOs) appear to be causing problems for other animals, and I feel the research may be extrapolated to horses. As an example, Dr. Judy Harman of Australia was part of a group of collaborating investigators that produced a peer-reviewed study after following 168 piglets through five months of genetically modified (GM) feeding. Pigs have a digestive system similar to humans *and* these pigs end up in the human food chain. The results were significant:

GM-fed females had on average a 25 percent heavier uterus than non-GM-fed females, a possible indicator of disease that requires further investigation. Also, the level of severe inflammation in stomachs was markedly higher in pigs fed on the GM diet. The research results were striking and statistically significant.

In some cases, animals eating GM crops are very aggressive. This is not surprising, given the scale of stomach irritation and inflammation now documented.[4]

4

Judy A. Carman, et al, reported in their study "A long-term toxicology study on pigs fed a combined genetically modified (GM) soy and GM maize diet" that pigs were harmed by the consumption of feed containing genetically modified (GM) crops (http://gmojudycarman.org/ new-study-shows-that-animals-are-seriously-harmed-by-gm-feed/).

We recommend viewing the award-winning documentary, *Genetic Roulette— The Gamble of Our Lives* (www.geneticroulettemovie.com) directed by Jeffrey M. Smith, author of the world's bestselling book on GMOs *Seeds of Deception* (Yes! Books, 2003). It is an eye-opening account of what is happening now in our own food, as well as that consumed by our horses and other animals. We also recommend *The Future of Food* (Lily Films, 2013), which you can find at www.the-futureoffood.com. View these films and form your own opinion about GMO food. There are many different views and strong opinions on both sides of this debate.

The new science of nutrigenomics is the study of how foods affect our genes and how our genes affect the way we respond to food.

Nutrigenomics is very new, but I like the concept of fine-tuning diets based on genetic pre-disposition.[5] According to the NCMHD Center of Excellence for Nutritional Genomics (nutrigenomics.ucdavis.edu), "Nutrigenomics or nutritional genomics is a multidisciplinary science that studies how foods affect our genes and how individual genetic differences can affect the way we respond to nutrients (and other naturally occurring compounds) in the foods we eat. Nutrigenomics has received much attention recently because of its potential for preventing, mitigating, or treating chronic disease and certain cancers, through small but highly informative dietary changes."

Let's say you have a Warmblood that has a slow metabolism, and you feed him a diet high in sugar. It is quite possible he may fall prey to insulin resistance and other nutritional conditions, such as *equine metabolic syndrome (EMS)*. It would be very beneficial to be able to identify those potential factors in the horse using genetic specifics in order to determine the best way of feeding him over his lifetime.

In the 2010 paper given at the Cornell Nutritional Conference, "A Brief Review of Current and Future Applications of Nutrigenomics in the Horse," S.A. Brooks of the Department of Animal Science, Cornell University, in Ithaca, New York, states: "With the completion of the equine genome sequence state of the art genetic tools are now available for a wide variety of applications in the horse. Similar to many livestock species, maintaining healthy animals through a proper diet is a key concern for most horse owners. Some genetic traits have already been identified that can impact the nutritional management of the horse" (https://dspace. library.cornell.edu/bitstream/1813/37008/2/CNC_Proceedings.pdf).

NATURAL ≠ ORGANIC

"Natural" is not the same as "organic." In the United States, a product can be labeled "natural" if it contains any naturally occurring compounds, even if it has been altered synthetically. Currently, the "organic" food label and seal is strictly regulated by the National Organic Program, which is administered through the United States Department of Agriculture (USDA), and foods and products with an organic seal are *certified organic* and contain at least 95 percent organic content.

To me, epigenetics is an even more exciting field.

Epigenetics is the study of the impact of various stimuli on the biochemical reactions that may affect genetic expression of genes. It also may reflect on the impact of nutrition, thoughts, beliefs, and a holistic approach on our own health and perhaps, the health of the animals under our care. "As an organism grows and develops," reports the University of Utah Health Sciences, "carefully orchestrated chemical reactions activate and deactivate parts of the genome at strategic times and in specific locations. Epigenetics is the study of these chemical reactions and the factors that influence them."[6]

According to the University of Utah Health Sciences Genetic Science Learning Center, "The epigenome dynamically responds to the environment. Stress, diet, behavior, toxins, and other factors regulate gene expression" (http://learn.genetics.utah.edu/content/epigenetics/).

This reminds me of a discussion I had with a Tibetan lama who once stayed with me. He remarked, "When I grew up in Nepal, we didn't talk about organic food. We just ate...and everything *was* organic. Here, everything is stamped and certified organic, and it is expensive."

Not too long ago, if you had good hay and basic grain, such as oats, you could keep feeding your horse a simple diet because it worked. The soils were still good, the hays were not genetically-modified or sprayed with pesticides, and they were generally local. Most feed products were not transported so far that they lost their vitamins and minerals during the process. You usually were aware of your feed's origin, and that if your horse feed was coming from a selenium-deficient area, you would need to add selenium as a supplement, and other such simple things. It was all relatively straightforward. We never had to specify *organic*. It just was.

Now there are certain crops such as soy, corn, even alfalfa that are almost *all* GMO. Looking at the research showing what GMO food is doing to our bodies—and our horses'—makes the old-fashioned, "simple" method of feeding not that "simple" anymore. Though there are conflicting reports on the possible effects of GMO foods, you must look at the source of the information provided and see if there is a possible conflict of interest. As I mentioned back on p. 271, "Follow the money" has a detrimental effect on the food industry as it does on other areas of public interest. When the researchers publishing results of GMO testing receive funding from or are associated with transnational companies that produce GMO food, is it not reasonable to question the results of the research? The fact is, there are significant financial interests backing the proliferation of GMO foods, and we must all be conscious of the implications.

Know your feed suppliers. Know where the feed originated.
Know if it contains GMOs.

It is difficult to determine the source and quality of food for both you and your horse unless you are *very* aware of checking labels and constantly keep up with

BASIC SUPPLEMENTATION
FOR HORSES ON STORED FORAGES

When your horse does not have access to ample, quality pasture, it is likely there are vital nutrients missing from his diet, which may need to be supplemented. These may include:

- *Vitamin E.* Not synthesized by the horse, vitamin E (alpha-tocopherol) is an essential dietary nutrient. It is the primary lipid-soluble antioxidant that maintains cell membrane integrity by combating the effects of free radical production. It also enhances both humoral- and cell-mediated immunity. Supplementation is especially beneficial to young, rapidly growing foals, pregnant and lactating mares, stallions, and equine athletes. Note that according a piece by Ed Kane, PhD, in a 2004 issue of *Veterinary News*, "It is often difficult to distinguish between the signs of vitamin E and selenium deficiencies."

- *Beta carotene and Vitamin A.* For horses, beta carotene is mainly recognized as a precursor to vitamin A, but it can provide additional benefits, especially to those horses not consuming adequate beta carotene from lush green pastures. Beta carotene, like vitamin E, can serve as an antioxidant and enhance the immune system.

- *Vitamin D.* Though vitamin D plays a significant role in calcium-phosphorus metabolism (and therefore bone formation), equine dietary requirements are less understood for this nutrient than they are for others mentioned here. Because horses can produce vitamin D systemically, there are few, if any, reports of vitamin D needs for horses, especially those with access to UV sunlight exposure.

current information and research regarding food products. My preference, in general (and depending on your situation and what is possible) is as much as you can, *go local*. Be a "locavore," as we call it. Know the farmers in your area and develop relationships with them. Frequent local farmers' markets. When you live in a big city or an area where you do not have direct access to local producers, seek out information regarding Community Supported Agriculture (CSAs), which "allow city residents to have direct access to high quality, fresh produce grown locally by regional farmers," states *Justfood.org*. "When you become a member of a CSA, you purchase a 'share' of vegetables from a regional farmer. Weekly or bi-weekly, and seasonly, your farmer will deliver that share of produce to a convenient drop-off location in your neighborhood."

In areas where regional agriculture allows, it might work for networks of barns within a reasonable distance of each other to get together and form equine-specific CSAs in order to purchase and support locally produced hay and grain. When farms also produce crops and plants for human consumption, the equine CSA could expand to include human food. It is a win-win-win situation for horses, their people, and the local farms! Carrots for horses, and carrots for humans! CSAs are great for farmers because they ensure a steady, local customer base as income, and they are great for equestrians because they provide a source of healthy (preferably organic) feed for horses.

When your horse's basic feed is of high quality and you know where it has come from and how it has been produced, you may not need to consider as many supplements to ensure his good health. With horses, as with humans, when you feed lower quality food or nutrition-depleted food, the need for supplementation becomes greater.

Local, fresh food is best, both for your horse, and yourself. Good quality food reduces the need for supplements. If you must ship in your hay, the less distance it needs to be transported, the better.

With many regions experiencing drought or other weather extremes, the only way to find hay or grain may be to purchase what has, in fact, been transported long distances. This is where building an awareness of climate conditions, as well as areas in your region or country that produce quality equine feed, is of benefit. It is possible that equine CSAs could organize and span greater distances so as to acquire better quality hay from where it is available at better prices. The goal is to still know where the food comes from, how long it has been in transport, and to support those farmers who continue to produce pesticide-free, non-GMO crops.

TEACHING FUTURE GENERATIONS ABOUT HORSES, FARMING, AND CSA

In the heart of busy Vancouver, BC, Canada, is Southlands Farm, where University of British Columbia graduate Jordan Maynard, BSc. Agroecology, has developed a program for teaching "city kids" all about the growing, harvesting, and self-sustaining production of their own food and food for their animals.

Based at the family's active riding stable, the farm's Seasoned Farmers Youth Practicum consists of an educational experience for kids ages 8 to 13 to learn about the basic steps to grow and process food. Participants in a weekly after school-program during the spring learn the stages of food production, food processing, animal care, and natural cycles. Participants receive a plot of land at Southlands Farm, which they plan, plant, and tend to throughout the "season." The program engages young people with food systems in an experiential learning environment and empowers them to participate in decision-making about where food is sourced and how it is grown. Learn more at www.southlandsfarms.com.

I have seen the full spectrum of extremes when it comes to feeding horses. Some people overfeed and over-supplement to the detriment of the animal. Others underfeed or do not believe in supplementing at all, also detrimental to the horse when conditions warrant the proper additions of vitamins and minerals. As with everything, the middle path is often the most balanced perspective, and keeping compassion at the base of our quest for optimal equine nutrition is ultimately the best course of action in keeping our horses healthy.

Questions to Consider

BASED ON PRINCIPLE 16

1   Does the existence of GMO products in my horse's feed concern me?

2   Have I or am I currently experiencing any problems with feed quality and delivery due to climate change issues, such as severe drought? Do I have contingency plans if my feed supply chain becomes problematic?

3   What kinds of supplements does my horse receive? Is he getting all he needs? Things he doesn't need?

4   Is there a network of like-minded equestrians or riding facilities in my area who I can approach about creating a CCSA—Compassionate Community Supported Agriculture—for our horses?

CHAPTER SEVENTEEN

Interspecies Communication and Mind-Body Medicine

We acknowledge neurobiology and quantum physics as a foundation for interspecies communication, the Transpecies Field Theory, and the Compassionate Field Theory.

Susan Gordon:

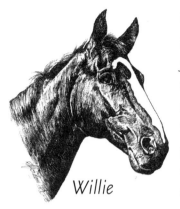

Willie

Willie and I experienced the kind of communication I had developed over the years with most animals. It just felt natural to me to talk to horses as though I was talking to another person, and I usually expected a two-way conversation. I can imagine many of you reading this have felt the same way, too, and have noticed that perhaps some horses and pets appear to be more perceptive and responsive to your verbal and nonverbal communication than others.

This story actually predates my experience with Willie. I learned a lot from animals when I was a child, but one of the most profound lessons was how to create reality from mental visualization—the power of intention. I believe everyone has this ability to create what he or she envisions. Your thoughts really can become your reality, so be aware of what you mentally create for yourself!

As an 11-year-old living in a town that was famous for its annual rodeo, I really got the "horse bug." Big time. My parents, especially my mom, knew I had a special gift for communicating with animals. She saw it with our dogs, cats, birds, and pet rodents. It was a stretch, however, for my parents to absorb the costs of a horse, and so all I could do was imagine having one. I saw "her" running alongside our car whenever we took a trip somewhere: a white horse, galloping beside me as I stared out the window. I had pretty much given up on ever having a *real* horse, when I asked my parents one last time. As it turned out, mom was ready to make the purchase. One of her dance students had a horse he wanted to sell: You guessed it... a big, white mare. This was White Cloud, the ranch horse I mentioned in the beginning of the book (see p. 25).

Over the years as I went from junior, to amateur, to professional, every horse I mentally created manifested in reality. I just *saw* the horses. There was no attachment as to where they would come from, how they would be acquired, where they would be kept, how long I would have them, or if they would be my own or a client's. They just came to me, one after the other. I was simply filled with gratitude at every new chance to ride a wonderful horse that came my way.

One of the most amazing horses I ever encountered was the young appaloosa stallion, Top Canadian, or "TC." One of my horse visualizations was a deep-bay Appaloosa with a classic white rump and black spots. When I was 16,

BELIEVING IS SEEING

We all know the familiar saying, "I'll believe it when I see it," or, "Seeing is believing." A more progressive intentional perspective on this is, "I see it when I believe it," or "Believing is seeing." Some books that review and explain the research behind the concepts introduced in this chapter and will help you believe in their validity and applicability include: *The Biology of Belief* by Bruce Lipton (Hay House, 2007), *The Genie in Your Genes* by Dawson Church (Elite Books, 2007), *The Spontaneous Healing of Belief* by Gregg Braden (Hay House, 2008), and *The Intention Experiment* by Lynn McTaggert (Free Press, 2007).

I found him at an Appaloosa Horse Club conference. For a special event he had been led through the hotel with another yearling, and they were standing like perfect little statues beside the hotel's swimming pool. It was the beginning of an extraordinary relationship.

Not only was TC a typically playful colt, but I was still just a teenager who could have gotten in *big* trouble trying to take on such a training project. To this day, I would *never* recommend a young person start a horse under saddle on his or her own, much less a stallion. Somehow, the level of communication and the remarkable bond I had with TC was quite unusual from the get-go, and I was lucky for it. TC demonstrated many times over that he could not only *think* and *reason*, but he seemed to have an uncanny ability to understand the English language. He even surprised me, along with other people who sometimes could not believe what they were seeing. Yes, I expected some type of communication with an animal, but not usually a verbatim understanding of a statement made in plain human-speak with no previous association to the words.

I had left him in a turnout pen one day, and when it was time to bring him in, one of the barn's grooms was also heading out to catch horses. As we chatted at the gate to TC's pen for a while, I noticed my horse had taken his halter off the fence post where I had left it and deposited it on the far side of the paddock. TC loved to be the center of attention and was standing quietly at the gate while the groom and I talked. I did not feel like walking all the way to the other side of the turnout to retrieve the halter, so I casually said, "TC, go get your halter."

Of course, I didn't *actually* expect him to retrieve the halter, as I assumed he had *no* idea what I was saying. I was somewhat stunned when he immediately turned around, made a beeline for the halter, picked it up with his teeth, and trotted back to the gate with it, dropping it at my feet. I looked at the groom who like me, was basically speechless. I just thanked the little guy, still not even under saddle at the time, put his halter on and took him back to the barn.

There were many such incidents with this particular horse, and I had to wonder what it was about him that made him so responsive to human communication. He was well socialized with humans as a baby. That probably helped. He had had no traumas that would have made him distrustful of anything. He had also been shown in conformation classes from the time he was 4 months old and had been weaned at an earlier stage than many foals are. He was a joyful a horse as could be, and his clownish personality was contagious, even amongst other horses that he often played games with. He made everyone smile until the day he passed away from colic, 24 years later. Whatever the combination of elements that allowed TC to achieve such a high degree of bonding and understanding when it came to humans, they certainly provided a fascinating set of circumstances that frequently led me to wonder about the "why" and "how" of interspecies communication.

"We humans are in the midst of a profound advance as a species to a higher form of global consciousness that has been emerging across cultures, religions and worldviews through the centuries. This awakening of global consciousness is nothing less than a shift, a maturation, from more egocentric patterns of life to a higher form of integral and dialogic patterns of life."

Ashok Gangadean, Professor and Chair of Philosophy, Haverford College, Founder and Director of The Global Dialogue Institute

---

It was training in meditation and energy-field healing, plus studies in neuroscience, that eventually provided me with insights as to how *the field of energy exchange* may have been occurring between me and my horses, especially with certain horses like TC. With years of study and practice, I learned this *field* is actually palpable, and a considerable amount of information exchange between species can take place when you become sensitive to that kind of energy. This concept is further explained by Dr. Schoen's Transpecies Field Theory (see p. 7).

Dr. Allen Schoen:

It is interesting to observe the emerging interdisciplinary approaches that are providing new research and documenting evidence of *quantum field information in human-human interactions*.[1] Ideas from Doc Childre's Institute of Heartmath®, transpersonal psychology, Dr. Dan Siegel's Mindsight, interpersonal biology, quantum physics, new biology, and neurospirituality, to name only a few, all acknowledge the impact of one person's thoughts and emotions on another. I have come to appreciate that these interactions may indeed relate to human-animal interactions as well.

Traveling barn to barn in my veterinary practice for decades, listening to audio books and other sources of continuing education on these topics, I began to ponder how they manifest in each small barn, large equestrian facility, or equestrian competition. Once I opened my mind to the possibilities, I began to see the microcosm of the equestrian world through the filters of these interdisciplinary approaches. And so I developed the term *Dr. Schoen's Transpecies Field Theory*© to explain my observations on human-horse interactions. (I briefly introduced this concept to you earlier in the book—see p. 7.) It seems that as Einstein said, "Energy is everything and that's all there is to it. Match the frequency of the reality you want and you cannot help but get that reality. It can be no other way. This is not philosophy, this is physics."

> Encyclopedia Brittanica *describes Quantum Field Theory in this way:* "A body of physical principles combining the elements of quantum mechanics with those of relativity to explain the behavior of subatomic particles and their interactions via a variety of force fields...The prototype of quantum field theories is quantum electrodynamics (QED), which provides a comprehensive mathematical framework for predicting and understanding the effects of electromagnetism on electrically charged matter at all energy levels. Electric and magnetic forces are regarded as arising from the emission and absorption of exchange particles called photons. These can be represented as disturbances of electromagnetic fields, much as ripples on a lake are disturbances of the water" (http://www.britannica.com/EBchecked/topic/486221/quantum-field-theory).

Each thought and emotion seems to have its own energetic resonance or frequency. For instance, angry emotions create a certain dissonant frequency that may not be beneficial to horses at times.

It does not seem unreasonable to extrapolate these theories to human-horse and human-animal interactions. This can be quite exciting as we realize that our thoughts, intentions, and emotions can have either a *constructive* or *destructive* impact on the field of energy that surrounds us. It would seem reasonable that we may want to be part of creating a more positive, happier, healthier, peaceful, fun, and constructive field versus the alternative.[2]

This takes into consideration the latest in quantum physics and transpersonal neurobiology and the data now available from the Institute of HeartMath, which shows that when one person slows down his or her heart rate, others in the vicinity also demonstrate slower heart rate.[3] My Transpecies Field Theory suggests the possibility of demonstrating the same connection between horses and humans. If you slow *your* heart rate down, *the horse's* heart rate will reflect your change in beats per minute.

The Institute of HeartMath's research has proven the existence of an electromagnetic field extending as far as 3 feet from the human body—and the field may be even bigger than that. When I think of a horse's heart, and how much larger it is than a human's, I wonder if perhaps so many people, especially women, relate to the horses the way they do because there is such a large "heart field" emitting from the horse, and it draws in the human "heart field" response.

2,3

In his article on Conscious Life News "Mind Over Matter: Princeton & Russian Scientist Reveal the Secrets of Human Aura & Intentions" (September 2013), Joe Martino writes, "A Russian scientist has been studying the human energy field and is claiming that people can change the world simply by using their own energy. While this idea is not new, not too many have taken the time to scientifically go about proving such ideas—although the field of quantum physics has shed some powerful light on the topic over the years. Dr. Konstantin Korotkov, professor of physics at St. Petersburg State Technical University, states that when we think positive and negative thoughts, each have a different impact on our surrounding environment" (http://consciouslifenews.com/mind-matter-princeton-russian-scientist-reveal-secrets-human-aura-intentions/1164859/#).

The Institute of HeartMath, founded by Doc Childre, is known for research-based programs, techniques, and technology to improve health and well-being, while dramatically reducing stress. HeartMath techniques are being widely used within hospitals and healthcare systems, academic settings, within the US military for resilience-building pre-deployment, and in veteran administration clinics working with emotionally wounded soldiers. Over 20 years of published research on HRV (Heart Rate Variability) coherence and clinical studies have demonstrated the critical link between emotions, heart function, and cognitive performance. These studies have been published in numerous peer-reviewed journals such as the American Journal of Cardiology; Stress Medicine; Preventive Cardiology; *and* Journal of the American College of Cardiology *(www.heartmath.org)*.

In addition, the latest research on *oxytocin* (a mammalian neurohypophysial hormone produced by the hypothalamus and stored and secreted by the posterior pituitary gland) and the *bonding process* has led us to be attracted to large equine eyes, which can resemble a human baby's (as can the expression of some dogs). This familiar "look" may somehow stimulate oxytocin-release in our bodies, furthering the bonding experience.[4] The bonding between horse and human, from my perspective, involves a biochemical, neurochemical, and neurohormonal connection, relating to the release of endorphins *as well* as oxytocin, combined with the horse-human heart interaction and electromagnetic field connection.

According to PsychologyToday.com, "Oxytocin is a powerful hormone. When we hug or kiss a loved one, oxytocin levels drive up. It also acts as a neurotransmitter in the brain. In fact, the hormone plays a huge role in pair bonding. Prairie voles, one of nature's most monogamous species, produce oxytocin in spades. This hormone is also greatly stimulated during sex, birth, breast feeding—the list goes on" (http://www.psychologytoday.com/basics/oxytocin).

Based on quantum physics, when two people's thoughts and fields of energy connect, they create a combined field.

Rupert Sheldrake is a biologist and author of more than 80 scientific papers and 10 books. He was among the top 100 Global Thought Leaders for 2013, as ranked by the Duttweiler Institute, Zurich, Switzerland's leading think tank. Dr. Sheldrake has discussed his theories on *morphic resonant fields* in animals and possibly between humans and animals in his book *Dogs That Know When Their Owners Are Coming Home* (Broadway Books, 2011).

If Sheldrake's theories of morphic resonance and others continue to prove to be valid, they may indeed shed light on some of the unexplained behavioral interactions and connections that we see between us and horses.

5

In 2000, Rupert Sheldrake and Pamela Smart published "A Dog That Seems To Know When His Owner is Coming Home: Videotaped Experiments and Observations" in the Journal of Scientific Exploration. *They write, "Many dog owners claim that their animal knows when a member of the household is about to come home. Typically, the dog is said to go and wait at a door, window or gate while the person is on the way home (Sheldrake, 1994, 1999a). Random household surveys in Britain and the United States have shown that between 45 and 52 percent of dog owners say they have noticed this kind of behavior (Brown & Sheldrake, 1998; Sheldrake, Lawlor & Turney, 1998; Sheldrake & Smart, 1997)" (http://www.sheldrake.org/Articles&Papers/papers/animals/dog_video.html).*

One day there was a fire in a stable in the area where I practice. I had just heard about it. By the time I arrived at a barn just a few miles from the one that was on fire, most of the horses in this facility were demonstrably anxious and seemed to want to get out of their stalls. Many were snorting, whinnying, and stamping their feet. Neither the barn manager nor the grooms nor anyone else had heard of the fire yet. Somehow, the horses seemed to know. Other barns that I saw in the area that day also remarked about the inexplicable angst that was going through their horses at the time. Coincidence? The horses at the burning barn and the other barns nearby may have been exhibiting what Dr. Larry Dossey (author of *One Mind*, published by Hay House, 2014, among others) refers to as "nonlocal mind"—that is, "consciousness is not confined to one's individual body."[6]

Dr. Dan Siegel approaches the concept of interconnectedness through the experience and eyes of a neuropsychiatrist. Based on his decades of clinical experience and his own studies, he has developed a theory within the field of interpersonal neurobiology that he calls "Mindsight" (see his book *Mindsight*, Bantam, 2010). It is based on the concepts of mindfulness meditation and how developing mindfulness can impact not only on you, but others as well.

Dr. Siegel's Mindsight approach applies the emerging principles of interpersonal neurobiology to promote compassion, kindness, resilience, and well-being in our personal lives, our relationships, and our communities. At the heart of his ideas is the concept of *integration*, which entails the linkage of different aspects of a system—whether they exist within a single person or a collection of individuals.[7] It is not unreasonable to believe this inter*personal* neurobiology may also be expanded to include inter*species* neurobiology—that is, when a single person chooses to be a certain way, that may have a beneficial impact on his or her horse, and your horse, as well.

> *In his book* Reinventing Medicine *(HarperOne, 1999), Dr. Larry Dossey discusses three periods or "Eras" in medicine: "Era III goes even further,"* *he says, "by proposing that consciousness is not confined to one's individual body. Nonlocal mind—mind that is boundless and unlimited—is the hallmark of Era III. An individual's mind may affect not just his or her body, but the body of another person at a distance, even when that distant individual is unaware of the effort" (http://www.dosseydossey. com/larry/QnA.html).*

> *Dr. Daniel J. Siegel is a bestselling author and executive director of the Mindsight Institute, an educational organization that focuses on how the development of Mindsight in individuals, families, and communities can be enhanced by examining the interface of human relationships and basic biological processes. He is a pioneer in the field called interpersonal neurobiology, which "seeks the similar patterns that arise from separate approaches to knowledge. This interdisciplinary field invites all branches of science and other ways of knowing to come together and find the common principles from within their often disparate approaches to understanding human experience" (http://www.drdansiegel.com/about/ interpersonal_neurobiology/).*

Being mindful can help us become more compassionate.

Research done by Dr. Dan Siegel and others has shown that mindfulness meditation (see suggested exercises on pp. 70–73) stimulates the growth of integrative fibers in the human brain. Carolyn Gregoire's May 2014 article "What Neuroscience Can Teach Us About Compassion" on the Huffington Post's Third Metric asks if *compassion* can have the same effect on the brain as *mindfulness meditation*. Gregoire cites a 2013 study from Harvard and Northeastern University that demonstrates "that meditation can improve compassion and altruistic behavior. The researchers found that participants who had meditated were more likely than non-meditators to lend a helping hand to an actor with crutches who was pretending to be in pain. A 2012 Emory University study suggested that compassion training derived from ancient Tibetan mindfulness practices may boost empathy, and other research has found that loving-kindness meditation could increase positive emotions and lead to more positive relationships over time. The bottom line? Mindfulness and loving compassion are the techniques that integrate our mental systems."

With the understanding that our conscious thoughts, intentions, and emotions may have effects on our horses (and other species), as well as people, intertwined with my past 35 years as a veterinarian, I have realized that perhaps we are actually *creating a Transpecies Energy Field* whenever we interact with a horse or horses. Looking back over the years, I think I have long been aware of this, consciously coming into a quiet space and meditating before starting my workday. As you now know, I always try to *slow myself down* and *breathe* before working with horses and horsepeople. I change my neurophysiologic and general physiologic state by becoming quiet, calm, and peaceful. I bring intention because it has been shown that personal intention impacts every other being's intention (see QFI, p. 8). People often comment on how calm horses are around me. Certainly that is not always the case, but I try to do my best to be as aware as I can be so it is the "norm" rather than the exception.

The horses that already know me associate me with feeling good. They know my voice so there is an immediate *release* and *relaxation* as I approach them. Every horseperson recognizes that when you have a nice relationship with your horse, he hears your voice and his happiness in seeing you is indicated by a whinny or nicker and a friendly expression. Some of the reaction may of course be food-associated, and part may simply be the horse watching and responding to visual, auditory, and other sensory cues. However, I am convinced there is far more to this connection.[8]

8

In his April 2014 article in The Atlantic *"Dogs (and Cats) Can Love," Paul Zak explains how "Neurochemical research has shown that the hormone released when people are in love is released in animals in the same intimate circumstances. That animals of different species induce oxytocin release in each other suggests that they, like us, may be capable of love"(http://www.theatlantic.com/health/archive/2014/04/does-your-dog-or-cat-actually-love-you/360784/).*

HEALING ENERGY

According to the International College of Medical Quigong (medicalquigong. org), *Qigong* is a combination of two ideas: *Qi* (pronounced "chee"), means air, breath of life, or vital energy that flows through all things in the universe. *Gong* (pronounced "gung," as in" lung") means the skill of working with, or cultivating, self-discipline and achievement.

There are renowned Qigong masters from China who can reportedly help heal individuals or groups of individuals with their intention, creating a transpersonal healing energy field.

Engineer and inventor Nikola Tesla said, "If you want to find the secrets of the universe, think in terms of energy, frequency and vibration."

Upon realizing we create *Transpecies Fields* when we interact with horses, I began noticing how when I visited certain barns, I felt a certain "vibe." These could be "good" vibrations or "bad" vibrations. My preference was and is that I really do not want to go into some barns—where, for example, the trainer or owner appears to be an angry person, or if there is a history of alcohol or drug issues, or when there are inconsistencies in behaviors and circumstances that make for an unpleasant atmosphere for everyone. I find that when the owner, trainer, or barn manager has significant personal issues, it may create a dissonant vibrational frequency in that entire field in the barn. Everyone seems to be walking on eggshells because they never know who is going to be short-tempered, hurtful, or yelling at the horses or other riders or barn staff. It is this kind of negative behavior and emotion that creates those "bad" vibes and an atmosphere that has a very detrimental effect, not only in a general sense, but which may trigger extreme stress in younger riders, adults who are children of alcoholics and substance abusers, and horses that have experienced a traumatic event. I remember one barn in particular that I always felt "strange and uneasy" going into, feeling the cognitive dissonance of an unhealthy vibration. I later found out that a significant number of the people working at the barn had serious drug and alcohol issues (see p. 91 for more on this subject).

What do we do when we find ourselves in the midst of "bad" vibes or a "negative frequency"? In this type of situation, we need to remember the difference between "response-ability" and "react-ability" (see p. 49). Our response-ability is to manage *our own* thoughts, emotions, neurophysiologic state, "heart field," and energy field, and how all of these impact our horses and others. We have a response-ability to enter the barn and impact the Transpecies Field with our intention. People will note the energy of the entire place changes when you enter with calmness and peace. Each and every one of us has the ability to create that shift. This is where the Transpecies Field Theory comes into effect. Part of *The Compassionate Equestrian* approach is to produce happy, humane, peaceful barns by developing individual awareness of how our own fields impact those of all the beings around us.

Transpersonal psychology states that your personality and your energy field extend well past your physical self. The *transpersonal* is defined as "experiences in which the sense of identity or self extends beyond (trans) the individual or personal to encompass wider aspects of humankind, life, psyche, or cosmos." It has also been defined as "development beyond conventional, personal, or individual levels." But to me, it is *beyond* transpersonal—it is *trans-species*.

EXERCISE IN COMPASSION

Feeding with Intention

New research is showing the positive results of mindful intention in *everything* you do—even the most fundamental of activities, such as eating and drinking. Consider the following human experiment: Yung-Jong Shiah, PhD, and Dean Radin, PhD, tested, under double-blind, randomized conditions, whether drinking tea "treated" solely with good intentions would enhance mood more than drinking the same tea "untreated." Three monks experienced in meditative practice mentally directed the following intentions toward the tea for 22 minutes: "An individual who consumes this tea will manifest optimal health and functioning at physical, emotional and mental levels, and in particular they will enjoy an increased sense of energy, vigor and well-being."

The results of the study showed that those who drank the tea "treated" with the monks' good intentions showed a greater increase in mood than those who drank "untreated" tea. In addition, change in mood in those who *believed* they were drinking "treated" tea was much better than those who did not believe, indicating that belief and "intentional enhancement" interact (http://deanradin.com/evidence/Shiah2013.pdf).

Now, try this experiment in your own barn!

1   If you are not the one who feeds your horse, see if you can engage those responsible for this aspect of his care in being part of your "study."

2   Follow the same procedure for treating your horse's hay and grain as the monks did for treating the tea. If you are practicing *The Compassionate Equestrian's* recommended 10 minutes of QFI (see p. 46), you can apply this same method but direct your intentional focus toward your horse's feed, adding beneficial intentions as your breathe slowly in and out. For 22 minutes (or however much time you can spare) say the following: "A horse that consumes this hay and grain will manifest optimal health and functioning at physical, emotional, and mental levels, and in particular he will enjoy an increased sense of well-being and contentment."

3   Practice this feeding of hay and grain "treated" with beneficial intentions for one week.

4   Observe your horse after one week. The good thing about horses is that they do not have a individualized "belief system" like humans do, so there is no confirmation bias as to whether they feel better or not. They are "present-moment" creatures with good memories. To make the Feeding-with-Intention Experiment effective, it is up to the human observer to decide if hay and grain treated with good intentions seems to have a beneficial effect on the horse's overall mood and well-being. If the horse being given intention-enhanced feeds is already in good flesh, fit, healthy, shining, and well-balanced emotionally, you may not notice much difference. If your horse is underweight, coming back from illness, or prone to stress-related behaviors, it would be interesting to see if the treated food noticeably improves his condition,

Continued →

(Cont.)

calms him, or uplifts his mood or energy level. The goal over time would be to create a more contented animal.

Note: There are a number of variables that may affect the results of this simple exercise, such as: Did the previous mind training of the monks and their accrued power of intention have an impact on their ability to treat the tea in the human experiment? Can we come close to approximating this with our lesser experience and power? Did the amount of time the monks spent projecting their intention impact the results? Do we need to spend a comparable or longer amount of time? We look forward to hearing the results from Compassionate Equestrians everywhere!

Questions to Consider
BASED ON PRINCIPLE 17

1   Do I believe the concepts and theory proposed in this chapter?

2   How do I see the ideas of the Transpecies Field Theory impacting my horse-keeping and my barn? My interactions with others in the industry?

3   How can I envision myself improving the Transpecies Field with my own thoughts? Intentions? Emotions?

CHAPTER EIGHTEEN

Transcending All Breeds and Disciplines

We acknowledge that compassion is the common foundation shared in the world of equestrian activities. Grounded in individual responsibility, respect, loving-kindness, and a true willingness to alleviate another's suffering; compassion is the unifying force that transcends all labels, beyond breeds, discipline, health care, and medications. The essential question is, "What is the most compassionate choice for our horses and all involved?"

Susan Gordon:

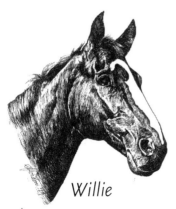

Willie

My interest in Willie started because of his breed. The Hanoverian was a favorite "type" of mine. As you've read, Appaloosas were my choice as a youth. And I also developed a love of the Thoroughbred after all the OTTBs I helped transition.

I can almost hear the thoughts of all the readers out there, weighing in with their breed preferences! We love what we love for our individual reasons. The horse world gives us a tremendous smorgasbord of wonderful breeds and breed types to enjoy. Then again, this preference is such a "human thing." So far as I can tell, horses are just horses to each other, and they do not discriminate between breeds and types. Willie was just as happy to take care of a colicky Quarter Horse as he was to keep an eye on Oldenburg babies.

It was a humbling experience to finally have a horse of the breed I adored, yet have him be so broken down he would never be the fancy show horse he once was. At the breed shows of my youth, everyone was proud of "their" breed to the point of a kind of "nationalism." Some would even openly voice their disdain for others as we were waiting at the in-gate for our classes. The comments could be hurtful and discouraging. I would imagine those same people were equally disrespectful toward other humans, too, based on far more troublesome characteristics than the type of horse they preferred.

Willie could have cared less, of course, when people made comments about his lack of refinement or beauty. I defended him regardless, noting the draftier type of Hanoverian was the kind I admired most. They were huge, magnificent horses that could still float like butterflies and sail over enormous fences.

Eventually, I learned to shrug off the negative comments about my beloved horses. I heard everything about why people did not appreciate "my" breeds—the Appaloosas, the Thoroughbreds, the Hanoverians—as much as they lauded "their" breeds. It is easy to see why people become defensive and possessive of "their" breed. It is all about the labels and what they mean to each individual, but it divides us. Put a Hanoverian in the pasture with a Quarter Horse, a Thoroughbred, a Lipizzaner, an Arabian, a Morgan, and a Mustang, and they will figure out the dynamics of that particular herd and live accordingly. They won't insult each other or hurt each other's feelings or *fail to ease another's suffering. They don't care how much the others cost or what their bloodlines are. They are simply One Herd.*

Acquiring a horse for his specific characteristics and as best suits the style of riding you prefer is often a good reason for selecting a particular breed. However, the breed is no guarantee of performance, given the number of variables that affect a horse throughout his lifetime. Willie was not branded with the famed "H" symbol, and as he was actually imported from Belgium, for all I knew his papers should have read "Belgian Warmblood." It did not really matter in the long run as he transcended it all when he packed a student around the ring or took on the care of whatever lonely or ailing horse was assigned to him. I was quite proud of him and the kind of horse he became in the days we spent together, but my pride had nothing to do with his breeding... that part was my luxurious little secret. I finally had "my" Hanoverian.

It is an extraordinary feeling when you gallop a horse to a 5-foot fence, fly over it, and charge onward to the next one. It is a melding of two species into one body, and involves a level of trust you come to rely on. One wrong step could put you both in danger of serious injury. It is the pinnacle of focus, discipline, athletic coordination, and power. It is a partnership of understanding and split-second agreements. It still amazes me to this day that we can reach this kind of coordinated ability and finesse in conjunction with an animal. We come to depend on him so greatly for not only exhilaration but for our very safety as he lifts all four feet high off the ground, leaping over obstacles of a shape and complexity that make little sense at all to his inborn nature.

Jumping, dressage, reining, barrels, hippotherapy... we are all in this for one unifying reason—the horse.

You cannot *make* a horse jump if he does not want to—at least not for very long. He has to be brave and willing to go forward. He must also be happy and comfortable, even exhibiting extreme joy and excitement about what he's being asked to do. This rule applies to whatever sport or activity you participate in with your horse. Some horses are so thrilled about jumping, racing, cutting a cow, or otherwise "putting on a show," they will continue to perform, even when they are hurting. In the midst of athletic competition and group events, it is easy to get caught up in the, "Go for it!" attitude. Our tendency may be to forget about how the horse might be feeling. The temptation might be to push the horse in the chase for that ribbon or prize money. I've been there myself, and I regret having jumped through another class when it would have been more appropriate to withdraw the horse.

Beyond our personal preferences regarding breeds, disciplines, and competitions, let us see how responsible we can all be for equine welfare, at every level of equestrian sports and recreation.

Compassion at the elite level of equestrian sports is both highly evident and painfully absent. If it is not there, sooner or later the trainer or rider will make a big enough mistake that others will take note of rough or unfair treatment of a horse. There are some competition rules in place that can stop someone in his or her tracks if caught abusing a horse, but the rules need to be enforced, too.

A case for debate in many different areas of the show and racing worlds is whether or not to continue showing and racing horses if they are being medicated for pain. In bigger competitions, many medications are banned (not always the case in the sport of flat racing in the United States). But as stated, enforcement is often a question and there is always the possibility of riders, trainers, and veterinarians working around regulations.

As we've mentioned, it is often quite difficult to convince owners of the amount of time an injured horse may need to rest *without work* to allow an injury to heal or to recover from illness. Understandably, riders are often anxious to get back in the saddle or a livelihood is at stake. Similarly, human athletes get frustrated waiting for their own injuries to heal and often end up reinjured due to impatiently returning to activity too soon, or training through pain and medication.

Riding, showing, or racing a horse that is being actively medicated for pain can lead to long-term chronic problems that may end or dramatically alter the horse's career. If you are medicating your horse for injury-related pain, but still working him at the *same intensity* that may have caused the pain in the first place, you are setting the horse up for further, more severe injuries.

Training professionally became somewhat discouraging over the past couple of decades—in all the disciplines and breeds I was involved with.

ELIMINATING BANNED SUBSTANCES FROM SPORTS FOR HORSE AND HUMAN

The FEI Clean Sport policy includes an affiliation with the World Anti-Doping Agency (www.wada-ama.org) for human athletes in an effort to eliminate banned substances from *all* sports. Not only is the use of performance-enhancing drugs cheating, it can be physically and emotionally damaging to all involved over time. Of course, horses have no say in the matter if they are being drugged for performance. Humans can at least make a conscious choice as to what they put in their bodies—although addiction can play a significant role in that decision. The rampant use and abuse of drugs has become one of the major policy issues in equestrian sport.

In spite of new research in regard to horse health and the high-tech modalities with which to diagnose and treat a wide range of conditions, many horse owners are unwilling or unable to pay for extensive diagnoses and treatment, particularly when the horse is used primarily for recreational purposes. For all the improvements in equine medicine, I see more lame horses with chronic conditions than in the past. Horses of all ages, of all breeds and types, in all disciplines, seem to be very susceptible to congenital defects and breakdowns, even at an early age. Good conformation and good bone with strong hooves used to be hallmarks by which to gauge the potential for a horse to stay sound. Yet horses today are often surprisingly weak in one or more critical areas.

Compassion, respect, and love for these animals hasn't, in itself, been enough to fully alleviate the suffering of masses of horses or prevent them from ending up in painful and compromised situations. It is a real dilemma as a trainer to go to shows or large barns and witness the amount of general discomfort horses actually put up with. Many well-meaning people who adore their horses have at the same time committed their horses to activities that cause them pain or stress. This, again, isn't limited to any particular breed or activity. It is universal within the industry.

If you have made a mistake when it comes to your horse, as we all do sometimes, forgive yourself, and proceed to take care of him in the future to the best of your abilities.

Awareness of how a horse responds to pain and excessive pressure is part of developing a level of compassion that will be retained through more intense phases of training and competition. Understanding methods that help compassion become a continuous part of *all* your equine-related activities will help ensure the most appropriate response in the moment. For example, a horse that is hard to handle due to excitement or because he's been stall-bound may require some strength to keep under control, but he does not have to be punished unreasonably for his behavior. As we've noted in this book, having compassion includes being able to control a horse in the safest way possible, communicating with him in a way he understands, so that nobody gets hurt.

It also means listening to what your horse *would* say to you if he *could*. A runner can say to him or herself, "Hey, that race last weekend took a lot out of me, I need an extra day or two to rest." Your horse *cannot* say, "Hey, you jumped me in six classes last weekend and my legs still hurt. I need another day or two of recovery time."

Even when horses are only used in non-riding programs and workshops, their physical abilities might be limited. It would be in the best interests of the horses if their stress and fatigue levels were carefully monitored. Spending time in round pens or doing a lot of ground-based exercises still requires a handler be mindful and check legs for heat and swelling, shoes and hooves for fit and trim, as well as the overall body for soreness, illness, or injury. "Pasture ornaments," rescues, and other horses that are not ridden cannot be neglected in terms of health issues—their special needs must be properly addressed, just as much as a horse that's regularly used for driven or under-saddle activities.

Horses are serving humans in new and wonderful ways that have been tremendous in developing the horse-human bond.

Since the manufacture of the automobile changed the role of the horse in society (as we discussed in chapter 11), horses have become part of the human existence in many different and—from our perspective—meaningful ways. These developments have been wonderful for humans. That said, we *still* have to consider what it means to ask the horse to participate in sessions that focus primarily on a *person's* emotional development, perhaps occasionally at the expense of the horse's welfare.

All disciplines and activities involving horses are a *two-way exchange*. The horse can be so valuable in helping ease the turmoil of the human psyche, soothe emotional wounds, build up self-esteem where there is none, and provide goals and a general sense of purpose in life, but we must always be considerate of the amount of time he is asked to "give" to our needs and perform certain tasks. We must be willing to shape training sessions, alter riding programs, adjust competitive ambitions, and customize the horse's general work schedule around the natural rhythms of equine behavior and his limits for tolerance, both physical and mental.

Maintaining compassion in all types of training programs and equestrian environments reaches well beyond the individual, the local barn, or regional show grounds. It extends beyond individual preferences in terms of breeds and discipline. We must help each other, help our horses.

Dr. Allen Schoen:

There are various approaches and techniques in different equestrian disciplines that have been questioned as being unethical or potentially harmful. Issues include (but are not limited to) inappropriate or excessive medications and training techniques that may be considered inhumane. With this in mind, it seems we should ask ourselves and our peers within the industry:

1 Is this a healthy, humane choice for this horse?

2 Is this accepted protocol in this particular breed or discipline? Should it be? Is it time to challenge the belief system of this breed or discipline?

When you can bravely ask yourself and others these questions, and expect honest answers while harboring the willingness to act if necessary, then this can be recognized as a chance for positive change.

Breeds and disciplines are all about us as humans needing to fit everything into a category with its own specific label.

I've discussed my challenges with labels before (see p. 268). By identifying too strongly with a label, we may not be allowing, say, a particular horse to show up as what he *really* is because we have perceptions and expectations about him based on that label. For example, we can be continually surprised by the gap between our perceptions of what we think a horse might be like due to his breed or type, and what he might actually be like in reality, based on his own preferences and abilities.

The human mind likes to organize things and put them into "boxes." It is a way of interacting in this world. We tend to categorize and divide in order to organize, which is normal. However, can we transcend that to allow for someone or some horse to be different from the limited parameters of the "box" we would normally put them in? Isn't this the more compassionate response when it comes to trying to remove divisiveness and criticism from the equestrian industry? Aren't many of these problems the result of the labels we place on *everything*?

EXERCISE IN COMPASSION:

Defying Breed Blindness

1   Note the reasons why you love your favorite horse. His head? His color? His long mane? His athleticism?

2   Now name another breed that you are either quite unfamiliar with or maybe even think you dislike. Determine which characteristics you could appreciate in that kind of horse, too. Spend some time with what you imagine to be his best attributes. Focus on what you might like, not the unfamiliar or negative.

3   Consider what you like about your favorite horse and what you think you would like about the other breed. Where are there significant differences in qualities? Similarities?

Breeds, expectations, and the various disciplines within the equestrian world have been created for our benefit and enjoyment. But it is this that also ultimately divides us. If we can learn to let go of the labels and expectations we place on ourselves, our horses, and the disciplines we participate in, we can come from a more compassionate viewpoint of the entire industry and see the opportunity to increase welfare for all involved.

Across disciplines, there has been an exponential and unfortunate increase in the use and abuse of medications and performance-enhancing drugs. While most of these substances are synthesized compounds, concerns have also been raised over the definitions and use of herbal and so-called "natural" products.

There are many herbal products out there, and it is very confusing given the array of choices. Frankly, many of them are not in alignment with the best interests of the horse and some are unethically produced. When I use or recommend herb-based products, I try to work with companies where I know the people involved. I have to be able to trust at some level that the company is using ethical methods of production, checking the source of ingredients for pesticides and toxins, testing for purity, and that they understand and stand by the active ingredients. I use a very limited network of suppliers. Even then, I still have to trust in the integrity and compassion of someone else, and that the company and those that work there have the good of horse and horse owner at heart.

As an example, an unbiased herbal research evaluation company found when testing ginseng products for humans, that only a small percentage of the active ingredient the product claimed to contain was *actually* in it. And in 2015 an investigation of store-brand herbal supplements sold by particular retailers by the New York State attorney general's office found four out of five products tested did not include any of the herbs listed. In both cases, the product labels were unreliable.[1,2]

ConsumerLab.com has found problems with many ginseng supplements over the years. In the review of ginseng supplements updated in February of 2015, 25 percent of ginseng supplements selected for testing contained less ginseng than expected from their labels (https://www.consumerlab. com/reviews/ginseng_supplements/ginseng/).

In February of 2015, The New York Times *reported the New York State attorney general's office investigation of store-brand herbal products— including ginkgo biloba, St. John's wort, and ginseng pills—sold by GNC, Target, Walgreens, and Walmart. Not only did the products tested not include the herbs listed on their labels, they contained "hidden ingredients and contaminants that could be dangerous to people with allergies to those substances. That such well-known brands should be found to be fraudulent suggests that the problem infects the entire industry" (http:// www.nytimes.com/2015/02/07/opinion/herbal-supplements-with- out-herbs.html?_r=0).*

1,2

I have seen herbs help where drugs are not helping, and some herbs also have fewer side effects. However, there is a gray area when we consider the limitations, indications, and actions herbal remedies might be having, and I

AN HERBAL CAUTION

It is of note that the FEI Prohibited Substances List specifically mentions the use of herbal and "natural" products, and in fact, warns against their use:

"The FEI however cautions athletes, trainers, grooms and veterinarians against the use of herbal medications, tonics, oral pastes and products of which the detailed ingredients and quantitative analysis are unknown and could therefore contain one or more Prohibited Substances. Moreover, the persons administering herbal or so-called natural products to a horse or pony for health reasons or to affect its performance, who have been informed that the plant of origin or its ingredients do not violate the FEI regulations, may have been misinformed. The use of any herbal or natural product to affect the performance of a horse or pony in a calming (tranquilizing) or an energizing (stimulant) manner is expressly forbidden by the FEI regulations. The use of a calming product during competition may also have important safety consequences" (http://www.fei.org/fei/cleansport/ad-h/prohibited-list).

understand why the FEI has a stringent policy regarding the use of herbal or "natural" products (see sidebar, above). In my textbook, *Complementary and Alternative Veterinary Medicine*, I go through all the safety considerations of herbs and their various concerns. Again, it is vital to know your source, trust the quality of production and ingredients, and follow the rules of the governing body when it comes to administration in conjunction with competition.

Some think herbs and natural medicine do not work at all.

Various herbs have *known* pharmacologic effects. They tend to be dose-dependent, and results directly correspond to amount administered. Quality of the herbs, percentage of active ingredients, the source of the herbs, and other factors also play a role in its efficacy. Also, few products work on each and every animal in the same way.

One of the challenges with veterinary associations has been the claim, "Homeopathy does not work." But the very fact that these products are listed by the FEI and other governing bodies and regulated alongside other prohibited substances suggests that some individuals do acknowledge that they have physiological effects. They must come from FDA-approved facilities.

Homeopathy and herbal medicine are two different categories. Herbal supplements are regulated by the FDA but not as drugs or as foods. They are categorized as "dietary supplements."

If an herbal supplement or medication helps a horse keep going, ensuring the horse a home, is it unreasonable to use the substance? What are the ethics concerning welfare around this issue?

An important question concerning medicating horses is, if it helps the horse and rider work together, and therefore ensures the horse has a home, is it unreasonable to use it? I completely agree with the FEI regulations on "Clean Sport" that at the highest level of international competition, no, horses shouldn't be allowed to participate if they are on certain types of regulated medications. Yet when you go below the FEI level you find so many horses on painkillers, calming agents, and performance-enhancing drugs these days. Some medications or supplements may make a horse useful and safe in a particular situation, and without these things...what would be the fate of the horse? These are important questions to consider.

To some degree, I think it depends on each individual situation and weighing the risk/benefit ratio of the product in question for the horse and rider. For example, an older horse you use for schooling or unrated shows needs some medication for pain but still enjoys going to shows and jumping small fences occasionally, the medication helps keep the horse a valuable addition to the lesson barn, giving beginner riders a safe, enjoyable learning experience. And perhaps the horse enjoys what he gets to do, too.

This is that "response-ability" we've discussed before: deciding what the most compassionate choice is for the horse in a particular situation, while at the same time abiding by the rules and regulations of sanctioned competition. The issues discussed in this chapter look beyond individual preferences for breeds and disciplines and take into consideration the most compassionate approach, not only for horses and their activities, but the general body of equestrian sports and competition as a whole. Ultimately it's the welfare of the horse that defies breed, type, or color, and surmounts the questions raised when competing in a particular discipline. This is the unifying force behind all of us as a compassionate equine community.

Questions to Consider

BASED ON PRINCIPLE 18

1   When I let go of labels—of the "boxes" I like to put things in—do I see the world a bit differently? If so, how does that make me feel?

2   What are my thoughts and feelings regarding the use of medications and herbal supplements for my horse? For myself? How does that differ?

3   Do I consider all the potential ramifications of medications and/or supplements each time I choose to use them or not use them for my horse?

4   Can I look beyond my choice of breed and discipline and still ask if what I am doing with my horse is the most compassionate approach for him?

5   If I am pushing for standards that are beyond my horse's capability, am I willing to be flexible and alter my activity so my horse will be more comfortable?

CHAPTER NINETEEN

Compassionate Rehabilitation

We embrace compassionate rehabilitative programs.
A cradle-to-cradle equestrian model ensures a humane
life from birth to completion for all horses.

Susan Gordon:

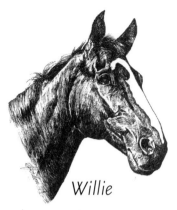

Willie

I rescued Willie out of compassion. Not really needing a horse at the time, I was initially more curious and "just looking" at him than I was interested in really buying him. My temptation to acquire a horse sprang from the fact that I had a backyard with an empty barn. My quandary was weighing how much I wanted a horse versus the questionable stability of the resources necessary for his care. For me, the fact that he was going to be sent to the slaughterhouse made it a different story.

You might wonder what kind of motivation is behind the decision to send a horse "down the road," so to speak. For the many horse lovers, it would be unthinkable. For others, they may feel they have no other choice if they can no longer afford to feed or care for a horse that is aged or unrideable. I don't know exactly why Willie's owner considered ending his life in such a way. The man did not appear to have the skill to ride or rehabilitate the big Hanoverian correctly, and he certainly was not feeding Willie well. It was likely quite simply the truth when the man told me nobody else wanted him.

As with the ex-racehorses I'd ridden for many years, this was a traumatized horse. It was a different kind of trauma than what the track produces, but a protocol of short, productive sessions still proved to be the most effective way to rehabilitate Willie. Restoring his health and well-being was my first priority.

If you believe in those "meant to be" situations, this was probably one of them. From the first time I saw a beautiful Hanoverian in Calgary I wanted one, but I could never afford to purchase one of my own. So here was Willie, an "old style," big, drafty type of Warmblood, like those that originally won my heart, albeit a little beat up and well past his prime. He taught me a lot about compassion and the real value of an aged horse. My reward was his complete turnaround. From skinny and dull to muscled and shiny, he was, following his rehabilitation, a sight to behold.

You've probably heard many stories about rescued animals that appear to understand what it means to have a human save them from a bad situation. You might even have a rescued pet or horse yourself. Sometimes, their behavior seems to convey a sense of gratitude that they express in any way they can. After we got through his hunger and residual pain, Willie was one such animal. As I've mentioned, when he came "back to normal," he was happy to pack beginners around small cross-rail courses and became a wonderful babysitter and companion for youngsters and sick or frightened horses. What was critical in this case is that I was able to manage enough time and resources to get this horse back up to good mental and physical conditioning before even considering putting another rider on him. It was almost a two-year process, and you've been reading segments of that challenging journey throughout this book.

At the age of 42 I made the decision to stop riding full-time. I had a tough training project in the form of a spoiled, poorly started, three-year-old, 17.2-hand Thoroughbred filly. The day she took off across the arena with me was the last straw. Something deep inside said, "Enough." The pressure had become overwhelming and I made some quick, radical changes in my life as a result—some of which were probably more in the category of "reaction" than "response." My mother had passed away the previous summer, and my grief combined with the demands of the horse business was too much to bear.

I sold my precious jumping and dressage saddles, then had to make the decision as to what to do with my last horse, Willie. My personal and professional circumstances were such that I wanted him to leave the barn, too, and hopefully go to a quiet place to live out his life in a comfortable retirement. As luck would have it, there was a reputable rescue organization in the city run by a wealthy socialite, and she agreed to take Willie. I wrote a long note explaining what a special horse he was and prayed the right person or persons would adopt him.

All too frequently I'm reminded of the impermanence of everything, as I'm sure many of you are, too. The day I sent Willie off to yet another home was a sad one indeed. He looked back at me from inside the trailer with a final, grumpy, good-bye flick of his ears, and off he went. At 28 years old, he was guaranteed a forever home with two fellows who made it their mission to keep horses to their last day on earth. I was fortunate they were found through the rescue organization, although I would have definitely preferred to have kept Willie myself until his life ended.

My days of owning horses are over, but I am hoping to make good use of my time left on this planet to make others aware of what it means to be responsible for horses in every moment and through to the end of their days. We owe so much gratitude to them. They have served humanity well.

As I've shared with you already, after turning professional, most of the horses I rode were off-the-track Thoroughbreds in need of rehabilitation and reschooling. Horses come off the track with a variety of lameness and psychological issues, requiring a lot of compassion and patience in their transition to a new life. Many never find their way to the kind of person who has the experience, tolerance, and patience to help them through the rehabilitative process. Sadly, many end up in slaughterhouses for a very tragic ending to their lives—often at a very young age.

Horses can live upward of 30 years, which is a long time when considering a permanent home, a career, and a comfortable retirement. The most fortunate horses live out their lives on a farm with green pastures and appropriate shelters. They have competent caretakers who tend to their basic needs of feeding and health care. Such places are diminishing in number as development replaces many traditional horsekeeping operations. And so it has become imperative to consider a general model of sustainability for the entire equine world. As hard as it is to look at the numbers of homeless horses, there is a great need to raise public awareness regarding the welfare of all equines.

"Too many" horses on the planet is not sustainable. Currently, their numbers are greater than there are people who can afford to care for them properly. Visit your local equine rescue and rehabilitation programs and find out where the "homeless" horses have come from, and why. Find out if they are being success-fully re-homed or going to auctions where their future could be very dim, indeed. Everyone who loves horses could help by taking responsibility for the excessive numbers of horses bred and born every year. The life cycles of the ones who are already here deserve to be monitored for the quality of their care and well-being. This is an enormous task!

Visit an equine rescue and rehabilitation facility in your area. Volunteer or support them in any way you can. Introduce them to the 25 Principles of Compassionate Equitation.

Rescues are often overwhelmed by the number of horses they are asked to take in. Many equine operations experienced financial difficulty when the economy plummeted almost a decade ago, which added considerable strain to the situation. There was nowhere to go with low-to-mid priced marketable horses. Owners felt forced to let their horses go to auctions or for almost nothing.[1] Others felt compelled to euthanize healthy horses they could neither sell nor afford to feed.[2] And then there are all the horses that end up neglected, ill, and starving until authorities come to their aid. This situation is frustrating. And it is unacceptable. It seems like everywhere we turn there are cases of abuse and neglect in the news...and those are just the ones we hear about.

> *According to the Unwanted Horse Coalition, "Unwanted horses can be old or young, sick or healthy, purebred or grade, highly trained or barely halter broke. They are unwanted for just as many varying reasons—the horse may have become sick, injured, old, outgrown, dangerous, a burden, or simply too expensive to care for (http://www.unwantedhorsecoalition. org/resources/rehab_brochure.pdf).*

1,2

> *In Dr. Christy Corp-Minamiji's 2013 post "Under the Blue Tarps" on The-Horse.com, we see the stark matter of equine overpopulation from the perspective of the veterinarian who receives requests to euthanize the horses owners can no longer afford. "Modern reality holds too many unwanted and unusable horses: old, intractable, chronically or expensively lame, or ill," she writes. "Reality is high hay prices, high fuel costs, lost jobs, foreclosed homes, and low prices for marketable horses. Today, the horse reflects discretionary income that for many is dwindling. The wanted horse is a luxury; the unwanted horse, a burden" (http://cs.thehorse.com/ blogs/across-the-fence/archive/2013/01/22/under-the-blue-tarps.aspx).*

My eyes were opened to the extent of the problems in the industry when I was researching a documentary film I was making about horse slaughter in 2010. Even as a professional, I had no idea how many horses end up in the processing plants in Canada, or what a terrible end they experience. It is truly horrific. In the past, I had several horses in training that were pulled off trucks at the slaughter plants and rescued. Understandably, they exhibited post-traumatic stress symptoms throughout their newfound lives.

I wonder how many horses have previous owners who would be shocked to learn the fate of their old mounts. Or breeders who would be mortified to know their gorgeous stallion's babies ended up in a kill pen, perhaps thousands of miles from where their lives began. There are less conscientious people who do not seem to care about a horse's longevity or quality of life, and it would be preferable if they were not horse owners or breeders in the first place. As a compassionate equine community, we try to ensure that we and others in the industry maintain a high regard for equine life.

In my opinion, slaughter is *not* a humane way to end a horse's life. Nor does the horse deserve the kind of treatment he typically receives from the moment he lands in an auction house that sells to kill buyers. This is a cold hard fact of the equestrian business. Sometimes horses are transported over thousands of miles in cramped trailers without water and food. Many are injured before and during shipping, causing terrible pain and distress. For others, their suffering is prolonged when kept in homes where people cannot care for them properly. These are very real problems of "homeless" and unwanted horses, which still today have not been resolved.

"Typically, rescuers celebrate the lives that they are able to save, and grieve over those left behind at auctions where feedlot operators pick up their quota. Horse rescuers express regrets about the fact that more cannot be salvaged."

Canadian Horse Defence Coalition
(www.defendhorsescanada.org)

Having compassion for all beings inspires us to look at the poor, the rejected, and the homeless of our own species, as well as equines. How can we alleviate their suffering? Is there some way to prevent it in the first place?

Can we, as an equestrian community, come together to help rescue and rehabilitate those horses that deserve another chance? The numbers are astounding.[3] How many little girls out there would give anything to have contact with horses? How many senior citizens would love to live in a home that overlooked a beautiful pasture full of horses? Think of the myriad ways horses can be of benefit to human beings. What could you do in your community or region to help find a way to provide for unwanted horses? How *can* we work this out?

Willie's story, which you find throughout this book, is an illustration of the challenges and rewards of a compassionate reschooling program. One of the goals of *The Compassionate Equestrian* is to develop a worldwide database of Compassionate Trainers with enough skill and experience to help reschool and

PORTRAIT OF AN ANIMAL RESCUE

Brogan Horton is a dynamic young woman, still in her early twenties. She is the founder and executive director of Animal Rescue Unit, a non-profit rescue based at her family's 60-acre farm in Bridgeton, Maine. Her compassion for animals and humans knows no bounds, and she has set an example of caregiving and rehabilitation for horses that many of us would find hard to fathom. Brogan has witnessed the worst of what humanity can dish out to horses, but has done her utmost to counterweight the scales, turning many despondent lives into happy, productive ones.

A "day in the life" of Brogan could fill an entire book in itself. Managing a rescue, especially with the statistics in today's equine industry of "homeless" and virtually unrideable horses, is extremely difficult and taxing—emotionally, financially, and physically. Hearing what motivates her and keeps her going can be a source of inspiration for us all.

"I would have to say my motivation is the tremendous need that I see on a daily basis," says Brogan. "I get numerous phone calls and emails every day from people who either need to give up an animal or are reporting an animal in trouble. I could fill my barn many times over.

"There are several reasons for the large number of unwanted horses in Maine, as well as elsewhere in the United States. One of the primary reasons was the downturn in the economy and its slow recovery. Many horse owners were laid off or had to take a cut in pay...one day a horse trailer pulled into the yard, and the owners got out of the truck holding their foreclosure papers in their hands. They said they had to move immediately, and could not find anyone to take their horse. Although we did not need to take in another horse at the time, we knew they had more than enough on their minds, and thought it was the least we could do to help them out.

"Many of the horses we rescue come from bad situations and are very often traumatized. We have had many horses in the rescue that have gone to auction, which is truly a traumatic experience for any horse—the sounds, smells, and

Continued →

commotion are obviously very scary. We have also had many horses that have been mistreated by their owners. Starvation, incorrect farrier work, cruel and inexperienced handling—these are, unfortunately, also common in rescue horses.

"The most compassionate way to rehabilitate rescue horses varies from horse to horse. Proper nutrition, veterinary care and farrier work, as well as love and attention will bring most horses back to health.

"Further, there needs to be more horse owner education in order for there to be fewer horses in horse rescues, as well as in the 'slaughter pipeline.' Many people feel that if they have a yard in the back of their house, or a patch of wooded land, that they have room for a horse. We have seen over and over again, that if the owner sees green grass, he or she feels they have plenty of feed to support a horse, and that is more then likely *not* the case. Soon, the horse is breaking out of fences or losing weight, perhaps also difficult to ride, and off he goes into the buy-and-sell market. We have seen several horses with hooves that were 'home trimmed' by the owner, resulting in permanently damaged hooves. Often, this is due to new horse owners who are ignorant to the true cost of horse ownership and so cut corners on farrier work, vetting, or feeding. More horse owner education would greatly help in situations like this.

"We need to reduce the number of horses bred every year. This includes 'backyard breeders,' who might breed many foals, which turn out to be more then they can handle, or not what they wanted, and also the large horse associations, which promote breeding as well, looking for the next big thing. However, tens of thousands of 'average' horses are born each year, only to be bought and sold all their lives. Sad to say, very few horses end up in a 'forever home.'

"Animal Rescue Unit is working to promote awareness of these and other serious issues facing horses in the United States. Many people are still unaware that there are thousands of horses still being shipped to Canada and Mexico each year to be slaughtered for human consumption. There also continues to be an active black market for horse meat in Florida. The wild horses of the West are being cruelly rounded up, and many of those animals are often found in the auction ring, being purchased by dealers for slaughter. Raising public awareness is something Animal Rescue Unit remains dedicated to as we also continue to personally rescue as many horses as we can."

You can find Animal Rescue Unit on Facebook. For further information on organizations dedicated to helping educate the horse industry about the issue of unwanted and "homeless" horses, contact your local or regional rescue, or visit:

- *Unwanted Horse Coalition* in the United States, which comprises a broad alliance of equine organizations that have joined together under the American Horse Council (www.unwantedhorsecoalition.org).

- *World Horse Welfare*, established in the United Kingdom by Ada Cole in 1927. The mission statement of WHW is to work with horses, horse owners, communities, organizations, and governments to help improve standards and stamp out suffering in the UK and worldwide (www.worldhorsewelfare.org).

rehabilitate horses like Willie.[4] We would like to see a pool of individuals who can devote time and resources to re-homing rescued horses and matching them with appropriate situations. Of course, ideally, it would be best if every horse could be compassionately started by a good trainer and ridden by individuals committed to developing independent seats, as well as treating their horses in kind, tolerant, and forgiving manners, so as to prevent them from needing rescue and rehabilitation in the first place. That would be my dream for all horses and all people who wish to connect with them.

> *According to the Canadian Horse Defence Coalition (CHDC) website, Agriculture and Agri-Food Canada reported that 82,175 horses were slaughtered in Canada in 2012. These animals arrived at one of this nation's federally-inspected slaughter plants from a variety of directions. Many were so-called "culls" from breeding operations and industries (for instance, Quarter Horses and Thoroughbred racehorses) and many others were from private homes no longer able or willing to continue caring for their horses (http://defendhorsescanada.org/horse-protection-initiatives).*

> *New Stride Thoroughbred Adoption Society of Abbotsford, BC, is one of two Canadian adoption societies granted "aftercare accreditation." Since 2002 New Stride has found homes for over 120 former Thoroughbred*

racehorses (http://newstride.com/). Stateside, New Vocations Racehorse Adoption is the largest racehorse adoption program in the United States with three locations, offering horses "a safe-haven, rehabilitation, and continued education" in order to transition them to new homes. Over 5,500 Thoroughbreds and Standardbreds have been placed in qualified homes through New Vocations' efforts since its inception in 1992 (www.horseadoption.com).

The goal of writing this book is to illustrate the ways the horse industry would benefit from a paradigm shift—and this is in regards to general management, lack of rider responsibility, drug abuse, and the overproduction of stock, to name just a very few elements we should be willing to consider with a compassionate eye and readiness for change. There is no aspect of the horse industry, from the wild herds that roam various places around the globe to the upper echelons of the international show world, that is currently untouched by high profile, challenging problems.

But we maintain that if the 25 Principles of Compassionate Equitation are accepted and practiced, we might be able to have a sensible dialogue and at least *begin* the process of eradicating the biggest obstacles to equine welfare. In chapter 22, we suggest a life-cycle management program that follows horses from birth to their life's completion (p. 356). As a community, we could then develop further resources to assist in rescue, rehabilitation, and when necessary, humane euthanasia, making those resources available to *all* horse owners, regardless of breed, show, or organization affiliations, or geographical location. A simple commitment to developing the compassionate actions we have already discussed on previous pages can make a huge difference to our personal relationships with horses, to the horse industry itself, and to all horse people at large.

Dr. Allen Schoen:

According to Dr. Dan Siegel in Carolyn Gregoire's 2014 Huffington Post piece "What Neuroscience Can Teach Us About Compassion," "One way to build integration in the brain is through healthy, caring relationships with others. These relationships can make us more mindful and more compassionate, facilitating greater integration in the brain...a relationship can be defined as the sharing of energy and information flow. And when we understand how that energy and information flow is happening—it could be with words, with the body, with an attitude—we can feel it, and we feel it with each other."

Of course, as Dr. Siegel points out, "unhealthy relationships can have just the opposite effect on the brain. Abuse and neglect impair the integrative regions of the brain—as a treatment for individuals recovering from abusive relationships, adding mindfulness to a psychotherapy practice could be beneficial."

The rehabilitation process with a horse can be a process of two-way healing.

If you're caught up in your world—as a depressed or anxious person can be, for example—your mind and electrical *neural-net activity* is firing very tightly and flooding the amygdala with fear and anger.[5] There is a lot of electrical intensity, which draws the energy field *inward* versus radiating *outward* as it does when an individual is meditating, especially when meditating on compassion for all beings (see my discussion of the Transpecies Field Theory on p. 326). Research has found that part of the hypothalamus related to the sensory awareness of your skin "quiets down" in such meditation, and you begin to experience the feeling of being "connected with everything."[6] I hypothesize that if the energy field of the person and the field of his or her heart were measured, anger will "close down" and "shrink" the field, whereas thinking about love and love for others quiets activity, allowing the energy field to be more expansive (see p. 93 for more about energy fields of the body and the heart). I believe this could also be applied to horses.

Dr. Joseph E. LeDoux of the Center for Neural Science, New York University, New York, states that "The amygdaloid region of the brain (i.e. the amygdala) is a complex structure involved in a wide range of normal behavioral functions and psychiatric conditions. Not so long ago it was an obscure region of the brain that attracted relatively little scientific interest. Today it is one of the most heavily studied brain areas, and practically a household word" (http://www.scholarpedia.org/article/Amygdala).

According to Dr. Ananya Mandal on News Medical, "The hypothalamus is a small but important part of the brain. It contains several small nuclei with a variety of functions. It plays an important role in the nervous system as well as in the endocrine system. It is linked to another small and vital gland called the pituitary gland" (http://www.news-medical.net/health/What-is-the-Hypothalamus.aspx).

5,6

We cannot actually teach our horses to meditate, however, so there are ways to look at their physiology and determine which tools and methods we can use to help balance their autonomic nervous system (ANS). As mentioned previously, the ANS is divided into the *sympathetic* (flight or fight mode) and *parasympathetic* (calm and quiet mode). In a sympathetic response there is a release of adrenaline, which causes *vasoconstriction* to all the organs, decreasing the function of those organs. It wouldn't be unreasonable to assume there is also a decrease in electrical activity, causing the horse's energy field to shrink. Whereas a parasympathetic reaction produces *vasodilation*, increases heat, circulation, and so expands the energy field.

Whichever states the horse and human are in when they meet, their two energetic fields then merge into one.

As discussed, we have the ability to create a more *compassionate* Transpecies Field based on our thoughts and emotions. By doing so, we become a place where animals *want to be*. This is the Compassionate Field Theory at work. Part of creating this field is to first be aware of it by *bringing our thoughts into physicality*. Our thoughts, intentions, and emotions affect any external tools we use to work with horses.

If someone comes into the energy field of a horse that has been handled with compassion, and that horse radiates a field of compassion as well, depending on the person's sensitivity, awareness, and the clarity of his or her mental state, he or she will pick up on *the horse's* level of kindness and sensitivity.[7] What I am saying is that even if a person comes into a barn *without* an awareness of being compassionate, that particular horse can and will have an immediate impact on him or her. This is the gist of my Compassionate Field Theory.

7 *"'My bounty is as boundless as the sea,' says Shakespeare's Juliet. 'My love as deep; the more I give to thee, / the more I have, for both are infinite.' That's how kindness works too," writes Emily Esfahani Smith in her June 2014 article "Masters of Love" in* The Atlantic. *"There's a great deal of evidence showing the more someone receives or witnesses kindness, the more they will be kind themselves, which leads to upward spirals of love and generosity in a relationship" (http://www.theatlantic.com/health/archive/2014/06/happily—ever—after/372573/).*

The Institute of HeartMath (see p. 94) has a formula for measuring and monitoring the effects of such interactions between humans. We are looking to determine a system for measuring those fields as they occur between the *human and the horse*. Inevitably, I think that's part of the horse-human bond and why horses have such a calming effect on us. They are normally in a much calmer energetic field than we are.

We can see evidence of a Compassionate Field Effect given the circumstances of the same horse being treated by a veterinarian with compassion, and one without. I have experienced this, and over the years have noticed the different impacts of the two types of veterinarians. I've had clients remark how some veterinarians always have to sedate a horse to work on him, or how a horse does not like a particular veterinarian at all, whereas I rarely use sedation any more for acupuncture and chiropractic. Clients often call attention to how calm horses are around me and how they'll allow me to perform acupuncture without resistance. A veterinarian with a different mindset, who isn't calm and compassionate, will often have to sedate the same horses before he or she can get near them with an acupuncture needle. My point is not that the horses' reactions to me are unique—they do not have to be. Compassion can be part of every veterinarian's medicine bag.

The attitude, the energetic field, the psycho-physiologic energy emitted by the veterinarian, directly impacts how the horse reacts to that veterinarian.

I've had to treat horses that were first treated by another veterinarian who I know is quite tense, nervous, and angry, and on those occasions, I couldn't get near the horses with a needle. As I've mentioned on my website, when a horse has had a negative experience to a veterinarian administering an injection, either intravenously or intramuscularly, it is not uncommon for the horse to then become more and more anxious and fearful to *any* injections to a point of being extremely difficult to handle and even dangerous. This is what had happened with these horses: They had become completely "needle-phobic" due to the other vet's manner. I only performed musculoskeletal adjustments until they started to trust me and realize that I was helping them, rather than causing them pain.

You'll see similar responses when considering trainers and training methods, too. As we've mentioned previously, a horse—being a prey-animal—will generalize when it comes to danger. When he has been conditioned by a "non-mindful" veterinarian, or beaten up by a trainer, he will associate anyone who even vaguely resembles the individual who hurt him as having the potential to do him harm, and he will respond accordingly. The horse will "fire" that pattern of fear that's been "wired" and then react. This is indicative of post-traumatic stress disorder (PTSD), just as it is in humans. And "danger" becomes more and more generalized as time goes on.

Evaluate and treat a horse's medical conditions before beginning a rehabilitation program.

One of the key challenges in diagnosing the many conditions that can cause horses to react uncharacteristically with distrust and in a defensive mode is the possibility of a physical disorder. For example, head-shaking has many causes (one known medically as *trigeminal neuralgia*). Sometimes you do not even know exactly what the cause is until the horse actually responds to a particular treatment. Another example, as we've mentioned previously in this book, is Lyme disease (or tick-borne illness), an infectious as well as inflammatory condition that can cause the horse's personality to change due to chronic pain and also presents a challenge to many veterinarians in the diagnostic process.

As the 25 Principles of Compassionate Equitation state, always assume and rule out pain as the cause of a horse's behavioral problems, especially when his base personality has become more aggressive or altered suddenly (although this may not be apparent in a newly acquired rescue or rehabilitation project). Owners must get past their own personal issues in the denial of pain or other medical phenomena as a cause of behavioral or training problems with horses.

When pain has been ruled out, and the behavior remains, there are techniques that can help with desensitizing the horse to the cause of his defensive behavior. One approach that's been very successful in humans for retraining and rehabilitation is Eye Movement Desensitization and Reprocessing (EMDR) developed by Francine Shapiro, PhD, in 1987. The EMDR approach helps to "unlock" fearful memories that continue to elicit unprovoked panic and visceral responses "as if" they were happening again. When a traumatic event is not processed and integrated into normal memory patterns, it does not fade with time and continues to cause anxiety and panic. Psychoanalyst Vera Muller-Paisner adapted the EMDR protocol to Bilateral Equine Tapping (BET), for similar work with horses, as we mentioned briefly in chapter 15 (see p. 260). It has been successful in some desensitization cases.[8]

In the Spring 2010 issue of Spring: A Journal of Archetype and Culture, *Vera Muller-Paisner and G.A. Bradshaw's article "Freud and the Family Horse: Exploration into Equine Psychotherapy" states, "There are several methods by which thoughts and feelings associated with trauma can be integrated and ameliorated. Often, it is the symptom presented which serves as the portal through which therapy can proceed....Among the approaches, cognitive behavior therapy (CBT) and Eye Movement Desensitization and Reprocessing (EMDR) are considered the most effective. EMDR was the treatment of choice (in its tactile form adapted for horses, Bilateral Equine Tapping for its application to horses (BET)" (http:// www.lifespanlearn.org/index.php/conferences/handouts/syllabus-2014/ gay-bradshaw/14-equine-psychotherapy/file).*

Muller-Paisner's battery-operated device attaches to the horse's halter or girth, depending on the target needed, and alternates the tapping mechanism from side to side. With the BET device in operation, the horse is carefully brought into the fear-inciting situation, using a specific protocol after a discussion with the owner and/or trainer. If the response is unsafe for horse or human, the situation is modified to a close association, and the tapping is adjusted on the horse while the horse is standing, until a sense of relaxation is seen. The horse then focuses on the tapping sensation, while the alternate tapping allows both sides of the brain to be available for the possibility of experiencing the fearful event differently. In this way the experience changes, the rewiring begins, and the horse doesn't break into fear mode.

We've been successful using this method in a couple of cases of horses with needle-phobia. Whether a hypodermic needle or an acupuncture needle, if there has been a negative experience with needle administration by someone and that person caused the phobia, BET seems to have been able to retrain the horses and resolve their post-traumatic stress to where they would accept needles again.

Yet another horse was a confirmed bucker who had frightened his rider to the point where she was afraid to get on him. Muller-Paisner's EMDR and BET therapy worked with both the horse and rider in this case and got them both over their fear of each other. However, it is important to note that we *first* had to resolve the underlying cause of why the horse was bucking, which was, in fact, a pain issue.

This horse had *three* different sources of pain that were setting off the bucking. We had to peel away each issue and treat each one, none of which had been previously diagnosed:

1   The horse had Lyme disease, so every time the saddle was put on, he was in pain and uncomfortable.

2   The saddle was poorly fitted.

3   The horse had hock problems. (The hock issues may have been further exacerbated because of the Lyme disease.)

With all three issues combined the horse was in considerable pain and discomfort. The Lyme disease was resolved with appropriate antibiotic therapy, the hocks were injected with conventional medications, and a properly fitting saddle was found. After the pain was relieved the horse still had a mental block and concerns leading to fear-related behavior responses. EMDR and BET were then brought in as the final tool to help rehabilitate both horse and rider in terms of their respective fear issues. Happily, they have been able to reconnect for an enjoyable riding experience.

If both horse and rider have had a bad experience with each other, after appropriate veterinary treatment and resolution of underlying issues, behavioral modification may involve specialized rehabilitation methods for the rider as well so the pair may work together once again.

We have the tools to aid in the resolution of such pain and trauma issues when simply having compassion for the animal (or human) in itself is not enough. Whether or not we need to engage those tools depends upon the severity of the conditions. Sometimes simply changing attitude and intention may be enough to solve certain issues. To the other extreme, there may be so much damage that no matter what you do, you cannot turn things around for a particular horse. In between those extremes are many opportunities to successfully reschool and retrain a rescue project.

While a horse is healing from past trauma, the "field integrity" of the people surrounding him is important. We need to understand that part of understanding the horse's response to us is being able to recognize our own energy field and what it is radiating toward the horse. Creating the intention of loving-kindness can help to create a more Compassionate Field, where a sense of calm permeates

EASING ANXIETY IN A RESCUE HORSE

I use different Traditional Chinese Herbal formulas that often help with stress and anxiety in a horse that is being rehabilitated, and they can help tremendously. The herbs can be used as the horse is being desensitized, and then eventually, the horse can be taken off the herbs—although some horses are so traumatized an owner may decide to have them remain on the supplements for the foreseeable future. It is possible to do so as many herbs seem to have few known side effects. Note: It is vital to know your source when using herbal remedies—see p. 311 for a discussion related to this subject.

Other nutritional supplements are available as well that can help "tone down" a rescue horse's stress and fear response. SmartPak® has one with magnesium that works well called Smart Calm (smartpakequine.com). Some people try valerian root, Rescue Remedy (Bachflower.com), or resort to tranquilizers in appropriate cases.

you, your horse, and everyone interacting with you. Integrating this awareness can be part of great benefit in equine rehabilitation.

Questions to Consider
BASED ON PRINCIPLE 19

1   Have I ever rescued or considered rescuing a horse? What are my thoughts and feelings on this subject after having read this chapter?

2   Am I aware of how past traumatic incidents (mine or his) may affect the relationship I have with my horse?

3   Do I understand how beneficial it is for me to work with my horse within an energy field of loving-kindness?

CHAPTER TWENTY

The "Response-ability" of Compassion

We choose to restore compassion to the center of all equine-based facilities, horse training techniques, and equestrian sports, and to clearly understand and acknowledge the difference between what constitutes kindness to horses and what does not. We cultivate responsible compassion toward all horses, including those deemed feral, unwanted, "homeless," aged, or unrideable for any reason.

Susan Gordon:

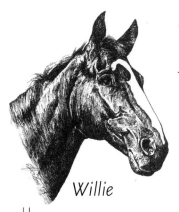

Willie

As you've learned, I had to decide what the best situation would be for Willie once I had taken responsibility for his future. The veterinarian who had cared for him at his previous owner's place told me he was only called out once, and that was because Willie was choking on something. He did not have much information otherwise, and couldn't shed light on what might have caused the unusual lumps under Willie's jaw and neck. The horse was not obviously lame, but he would not have passed a standard pre-purchase exam either. He was old, possibly unrideable.

As it turned out, bringing a broken down, beat up horse into my backyard was the catalyst for healing for both of us. Through Willie, I developed respect and compassion for older horses. I had the chance to spend quiet, reflective time together with him in the privacy of our beautiful home, and remember why horses had always been so important throughout the course of my life.

When the time came that we had to introduce ourselves to the boarding barn world and ride in the company of others, we were both tested as to just how far our "buttons" could be pushed and how much we wanted, or didn't want, to return to the world of competition. We both were invited back into the proximity of upper-level horses and riders, and it was very satisfying. In the end, we had journeyed together from "kind-of broken" to "restored," until it was time for both of us to retire to the latter portion of our lives.

Willie and I became "buddies" of the best kind. If he was suffering prior to being under my care, I can only hope that I did my best to alleviate that in the years we had together. I believe he understood that I was trying to help.

Compassion is a choice. We decide at a personal level if we feel sensitive enough to others' needs to *want* to alleviate their suffering, even after realizing we cannot actually alleviate the suffering of *every* person and *every* animal in the world. I believe most horse people would prefer optimal care and concern for horses at every equine facility and in every training program. But the task is monumental given the diverse personalities, backgrounds, and education of those in the equestrian business, and when we consider horses in developing nations, as well, where they are often still used for transportation and agriculture.

By now, most people are familiar with the ethical questions that have been raised regarding the North American racing industry, yet thousands of Thoroughbred foals continue to be born every year with the track their only hope.

Thoroughbred babies are sometimes passed on to nurse mares (whose own foals are taken away early) so the Thoroughbred mares can be bred back sooner. Youngsters are trained and run before their bodies are developed enough to handle the repetitive stress. The industry continues in the endless cycle of news-makers and money, as well as the drugs, breakdowns, and dark side of the backstretch, which we have all had a chance to see in numerous exposés over the past few years. This does not mean there aren't compassionate horsepeople in the Thoroughbred industry—in fact, there are many who care about their horses immensely. However, there remain negative aspects of the racing world that certainly need changing, and it has never done well by the huge numbers of horses bred and birthed in the search for a "star" that in the end cannot run fast enough to pay their way.

If it were possible to turn every Thoroughbred deemed "not a winner" out to green pastures and a life of ease, I am sure many people would be happy to comply. In the perfect equine world there would be rescue facilities in every country with enough financial backing to ensure satisfactory retirement for every horse, even if he could not run fast enough, was not up to breed standards, or was injured and worn out after a lifetime of service.

"Response-ability:" whether it is your own horse or a lesson horse, we owe them good care, a safe, healthy environment, and the trust instilled by correct, compassionate riding.

As we already covered on p. 165, at the basis of classical, correct equitation is the proverbial "good hands and seat." A compassionate equestrian aspires to develop these qualities on a well-schooled horse, and has a sense of responsibility to assess his or her skills and methods on a regular basis. Bonding, ground-work, and learning the horse's language comes from a tremendous amount

COMPASSIONATE HORSE CARE CHECKLIST

Being kind to your horse means:

- Giving regular, thorough grooming that checks every square inch for potential problems.

- Providing appropriate hoof care.

- Arranging qualified veterinary care.

- Ensuring equipment fits correctly and is not causing discomfort.

- Keeping stalls and paddocks clean and free of biting and irritating insects.

- Minimizing loud noise around the barn.

- Understanding how inherent herd psychology might affect behavior.

- Making sure your seat is balanced and your aids are correctly applied so as not to confuse the horse, disturb his balance, or inadvertently cause pain.

of time spent grooming, leading, and managing other tasks around the barn. "Response-ability" means the basic needs of your horse are first and foremost. For example, teaching your horse tricks but leaving him with a rough coat and unpicked hooves is not good horsemanship. If we are going to insist on keeping these animals in captivity, we owe it to them to pay attention to their health and welfare above all else.

What do we do with an "unrideable" horse?

Horses can live for 20 to 30 years or more, and those kept in barns and paddocks have a considerable "footprint" on the environment in a way that is different from the wild horses that still roam free. No horse—even if aged and unrideable—can simply be ignored or discarded. Just as we care for aging parents, we must find suitable answers to care for the large number of horses currently filling up rescues and rehabilitation centers, as well as endangered wild herds.

Cultivating compassion toward *all* horses includes developing an awareness of what happens to the horses we want the least to do with. This is especially true when the economy and shrinking availability of pastures and grazing land affects the industry in a negative way. If Compassionate Trainers were to become more prevalent, there might be fewer horses that are difficult to re-home.

It is impossible to save all horses from neglect and tragic endings, but if more equestrians can open their hearts to the needs of *all* horses, including those that have fallen through the cracks or might be considered "worthless" by some, then we will become known as a compassionate industry that cares deeply for all it calls its own.

UNRIDEABLE BUT NOT WITHOUT PURPOSE

When caring for a horse deemed unrideable for any number of reasons, be sure to check with your veterinarian to confirm whether pain is what has caused the horse to be unrideable, and if so, if something can be done to ease the pain. Your veterinarian can also help you determine activities other than riding that may or may not be appropriate as potential sources of exercise and entertainment for your horse, such as:

- Horse agility (in-hand and at-liberty obstacle coursework)

- "Babysitter" (a "buddy" horse used to accompany frightened, recuperating, or young horses)

- "Lesson model" for beginner riders to learn about grooming, handling, anatomy, or tacking-up (great for old horses who tie well and enjoy being groomed)

- Equine Assisted Learning (a program that uses horses to benefit human psychology)

- "Pony companion" (ponied off a green horse in training)

- Art or photography class model (art students always appreciate live models!)

- Animal visitation programs at hospitals, elderly care homes, and with trauma victims (especially great for miniature horses and friendly ponies)

- Therapy for Alzheimer's patients (a recent study found symptoms of dementia eased to a great extent when patients cared for a horse under supervision)

Dr. Allen Schoen:

In my current practice most of my clients are quite compassionate. Before I sold a part of my practice, however, it was much larger, and I had other veterinarians working along with me. At that time I did see a few horses being ridden that I would have said were ready for retirement.

There are many layers to the question of when to retire a horse because of the emotions of the rider. There might be finances involved—perhaps it is more viable to keep a horse on "bute" (phenylbutazone) or other anti-inflammatories or analgesics because he is useful and paying bills, as might be the case with a good school horse. The horse is "earning his keep," so to speak. The more delicate situation, I find, is when the client and the horse are strongly bonded, and he is the only horse the client can afford. Then the client tends to want to keep the horse going as long as he or she can.

There is also the transference of awareness and perception to the horse—that is, thinking that he *wants* to keep on working. Let's say the horse loves to jump. There may be truth to that. He might get quite psyched up about it, like a human who loves to participate in sports. Then he tries, and says, "Oh, ouch, I can't." He cannot do what he used to be able to do due to age, injuries, or disease. Will the horse push himself in such situations as a human might?

I know about this inclination firsthand. Recently, a couple of friends who are in their thirties said, "Let's hike up the mountain in the full moon." I thought I could do it, and I did, but on the way back down it was completely dark and the trail steep. I should have at least had a headlamp, but all I had was a belief that suggested I *could* keep up with the 30-something friends, and I paid for it later.

Do older horses do the same thing? I think some horses do. They get all revved up and try to clear jumps like they remember doing in the past, then suffer the consequences. And there's the other player in that story: the owner who may say the horse still *wants* to jump (which may or may not be true), and can do it as long as he has a little "bute." Of course, *that* is the difference between horses and humans...the judgment over whether they can do something or not. Horses have someone else making the decisions for them while humans can make up their own minds regarding the limitations of their bodies.

As with so much else, the answer here is individual to every situation. The Principles of Compassionate Equitation suggest taking a step back, weighing all the different pros and cons, and asking yourself if continuing an activity or work is the best, most considerate choice for *this* horse given his age, condition, and other factors. Do you inject the joints *one more time*? Do you do the "dance" over the amount of "bute" or other painkillers to give him? If a little is good, is more going to be better? If your horse starts having ulcers, and therefore different pain in a different place, is increasing the "bute" the compassionate choice? We must always be open to asking what the best, most conscientious act is *in that moment*. In addition, we need to be prepared to re-evaluate the situation regularly—maybe a month ago, the horse was fine, but 30 days later he's ready to spend his days under a shady tree in the pasture.

Sometimes the horse really does seem to want to keep working. He will try, but if he cannot perform as he used to, are you aware of what your options might be for his optimal comfort?

You always want to find the right job for your horse appropriate to his age and condition. I have had to readjust my own schedule to accommodate these factors. I cannot work on as many horses now as I used to five years ago, or even a year ago. It is about being flexible moment to moment and being ready for a change when it is needed.

I used to treat a lot of older, semi-retired reining horses that moved over to trail riding and backpacking trips. Integrative approaches helped keep these horses with musculoskeletal conditions as comfortable as possible, including

EXERCISE IN COMPASSION
_____

Tough Questions

There are certain tough questions we need to ask ourselves as horse owners, and it can be better to consider our answers *before* a decision has to be made. Take a quiet moment to ask:

- Will you know when it is time to retire your horse for good?

- What are your plans for your horse when he can no longer be ridden due to age, illness, or injury?

- Will you be in a position (psychological, financial) to make the most compassionate choices for your horse? What might those be?

joint injections, acupuncture, chiropractic, and all the related approaches for relieving pain and discomfort so they could keep moving and stay active.

It is a hard thing to keep your own judgments and perceptions out of the way as you manage your horse's care according to your financial capabilities. You can face challenging questions. I have a friend who was always asking me about her old Appaloosa. She continued to do everything she could to keep the horse comfortable, and you could see he really *wanted* to work. My friend was looking at the horse's mind, while I was looking at his body. Unfortunately, the Appy finally had an injury that made the decision a black and white issue.

After a year and a half off, the horse "appeared" sound enough to ride again; the owner asked if she should. Knowing the extent and severity of the injury, I had to say, "No, it would only be asking for trouble." The horse was also very happy and comfortable just living in the field. If she had gotten back on him, there was a chance the injury would recur quickly, and then she would be left with a horse in worse condition, and potentially not as happy and comfortable in his retirement. This is not the kind of risk an owner should take, knowing how debilitating it could be to the horse.

We need to reduce the numbers of unwanted and "homeless" horses.

The overpopulation of unwanted horses is an issue that needs to be dealt with, and we do have a number of potential avenues for change. "Closing down" parts of the equine industry may be extreme, but it is reasonable to suggest and instigate reform where possible. We need to breed fewer horses. We can increase the age that horses begin racing in North America, as exists in Europe, which might immediately help reduce breakdowns due to Thoroughbreds starting too young. More diligent training in the workload of all young performance horses would be helpful so their joints, tendons, and ligaments have a chance to mature. So many horses break down at an early age due to overwork or poor training.

Some people still think of horses as "livestock," with the "extras" labeled "salvage livestock."

For those who believe horses are not sentient beings and have no thoughts and emotions, it is black and white as to whether horses should keep working, regardless of age or condition. When the horses are "done," in these cases, they are not necessarily "disposed of" in a humane way. Such a mindset allows for overbreeding. The "extras" are just "salvage livestock."

Is this about compassionate choices? No, it's completely contrary to the foundation of this book, where with the very first Principle we recognize horses as sentient beings with the ability to feel pain and pleasure. People who do not follow Principle 1 may feel they can do whatever they want with horses. Frequently, *financial interest* becomes *primary interest*.

In some ways, it seems like this is the *modus operandi* for the whole planet right now. Big financial interests do not seem to look at *any* being as though it is a sentient being. Everything is just data and expendable commodities. It boils down to a basic difference in awareness, consciousness, and core central belief system. Are living beings conscious and sentient, experiencing pain and suffering and having thoughts and emotions? Are such allowances limited to just humans or applied to all animals? Where do *you* draw that line? One of the goals of this book is to help shift a sense of compassion to as many people as possible.

CONDITIONS THAT ARE POTENTIALLY CAREER-ENDING

- Severe joint disease that decreases range of motion.

- Severe ringbone, which may not look that bad, but the way it rotates can make it permanently debilitating.

- Severed tendons.

- When the level of reasonable, safe, pain relief is no longer able to ease the horse's discomfort and what remains is resorting to more drastic measures, that's when you really need to ask the question: Is it time to permanently retire this horse?

Questions to Consider
BASED ON PRINCIPLE 20

1   Is my compassion limited to my own horses, or those of financial "worth," or can I develop compassion for *all* horses, included the feral, aged, unwanted, and "homeless"?

2   Is my horse currently healthy and working? If so, have I made plans for his comfort and care during retirement?

3   What do I think can be done about the excessive numbers of horses still being bred in spite of fewer available homes and a lack of appropriate lifespan care for the horses already on this planet?

4   If my horse sustained a career-ending injury, what would I do?

CHAPTER TWENTY-ONE

Compassion for the "Global Herd"

We allow for an authentic bond based on compassionate care to form between horses and humans, leading us into a new paradigm of training and understanding that brings our worldwide community of horse lovers together with peace, awakened compassion, and loving-kindness, for the good of all.

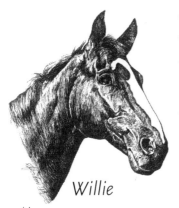

Willie

Susan Gordon:

Willie's story was international. In fact, when we met, Willie had led a more well-traveled life than I had. Prior to his arrival in Los Angeles, California, somebody flew to Belgium, coordinated a deal between the American purchasers and European trainer, then arranged flights, veterinary certificates, export/import papers, quarantine, and other such details. The horse industry is, without a doubt, a global network of business people with considerable influence in many sectors of society.

We, the horsepeople of the world, are the ones who decide how the welfare of equines will be managed in the future. Willie went from being a very expensive, imported show horse to barely escaping a one-way trip to a processing plant. How could we possibly let this happen to any horse? In this case, the owner appeared to want to get some of his purchase price back for Willie, even just a portion of it. This is why I think horses end up at auctions or being sold for slaughter—it offers some kind of financial return to the owner. Standing back and looking at this situation with a compassionate heart is a challenge. Sacrificing such a wonderful animal for a few measly dollars does not seem suitable or acceptable.

Imagine Willie's life in one big picture. From a happy little colt at his mother's side in a pasture, to being loaded on a plane and flown to California, to competing in huge jumper classes and advanced events, to a thin, grumpy, worn-out gelding, rejected by almost everyone. What different set of options could have been offered to this horse as he aged and refused to jump any longer? Who could have been keeping watch on where he went, and what his fate was? Willie's lifecycle predated the widespread use of the internet and the social networking capabilities now available to us. The movement of horses internationally was not as easy 30 years ago as it is now, either. Willie was just one of tens-of-thousands of horses sold and traded every year that could potentially fall into the wrong hands and eventually meet an inhumane end.

I'm certain Willie would wish for all of his "Global Herd" to have peaceful, compassionate completions to their lives. We are all connected. When Willie was content, so was I. If the Global Herd can be cared for with loving-kindness and peace, we will all feel a little more at peace ourselves.

When we bond to another being from a place of compassion, we find an authentic and long-lasting stability within our hearts. Gradually, we calm the emotional pendulum that causes so much distress throughout our lifetimes. Nothing is permanent, and attachment and desire cause psychological stress. Accepting this can bring us to a point of much greater balance and clear thinking when things change in our personal lives.

The influence of parents, friends, siblings, and spouses on our personal development is significant. In spite of external influences, the extraordinary thing about all humans is that we have the ability to raise our consciousness and pursue a path of compassion, no matter what circumstances have affected our lives. Great figures, such as the former president of South Africa, the late Nelson Mandela, have proven that concept throughout history. If you have been less than kind and loving toward others, or not mindful of how much stress or pain you've caused your horse, *forgive yourself* and begin to find a new way forward starting now.

If your awareness has opened your heart and mind to where you feel overwhelmed by the suffering of others, this is an area of caution. Those who have overextended their capacity for caregiving of others while not taking care of their own emotional needs are not in a position to be of the most benefit to other beings, especially themselves. In an authentic mode of compassion, it is important that *joy* be present and radiant, as that alone is healing for all others. The effects of *compassion fatigue* are seen a lot in the medical and veterinary fields.[1] The constant need and desire to heal all those who come by the way of the practitioner can lead him or her into a perpetual state of stress. People are generally unaware of the amount of time caring medical practitioners devote to thinking about how to help as many people or animals as they can.

> *Patricia Smith, founder of the Compassion Fatigue Awareness Project (CFAP) says, "Affecting positive change in society, a mission so vital to those passionate about caring for others, is perceived as elusive, if not impossible. This painful reality, coupled with first-hand knowledge of society's flagrant disregard for the safety and well being of the feeble and frail, takes its toll on everyone from full time employees to part time volunteers. Eventually, negative attitudes prevail" (http://www.compassionfatigue. org/pages/compassionfatigue.html).*

1

To those who are in need of care, it is also the cause of considerable stress when their caregivers are overworked and perpetually fatigued. As a society, we do not pay much attention to issues faced by ill, incapacitated and elderly people or animals until we have personal experience that raises our own awareness. Some people are disturbed by sadness expressed by those who are ill or elderly. This is more apparent than ever as our population shifts to a senior-dominant demographic. This includes old animals—our pets, too, are living longer than ever.

As we age, wouldn't we prefer to be cared for by those who have compassion for us, rather than those who find us to be a burden?

Many horsepeople are also caretakers of dogs and cats, and some have other farm animals. As research has shown, pets of all kinds can relieve stress, yet caring for them can *cause* stress, especially when finances are tight.[2] Finding balance in life is challenging in so many ways. A key to good health for everyone, including the animals in our care, is to look into our own hearts to find the

EXERCISE IN COMPASSION

Find Your Heart Center

As we learned in chapter 6, a field of energy radiates from your physical heart. Your heart center is a powerful energy center and the "space" we come home to. Finding our way there helps us feel safe, self-loved, at peace, and free of the pain of the outer world.

1   Sit with your back erect, but comfortable, breathing slowly and deeply. Place your attention on your "heart area" in the center of your chest. Close your eyes or leave them open, but soften your eyes and gaze (see p. 133).

2   Place your fingertips, or both hands, one on top of the other, in the center of your breastbone.

3   With your fingers or hands, feel your breath going in and out gently; feel the energy from your loving heart, and allow this to expand around you.

4   With each out-breath let all tension, fear, or any sense of negativity release.

5   Place your hands in your lap or the top of your thighs. Stay and rest in your heart center for a few more breaths.

balance point—meaning, we always come back to our "heart center" as described in the sidebar on p. 346 when we feel overwhelmed or confused—and catch ourselves when we try to take on too much.

> *Kathleen Doheny's WebMD article "Pets for Depression and Health" states, "Studies show that animals can reduce tension and improve mood. Along with treatment, pets can help some people with mild to moderate depression feel better" (http://www.webmd.com/depression/features/pets-depression).*

Assisting individuals who may have challenges when it comes to the ability to take care of their horses and other animals is a fundamental concept to functioning as part of a global community of Compassionate Equestrians. I believe it would serve us well as an industry if everyone could be taught to change from a passive "not-in-my-backyard" mindset to stepping boldly forward and actively preventing abusive, neglectful situations for horses as often as possible.

"We cannot change our past. We cannot change the fact that people will act in a certain way. We cannot change the inevitable. The only thing we can do is play on the one string we have, and that is our attitude. I am convinced that life is 10 percent what happens to me and 90 percent how I react to it. And so it is with you. We are in charge of our attitudes."

Preacher Charles R. Swindoll

As the market for horses fluctuates with the global economy, it is imperative to make wise decisions for the sake of the equine community's future.

The equine community can hopefully find a way to educate and assist in the proper re-homing and retraining of unwanted horses. And we need to do this without placing judgment on our fellow equestrians and how or why they may need help finding new homes for their horses. We will see them with loving-kindness, without levying criticism regarding how they and their horses have ended up in less than ideal conditions.

Globally, the horse industry is as diverse as the many different types of people who care for horses and use them for work or pleasure. In some parts of the world horses are still beasts of burden and a primary mode of transportation.[3] There are people who may wonder what all this "compassion for animals" is about, when people all around them are suffering. We can choose to remember that *everyone* suffers in some way. Having compassion for others is the desire to alleviate their suffering. When we make the positive decision to place our focus on the "Global Herd," it does not matter which aspect we choose, what matters is that we pay attention to some small part of it.

3   *According to World Horse Welfare, "There are around 100 million working equines in the developing world that fuel the economies of countries in Africa, Central America and Asia. Working horses lead demanding, exhausting lives made worse by the wounds and injuries they suffer through inadequate shoeing, harnesses and nutrition" (http://www. worldhorsewelfare.org/International-Work).*

We are fortunate in wealthy, developed nations to have access to almost everything we need and anything we can imagine. Dr. Schoen and I are ever so grateful to live and write this book from one of the most beautiful, peaceful places on Earth. Yet we still see the suffering of animals and people in our small island community. No place is immune. Every day we can sit in our quiet, thoughtful places and take a few moments to do whatever we can to help others as well as focus our intention for loving-kindness and compassion for all beings, including those horses who may be far beyond our own shores and their caretakers who may be living in circumstances quite different from our own. Yes, we must help on a local level too. We are all connected.

Dr. Allen Schoen:

Animal behavior and human neuroscience studies continue to acknowledge our similarities rather than differences. This enables us to have more empathy for horses because we recognize that we have very similar emotional responses to situations: such as pain, trauma resulting in PTSD, or a loss of identity and balance in our lives. The thing is, once we recognize our similarity, we can overextend ourselves by having compassion for all the suffering that is going on in the equine world, as well as the human world. You may find you empathize so much with abandoned and abused horses that it *overwhelms* you. Just as an overcrowded horse rescue or sanctuary can become more harmful than helpful to the horses and people involved, when we suffer *compassion fatigue* as individuals, we cannot ease the burdens of others.

At the peak of my career I had lost a sense of balance. I was an assistant professor at two veterinary schools, writing and editing two books, managing my own practice, and traveling to lecture around the world, which certainly had a way of skewing my work/life balance. I was pioneering my approach, integrating the best of all conventional therapies with the complementary therapies of acupuncture, nutritional and herbal supplements, and manual therapies, so I ended up being called in for the worst off, most hopeless cases. People would say, "You're the last hope for my horse or my dog or cat. Nothing else has worked, I have been to x-number of veterinarians and I do not know what else to do." Wanting to be of service, I kept fitting them all in. It got to the point where it would be nine o'clock at night and I would call a client at a barn to ask if he or she wanted to reschedule, and it was always, "No, we're all here waiting for you."

It is harder to feel compassion for the "Global Herd" when you have exhausted yourself by overextending your kindness and giving nature to the point that it has become overwhelming. Leave space for yourself.

No matter how late it was and how long my days were, I would fit everyone in, and I was utterly exhausted. I was not always at my absolute best as much as I wanted to be. I kept focusing on being present in the moment, being present for each animal and each person, but by doing that, I was so exhausted by the end of the day, the week, or the month, that I was not taking care of myself. That impacted my personal life, my health, and everything else.

I know that in myself I have experienced compassion fatigue firsthand, borne of not being aware of how to create healthier personal boundaries and not being able to say, "No." There is an old Taoist saying, "One *no* is worth a thousand *yeses*," because it creates space for other opportunities. It was a big teaching for

REASONS *NOT* TO BREED

One sad situation that I have seen more often than I would like to is when people say something like, "Well, my horse is too 'mareish' (or some other behavioral condition), so I figure I might as well just breed her." Breeding horses that may have a predisposition to certain issues, diseases, or lameness not only produces more horses in a world that already has an *excess* of horses, it produces horses prone to problems, illness, and injury. This is a good example of what is *not* the most compassionate choice for *any* horse. It is not sustainable.

me, learning the word "No," because I was not very good at it. I just wanted to be of help. I wanted to be of service. It was noble, it was kind, but it took its toll on me. I could not be in each place as long as I would have liked to be. I was booked six months ahead, and I could tell you every day which barn I would be at, or which animal hospital, or where I was teaching or lecturing. I became exhausted just thinking about it. My own personal experience with compassion fatigue became significant, and it is the background from which I have developed my workshops on the topic for veterinarians and other health professionals.

The key lesson here is to learn the balance of compassion. There are many stories from various perspectives on compassion fatigue and its effects. For example, how many people do we see who take in every horse that needs rescuing, only to then be put in a compromising position when decisions have to be made around finances? Then the authorities get called in to deal with "horses that are being starved," but it is the *rescuer* who is at fault, and he or she had every intention to maintain the horses properly, before he or she was literally overwhelmed by his or her compassion.

A pastor was once called in to lecture at Harvard University on compassion, and he talked about "the noble attempt" to be there for everyone, but how then *unfortunate reality* made it impossible. Then what do we do? We usually beat up ourselves for not having the ability to care for everyone, and in our case, for not caring for all the horses that end up starving or abused, as well. But if we get so down on ourselves about our inability to help everyone that *we* need help, it becomes a vicious cycle.

We are all one herd with similar neurochemical processes, imprinting and programming. We need to care for others and ourselves without going to an extreme—there needs to be balance between caring for others and ourselves.

Each animal that we rescue or save can be an opportunity for emotional and mindful awakening, or an opportunity for distraction. It is up to us in each and every moment to decide if it is really the animal we are rescuing, and why. We need to be sure the effort is an opportunity for opening and awakening in ourselves rather than a distraction from ourselves. We want to be mindful in each choice we make.

I saw Livingston Taylor (brother of James) play at a coffeehouse in New York once—at the Town Crier Café. He began with a few words to introduce a song, "How many times do we do something that seemed like a good idea at the time?" That stuck with me and is relevant now because part of compassionate care for the Global Herd is to ask, "What are the implications for this choice?" You are never going to know what all of the answers are, but it is important all the same to find your heart center (see p. 133), slow down, and say, "What will my life look like once I say 'yes' to this situation? Is this the healthiest thing for the horse, and for me, and for my family? If I truly want to help, what are different options that are beneficial to all involved?"

EXERCISE IN COMPASSION

Determining the Compassionate Approach

Create a mental list of how you would like to enact compassion in your life in a balanced way. For example:

1 Be empathetic to the suffering of horses.

2 Through that empathy, have compassion for yourself. Ask yourself, "Do I have the financial means to appropriately care for the horses I have now and any I wish to rescue in the future?"

3 If not, determine what might be *other* actions that would be of benefit to the Global Herd.

I offer workshops on compassion fatigue for health care professionals and consultations for guidance and support, speaking from personal experience and advanced training, as well as retreats and programs on mind-body medicine for veterinarians and animal lovers. We invite you to open the dialogue with us so that you may open your own doors to the needs of the "Global Herd" with the wisdom and skills to maintain your own personal balance and self-compassion.

Helping Another without Judgment

If you were aware someone was struggling to properly care for his or her horses, what would be the most compassionate choice in helping both the individual and the horses in his or her care? Consider the following questions *before* becoming involved.

- Are you creating more problems than solutions by getting involved in this way?
- Is it best for you to get involved hands-on or with financial or some other support that would be beneficial for all?
- Can the person you are trying to help let go of his or her own ego and genuinely accept support from you or another expert?
- Who decides what a "reasonable quality of care" is for these horses?
- Is the issue serious enough for a regulating body or humane authority to step in?
- Who is actually rescuing whom? As we discussed early in the book, and do again on p. 350, a lot of rescuers actually want to be rescued themselves.
- When *you* consider rescuing an animal, is it for the highest good of all involved?

These questions are not intended to discourage altruism, but merely to help us ensure that our motivation to help comes from a compassionate place, and not an egoic one.

Questions to Consider
BASED ON PRINCIPLE 21

1   Do I feel overwhelmed when I think about issues concerning equine welfare around the world, or do I feel as though I can expand my own vision to include the Global Herd?

2   Have I ever felt overextended while caring for another person or my horse? Have I practiced self-care in those moments?

3   Can I create a healthy, balanced situation where I feel I can be of benefit to others in some way, along with caring for myself and my family appropriately?

Birth to Completion Life-Cycle Management

22

We recognize the importance of applying a life-cycle assessment and sustainability model to the equestrian industry.

Susan Gordon:

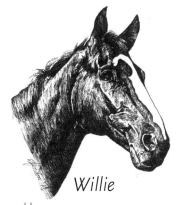

Willie

One of the biggest concerns I have for all the horses I have cared for over the years is how their lives may have come to completion. I have observed both horses and humans going through the transition process, leaving all things of the Earth behind them. They were fortunate ones who had a relatively peaceful passing, knowing there were caring hearts and loving arms nearby, keeping them safe while they made their journey to the other side.

I did not keep the contact information for the people who adopted Willie when I had to give him up. I don't know why. Maybe I did not want to know in case I had to rescue him again and simply could not do it. My friend used to check on him at his last home and reported that he looked just fine. I retain some guilt about not keeping track of him, as I don't know what year or day he passed away, or how his remains were disposed of. I would like to know that. Part of me just wanted to be discreet and not bother the fellows who adopted him, especially if he was seemingly safe and healthy in their hands. He was their horse, after all. I had surrendered him to their care via the adoption organization.

Willie's story and many others like his have inspired my desire to bring a citizen-based tracking method to all equestrians. What if I could just log in to a social network and find out what happened to Willie without having to disturb his owners? Usually such information is private and many people do not make public announcements about the passing of their horses unless they own a famous one. But what if we just want to make sure our old horses had humane completions to their lives? What if there was a privately maintained service whereby conscientious, compassionate equestrians could post as much or as little information about a particular horse, away from the general public's eye? In Willie's era, this was not possible. Today, it is. The technology exists to put an entire community on private servers, available only to member-users if the industry is receptive to such an idea.

Meanwhile, our interconnectedness as a community on Facebook, Instagram, and other social media sites is proving to be a great way to let people stay in touch and keep virtual-watch on the horses they once owned when the parties are in agreement to be "friends" and "followers." I would have loved to have had this kind of connection to Willie via those who adopted him, just *so I could take a peek every now and then, even from a distance, to see how the old boy was doing.*

Dr. Allen Schoen & Susan Gordon

The term "cradle-to-cradle" was first coined by Walter R. Stahel in the 1970s. Cradle-to-Cradle® is an approach to the design of products and systems, based on nature's cyclic processes, developed by William McDonough and Michael Braungart (2002).[1] It is a certified protocol (Cradle to Cradle Products Innovation Institute) designed for products that has not been applied to living beings. We are suggesting it may be possible to apply the life-cycle assessment model to our equine world. For the purposes of *The Compassionate Equestrian*, we are converting the word *product* to *horse* and structuring the program to apply to the birth-to-life's completion assessment and tracking of equines. The purpose is to prevent excessive numbers of horses from entering the market, and to assist owners in ensuring horses meet with humane death and disposal. It is up to all of us as equestrians to monitor the condition of the industry and plan for responsible breeding, training, and humane endings for as many horses as possible. We acknowledge the necessity to work together as an entire community to educate horse owners and prevent the cycles of neglect, abuse, and ignorance that lead to equine suffering.

In 2002, William McDonough and Dr. Michael Braungart published Cradle to Cradle: Remaking the Way We Make Things, *encapsulating a journey of discovery about materials as biological or technical nutrients and their use periods and evolution. They created a framework for quality assessment and innovation: the Cradle to Cradle™ certified program, a systemic approach to product innovation that spurs the creation of truly beautiful, high-quality products, and transforms the production of consumer products into a positive force for society and the environment. The Cradle to Cradle Certified Mark provides consumers, regulators, employees, and industry peers with a clear, visible, and tangible understanding of a manufacturer's commitment to sustainability. In 2010, McDonough and Braungart created the Cradle to Cradle Products Innovation Institute™, a nonprofit intended to bring about a new industrial revolution that turns the making of things into a positive force for society, the economy, and the planet (http://www.c2ccertified.org/about/what_is_cradle_to_cradle).*

"You never change things by fighting the existing reality.
To change something, build a new model that makes the
existing model obsolete."

Buckminster Fuller, Neo-Futuristic Architect and Inventor

Consider implementing a "Life-Cycle Management Policy" for your barn or equestrian operation. Sponsors, organizations, insurance companies, and industry-regulating bodies would do a world of good for all horses if they helped make this the new standard.

Part of our teaching of the 25 Principles of Compassionate Equitation is to instill awareness in horse people that when we come from a base of compassion in all equine activities, then we commit to keep watch and take care of our horses throughout their entire life cycle. We do not bring horses into being for the purposes of inhumane treatment and unethical means of disposal, so why are we so capable of turning a blind eye to those that are neglected, "homeless," or abandoned and left to die?

We feel that as we bring up a new generation of horse-loving youth we can make the choice to teach the importance of coming from a foundation of kindness, tolerance, and forgiveness in all equestrian activities. This includes education in how to take compassionate action that could potentially lead to a much safer, more sustainable world for horses. It starts with controlling the breeding stock and ensuring horsepeople have high standards for equine welfare, as well as a clear understanding of training methodology and general training goals. If too many people accept a lower quality of horse and poor training as the "norm" then we have a huge problem centering around horses that are difficult, lame, or unrideable from an early age, yet living well into their twenties or longer.

Equine Canada, for example, has acknowledged the concerns of their country's membership in addressing the need for a national policy with respect to the life-cycle management of horses.[2] A sport-regulating body such as Equine Canada can have considerable influence, not only on horse owners and every level of equine use, from recreation to international competition, but all levels of the country's government, as well. The organization is still in the early stages of educating horse owners about life-cycle management, but it is addressing the need to engage more of the equestrian world in paying attention to, and acting on, policies that will help horses maintain a good quality of life from birth to death. As more horse facilities are squeezed out of areas that were once low-density in population, our careful, considerate stewardship of the equine environment and the horses themselves is ever more critical to the very survival of the industry.

The following excerpt from Equine Canada's Equine Life-Cycle Management Policy, developed by the Life-Cycle Management Subcommittee of the Equine Canada Health and Welfare Committee, is reprinted by permission:

Our Policy Objective

To maximize the horse's quality of life and death through the following equine life-cycle management action steps, from birth to death respectively.

- *Working towards a balanced equine population in Canada.*
- *Working to ensure all horses are treated humanely throughout their lifetime.*
- *Fostering longer, healthier, active careers in industry.*
- *Maximizing opportunities for a secured retirement.*
- *Ensuring a humane death for all horses.*

These action steps would apply equally to all of the unique roles the horse plays in Canadian society, from companion animal to a valuable component of our agricultural/processing sector.

How We'll Implement Our Policy

The Equine Life-Cycle Management Policy will be implemented relying on the following CLEAR principles.

Communication: *The widest possible sharing of information.*

Liaison/Collaboration: *The use of all concerned organization's perspectives, resources and strengths.*

Education: *The development, promotion and provision of formal and informal training.*

Action: *The application of incentives and levies, subsidization of research and compliance supervision.*

Review: *The regular review of policy and programs on a defined basis.*

The Equine Life-Cycle Management Policy will be implemented using the Five R Program. This program will incorporate the popular and descriptive three Rs:

- *Reduce*
- *Reuse (Retain)*
- *Recycle (Retrain)*
- *Retire*
- *Respect*

The first Four Rs will develop a balanced and dynamic population base, which when coupled with better research, education, and supervision, maximizes opportunities for the policy's fifth R: Respect. The final R represents both respect for the final act of good equine stewardship—a humane death—and respect for good environmental stewardship, in the handling of the horse's body (http://equinecanada.ca/index.php?option=com_docman&task=doc_view &gid=6457&Itemid=88&lang=en).

We understand that thinking about end-of-life issues is a difficult, complex, and emotional subject for many people.

It is important to realize that we have options available when it comes to creating a new level of awareness and potentially new protocols that could significantly impact the equestrian industry. Sustainability within the world of horses, and the world in general, is not a topic we want to fall behind on, as the environment in which we keep horses is changing so rapidly. It is our hope that all nations affected by governing policies of equine welfare will join in one common voice, based on these new protocols, for the ongoing improvement and well-being of all horses, no matter what status that particular horse holds in the eyes of humans. May we treat them all as equal, and equally deserving of compassionate care throughout their entire life cycle.

Questions to Consider
BASED ON PRINCIPLE 22

1   Do I think there is a need to manage the numbers of horses currently in existence?

2   How would I propose we monitor the welfare of the many tens-of-thousands of horses that exist?

3   Would I be willing to contribute the time and effort necessary to maintain my horse's information on a private-citizen network for tracking the life of domestic equines?

4   Do I wish I had a way to find out how my former horses were doing and if they passed away in a humane manner? How do I feel about having this information available to me?

CHAPTER TWENTY-THREE

Healing Old Wounds

We acknowledge the importance of healing old wounds as an integral foundation of heart-centered horsemanship. Healing old wounds allows us to be the absolute best human beings we can be. Removing these harmful "filters" allows us to see the world with clearer vision, unobscured by destructive patterns and emotions.

Susan Gordon:

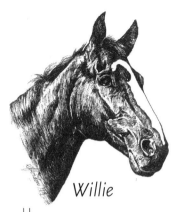

Willie

Willie was a wounded horse. Those on the frontline of a rescue operation know how far horses can go in an abusive situation and still be resilient enough to survive—even eventually learning to trust humans once again. The mental and physical wounds sustained by so many horses every year are the result of our equally wounded human psyches. Willie and I could have gone down each other's checklists of traumas and compared notes on the long-term effects, including developing defensive mechanisms to protect ourselves.

Not wanting to give up entirely, we both fought back to regain strength, dignity, and grace, perhaps with the intention to teach and help others based on our own journeys. Humans who have recovered from trauma or substance abuse are then often able to help others who are going through the same thing. Perhaps in a relative way, it is the same for horses. It is those who are most humbled who seem to be the most open-hearted and compassionate toward others.

I watched with great interest as grouchy old Willie's wounded personality and broken-down body healed and he turned around and helped other horses. His previously veiled gentle side reemerged. He appeared quite delighted with his job, especially as "babysitter" for two sweet, chestnut Oldenburg colts. Two-year-old Lancelot was a playful, athletic fellow with a personality full of joy. He bounced around Willie like a puppy, biting, kicking, and sometimes jumping on top of the big old horse. Willie patiently allowed Lancelot the freedom to cut loose until his enthusiasm threatened to do some damage. Then he would quickly plant a well-placed hoof on the youngster's body, letting him know the roughhousing had gone far enough.

With Arthur, the gorgeous yearling, Willie had a different mannerism altogether. Arthur was unusually quiet and polite for a young horse. He was like a shy but very happy child who had been taught good manners around adults. Lancelot and Arthur were not turned out together lest the bigger brother injure the little one. Willie would quietly follow Arthur around the turnout, and then they would both stand placidly at the gate. One day Willie decided it was time to incite the baby to play. At first I was somewhat horrified when Willie suddenly turned and grabbed the crest of Arthur's neck with his teeth. Arthur,

*caught by surprise, stood on his hind legs and struck at Willie, who casually
ducked out of the way, almost grinning at his success. I realized what the now
healthy old Hanoverian was doing and laughed along with him.*

*What joy do we find in helping others? It is so immense it is hard to put
into words. What is amazing is when horses also appear to find joy in their
own healing and are able to pass the benefits of their rehabilitative journeys
on to others of their own species.*

As we've discussed, when we take away the breeds, the disciplines, the methods of training, and the divisiveness of all those aspects of horsemanship that
separate us from others, we can see from our heart that we need to take care of
the planet, our horses, and ourselves as one *whole* collective of sentient beings.

It is time to remove the separateness and look at the science that defines
the boundaries of horses' comfort zones. Then we can translate the science to
an understandable, fundamental program that lays out a clear foundation for the
various disciplines and methods, keeping compassion as the base. Our goals
include educating equestrians, from beginners to the most advanced, to reach an
agreement on techniques that put equine welfare above all else. Horses cannot
speak as a collective for themselves, but we can have a voice for them.

We can all—humans and horses—benefit from heart-centered healing.

By inviting all horsepeople to examine and heal their own emotional wounds
through the 25 Principles of Compassionate Equitation and finding their heart-cen-
ter (see p. 346), we offer them a chance to develop a voice of loving-kindness.
We can learn to look at others without placing judgment or blame if they are not
acting in accordance with our limited viewpoints and understanding of their situations. All humans are on their own paths of development, and each one of us
has the ability to reach an awakened state of consciousness. This is something
we can choose to remember when riding and working with others, and requires
care in how we use language when addressing other people.

Oftentimes, people need more than self-compassion to heal old wounds
and destructive patterns. Choosing to work together with appropriate health
care practitioners can be extremely beneficial. An intervention might sometimes
be necessary to prevent the human from passing on his or her distress and
suffering to other people, or to his or her horse. In this case, however, it is suggested that you be certain the need to give advice or instruction to another is not

coming from your own ego. There is a line of demarcation between giving unsolicited advice and acting upon the need of another soul who may be suffering. In addition, sometimes it is impossible to diplomatically and peacefully deliver a message to someone who is in an abusive or agitated state. In this case all you can do is remain at peace with yourself and offer the energy of your mindful and loving thoughts and words. When someone puts you, others, or his or her own self or horse in a dangerous situation, however, it requires immediate action, and do not hesitate to bring up your concerns.

EXERCISE IN COMPASSION

Shift Away from Ego

Before you are tempted to offer someone "unsolicited advice," ask yourself why you want to give the instruction.

- Is it coming from your ego?

- Is it coming from an inner voice of compassion?

- Or are the horse and/or rider in a dangerous situation that needs to be addressed immediately?

If you *do* sense that your inclination to offer your opinion or guidance comes from ego, you can actually *shift that thought* quickly within yourself. Change your awareness and use the appropriate language whereby your motivation to "help" comes from the compassionate place within.

It is vitally important to distinguish genuine suffering *of a horse from* perceived suffering *based on opinion.*

Bringing the horse world together in a coherent community is easily fractured by differences of opinions. This is why the 25 Principles of Compassionate Equitation are backed by current research and peer-reviewed scientific papers that define what does and does not constitute equine suffering.

In many social equestrian situations, such as large boarding and training facilities, it seems like you often find ego-based commentaries from observers who do not realize what you are feeling when on a horse or what concept it is you are trying to convey to a student. People tend to pay attention to snippets of information that are interesting to them or those that support their viewpoints. We must remember that unsolicited advice, especially when coming from a place of ego and possible misunderstanding, may contribute to division and mistrust amongst others at the barn. In addition and in the worst case, it could even possibly cause an accident or injury to horse and/or rider if the advice given is inappropriate, not timed correctly, or misperceived. Riding is most productive when a rider is paying attention to his or her own instructor or trainer, the progression and development of the horse, and the advancement of his or her own skills.

"Compassion is the antidote to suffering. If you think of it this way, the cultivation of compassion has a direct effect on suffering. This applies at a personal level as well as at a global level."

Lama Tenzin Dhonden, the Dalai Lama's Personal Emissary for Peace and Founder and Chair of Friends of the Dalai Lama

---

When we observe others from a foundation of compassion and when the ego is no longer involved, the tendency to want to "correct" another's issues wanes greatly. It can be awkward, however, to observe less-experienced riders causing discomfort to their horses and still resist the urge to "help." How do we *really* know when to speak up, and when to remain silent under the circumstances? When most people, including professionals, ride without supervision, they will inevitably make mistakes that may be confusing or uncomfortable for the horse. Unless they are in extreme danger, or a danger to other horses and riders, it is important to think of the reasons that particular person and horse may be together in this lifetime, and what lessons they may need to learn from each other. If you are an excellent horseperson who has *earned* the respect of others, perhaps the errant rider will make the decision to come to you for advice or instruction.

In that case, be gracious and humble, and help them develop their Compassionate Equestrian nature, as well.

*Decreasing the destructive impact of egoic tendencies in a
very ego-based business, will be one of the biggest challenges
to unifying a global community of horse people.*

Letting go of the ego is imperative when we aim to take a more compassionate approach to how we work with all kinds of horses and riders. Becoming mindful of the need to unite around the common cause of solving issues, such as sustainability, may be a good starting point from which to encourage people to *envision a larger, more expansive healing perspective.* Can we take the time and have the courage to look within, and possibly work on healing our old wounds? Perhaps we can work together with a common vision as horse lovers with the intent to create a world where all our beloved equines can exist in comfort and peace. Isn't that really what we would like to see for humanity and ourselves, too?

Dr. Allen Schoen:

One of the foundations of being a Compassionate Equestrian is leaving any detrimental thoughts, emotions, and overly busy mindstreams out of the barn. Leave that kind of energy behind. Oftentimes, what we are feeling and thinking in the moment is not directly related to the current situation. It is usually based on our *old* neural emotional imprints and patterns—what some people call "old wounds." There is no judgment passed with that label, as most people have old wounds. However, as I've mentioned already in these pages, I find "labels" can often be divisive, and therefore I prefer to call these *old patterns*, or *old neural net wiring* based on past experiences.

*What old imprints and neural programming can you see in yourself
that might be hindering you from being the amazing, compassionate,
loving being that you really are? What do you see in yourself that, once
healed, could improve your relationships with horses and other people?*

Say to yourself, "This is a unique opportunity for me to heal those old patterns, reprogram my neural net, and release any destructive imprints." Our animals *can* be our teachers and healers if we allow for the opportunity to look at them from that perspective. One of the goals of the Compassionate Equestrian is learning to *not* bring our old baggage into the horse's space or onto his back.

> "To love and to be loved, one must do good to others. The inevitable condition whereby to become blessed, is to bless others."

> **Mary Baker Eddy**, Founder of Christian Science

This is the time to look at all our old "stuff" and consider how it impacts the horse. How it impacts the way we interact with him, and with grooms, trainers, veterinarians, farriers, and everyone else involved with our barns and competitions. Say, "From this moment on, I am going to do the best I can to leave all that behind and work on healing old patterns. I am reprogramming old imprinted neural nets in my mind, my heart, and my emotions." Finding appropriate, well-trained mental health care professionals can be of immense benefit in assisting you in your inner shift and making long-term changes.

There are many levels and potential depths of exploration of old patterns. It depends on how far down that "rabbit hole" you want to go. At the very least, there is scientific evidence for not only childhood wounds—they say from birth to the first few years of age is where so many influential events happen. But if you reference Bruce Lipton (author of *The Biology of Belief*, Hay House, 2007), you will find that he and others have shown that the neurohormones and neurochemicals you "bathed" in while in your mother's womb also impacted your development. For example, if your mother was highly stressed and reacting to life in crisis mode while pregnant, there was an overabundance of cortisol surrounding you in utero. Subconsciously, that then is what your body considers "normal." You may end up recreating stressful situations in your life to keep that cortisol level up because that's what your body craves. So yes, amazingly, what happened to you while in your mother's womb can affect your interactions with your horse.

Recent research in epigenetics (see p. 283) shows that the impact of stress and old patterns on our DNA can go back generations. This is a very profound awareness. For instance, if your grandparents, or great grandparents survived a traumatic war event, the holocaust, a global trauma, or even an interpersonal trauma, it can not only effect *them* but their children (your parents) and their children's children (you, your siblings) for generations to come.[1] It seems that if stress and patterns can affect human DNA, it is not unreasonable to think that it could affect the DNA of other species, such as horses, as well. The good news is that through epigenetics, we may also be able to heal some of those intergenerational wounds through various personal growth programs, EMDR (see p. 328), cognitive behavioral therapy, positive psychology, and other psychological approaches, creating a happier, healthier current generation.

When it is embedded deeply, is the stress identifiable enough and accessible enough that a person or horse can be reprogrammed?

At one barn where I treat horses, they adopted a Premarin mare. "Mommy," as they called her, was arthritic with both knees swollen, and she was stiff all over when I was first asked to see her. She limped out of her stall, almost three-legged. After treating her with acupuncture and adjusting her chronic misalignments, we watched her lower her head, tears began to drip from her eyes, her jaw dropped open, and she let out a deep sigh. The barn manager, grooms, and owner were all there with me to witness this "letting go" and release of old traumas. It literally brought tears of joy to all our eyes. It was like the first time Mommy could relax and feel such relief of the pain from the restrictions in her body.

Following her treatments, the barn manager said it was the first time the mare seemed happy and actually walked up to the front of the stall to be with people. We developed an integrative approach to help her heal, using many natural therapeutic options such as herbs, acupuncture, and chiropractic care, along with whatever else was needed. Mommy has continued to heal, come out of her "shell of fear," and become friendlier toward everyone; I think she actually seems to enjoy her new life.

There are many different therapeutic approaches to healing old patterns and neural-net imprints.

We cannot just "get over it." Healing takes practice. But the latest in neuroscience does actually show that there is *neuroplasticity*—the ability to change neural wiring—in our brains, and in effect, we can "rewire" our brains and change our biochemistry. We may be preprogrammed to create a certain level of stress in our lives, but the good news is by consciously changing our patterns, we start rewiring old neural programs in our mind and creating new ones. This is one example of neuroplasticity.

Various psychological approaches, such as cognitive behavioral therapy, EMDR (see p. 328), psychoanalysis, biofeedback, brainwave entrainment with bilateral bioacoustics sound waves, and many other therapies have been found to be beneficial. The U.S. Department of Defense is beginning investigative trials on neural implants to heal Post-Traumatic Stress Disorder (PTSD) in army veterans. Animal-facilitated therapy and even specifically equine-facilitated therapy have also been found to be of help.

It may seem to be a contradiction when we say we don't want to bring our old destructive patterns to the barn...and yet we are successfully using equine-facilitated therapy to help heal old patterns. In some ways, it *is* a contradiction. In equine-facilitated therapy programs, it is essential that the people running the programs are professionally trained and ideally have professional degrees in dealing with trauma and PTSD in humans. In addition, the practitioner needs to make sure the horses are appropriate for the task at hand and that they are continuously, carefully monitored for their own stress levels.

Yes, we all have imprints from childhood, but we should recognize there are also more recent imprints.

How often have you seen someone fall off his or her horse and then you or the instructor has said to get back on? With swimming, if someone has almost drowned, experts say it is best to get right back in the pool. "Getting back on" or "back in" is to prevent a *trauma pattern* from emerging.

WHAT IS PREMARIN AND PMU?

PMU stands for Pregnant Mare's Urine used in the production of the hormone replacement drug, Premarin®. The resulting foals are considered the "byproduct" of the pregnant mares and often processed at Canadian slaughter plants. There are rescue organizations in the United States and Canada that try to obtain the foals and put them up for adoption. While the drug has been implicated as a cause of cancer in women, it is still manufactured and prescribed. For further information visit www.savinghorsesinc.com/PMU_Nurse_Mare_Foal_Rescue.php.

The more we become aware of where these patterns come from, the more we can choose to work on healing them, and the more we can take personal responsibility for not bringing our "stuff" to the barn or to the horse. It gives us an incredibly great opportunity to see horses as our mirror, but a reflection *without* all our usual baggage.

The first step in healing is *becoming aware* of your patterns of thinking. By just reading this book, recognizing your old imprints, and becoming aware of your patterns, you will realize that you may have some challenges that you would like to deal with and you can ask yourself, "Where do I go from here?" There are numerous self-help programs that can help you literally create a new "operating manual" for your heart, mind, and body. As mentioned previously, sometimes you may need a combination of options for healing, so perhaps consider professional health care, as well. Each person is unique, and different support networks or programs may help one better than another.

As a Compassionate Equestrian, we invite you to look at what you might bring to the time and space you share with your horses and the potential for resolution.

Whatever your mood, whatever your behavior, there is a window of opportunity to become *aware*. Once you become *aware*, you can consciously "switch over" to a different state of being if you *choose to do so*. Of course, when an individual is in a state of anger, for example, it is very hard to get him or her out of it. This is when it is of utmost importance that other people around him or her or in the barn model "choosing the more compassionate approach." Their behavior may help the person who is angry catch him- or herself in the "gap" between thought, emotion, and response. *That gap* is where all the potential for change happens.

"Don't we know, only too well, that protection from pain doesn't work, and that when we try to defend ourselves from suffering, we only suffer more and don't learn what we can from the experience?"

Sogyal Rinpoche, *Glimpse After Glimpse* (HarperOne, 1995)

I saw one client realize what she was beginning to do—and catch herself in *the gap*—and take a few deep breaths, before starting to gently talk out loud to her horse. My client apologized to her horse, saying, "Oh, I am so sorry, I was so stressed when I came in here. Thank you, Mirabelle, for just giving me your loving eyes, and making me realize I need to leave my 'stuff' outside the door. I am so much happier here."

This can also work as a kind of intervention when you observe anger or anxiety entering your barn via another person's body. By speaking to *your* horse about your *stress*, but loud enough that the angry or anxious person can hear you process it, you can help *shift the energy*. Using a third party, non-confrontational approach may be the best way to not only heal your own old patterns, but others', as well.

Anger around horses can put you and others in danger. When you over-react and punish a horse in a rage, it can send that horse into a panic.

Anger solves nothing and is never a compassionate way to respond to the horse. This is particularly the case when a horse is being beaten on for a behavioral issue. It could, in fact, create a very dangerous situation. That said, there is a purpose to "righteous indignation" or a moment of sharper response when a person or horse is doing something that is dangerous. A swift wake-up call in that moment, even if it is just a quick, "Heads-up!" may keep a person or horse from getting hurt. We want to be clear in making that differentiation.

We should consider fear in a similar manner. There is a place for fear. For example, if your horse is about to be attacked by another horse, he needs to get out of the way. Quickly. While fear is an innate defense mechanism to help horses and humans escape from danger, it can also be extrapolated to other situations that might not be appropriate or necessary. It is a primitive behavior for a more natural environment.

Sometimes we have to let go and move on.

As I've described in other parts of this book, I have been to some barns that I do not really want to go back to. I tell myself in those moments, "I don't want to do this." I am responding to the Transpecies Field rife with anger and fear (see p. 113). In most cases I choose to try to go in and be of benefit to the horses, relieve their suffering, and shift the energy with compassion. But if after a number of times the bitterness remains, I may finally decide, "This is not going to change here."

I always feel sad about this decision. I feel badly for the horses and the people, but sometimes we have to let go and move on in order not to be adversely affected by the atmosphere. I used to ask myself, "What's wrong with me? Why don't I feel comfortable here?" This brings to mind one of my favorite quotes by Krishnamurti, who said, "It is not pathological to not fit into a dysfunctional society." Unfortunately much of society these days has become totally dysfunctional, and everyone is trying to adapt to the related stress and the anger. It is present in the microcosms of our horse barns all over the world, as well.

Even when a horse's behavior problems have been confirmed as related to pain, you may still be faced with an angry rider or trainer who is unwilling to admit that he or she was wrong, and was in fact, mistreating a horse that was hurting.

There was a huge Warmblood owned by an old client of mine. My client asked me to come have a look at the horse, as he was becoming dangerous and would not let anyone near him. His behavior had changed although a number of veterinarians and trainers had evaluated him without finding anything wrong. The horse was at a barn I do not really enjoy going to—one of those situations I have just described. The horse's ears were back as I did my evaluation, and based on the history, my physical exam, and my acupuncture and chiropractic exam, I suspected the horse had Lyme disease. I asked my client and the trainer about it, and they said that they had previously run a titer, and it was low (see p. 190 for my discussion of this issue). In the meantime, the trainer had continued punishing the horse for his behavior, claiming, "He's a bad horse."

Catch the Anger and Let It Go

1   The first step is to recognize your behavior. Identify it: "Ah-ha! I am bringing anger into this space." Fear is another example. Most emotions boil down to fear or love. When you *catch* yourself being angry or fearful, explore what it might be about; then you can take steps to resolve the reasons behind the behavior.

2   Model another way. Consciously act how you *want* to feel so you can get through that "gap" and change your *reaction* to a *response*. In this way, you can both *catch* anger yourself, and *deal with it* yourself.

3   Take a few minutes to calm down and be quiet. Let everything go, rest, and ask the question, "What old programming or patterning in me has provoked this?" Then say, "No, I do *not* want to bring this to my horse. I do not want to bring this to my ride. I do not want to bring this to everyone else in the barn."

Well, of course the more they beat on the horse, the angrier he got, to the point that you could barely get near him. I said, "Number One, it wouldn't hurt to run another Lyme titer, and Number Two, it wouldn't hurt to try and treat him with doxycycline." I re-examined him two weeks later. There was a 90 percent improvement in his behavior from being treated with doxycycline, an antibiotic for Lyme disease. It was dramatic. My client's horse was friendlier, less fearful and defensive, and he allowed people to touch him. He was much more relaxed and comfortable in his own skin. (Note: Some skeptics may say it was the anti-inflammatory effect of the doxycycline, rather than the anti-infectious effect; however, this horse had been treated with various nonsteroidal anti-inflammatory medications with no effect. What it shows is that the horse was in pain and discomfort.)

The thing was, the trainer was angry with my client for even bringing me in, or for asking for a second opinion, and for thinking it was Lyme disease when the trainer said it was not. The trainer did not want to acknowledge his role in the situation and became completely defensive. The client realized the barn was not the right place for her or her horse, and I judiciously supported them and gave them a list of other barns to check that would be more understanding of them both. They moved and the horse got better and better. The Lyme disease resolved completely; my client changed her training program. It took *eight months* of reprogramming the horse to no longer generalize all situations through a filter of fear. Now the horse is friendly, happy, healthy, pain-free, and has a whole different personality.

While a variety of factors were in play in this scenario, my client being aware of the unhealthy patterns in others, and being compassionate enough to know when it was time to remove her horse, made all the difference.

When a horse has been treated badly while in pain, resulting in behavior problems, the behaviors can be triggered again in the future, even after the horse has been rehabilitated.

Recurrence of behavior is always a possibility. It depends on how long a horse suffered pain, the depth of the negative experience, how that particular horse's mind integrated those negative experiences into his own mind and into his own life, and how he generalizes that out to other situations. I have seen cases where a horse has been completely healed, inside and out; where the trust comes back. On the other end of the spectrum, with some horses, you can never heal the fear and negative programming.

"Why do I consider it so crucial to balance the outer aspects of non-violence and compassion with the inner support of contemplative practice? Because in the end, all politics are local, and we cannot love life and humanity if we do not love each other, one on one."

Lama Surya Das, Western Buddhist Meditation Teacher

How to Heal Old Patterns

1   Do what you can for yourself so you do not bring negative "stuff" into the barn. Consider getting help from professional or medical support, or try self-help programs.

2   Do what you can for others to see if you can *shift their energy* when anger, fear, and other destructive emotions are present. Such action may assist you in identifying and healing unhealthy patterns in yourself.

3   Realize that once you may have worked on healing your own old patterns and you've done what you can for others, but your social barn or show situation remains a place of anger or bitterness, the compassionate and loving thing to do for yourself and your horse is to move or spend your time elsewhere. You may have to affirm: "I love my horse enough and I love myself enough that I am going to find another barn or a different local show that abides by the Principles of Compassionate Equitation."

Questions to Consider
BASED ON PRINCIPLE 23

1   What are some examples of old destructive patterns in other people that I have seen have negative impacts on horses and others?

2   Am I willing to explore old destructive patterns in myself that might hinder my relationship with my horse or others?

3   What kinds of patterns do I see in myself?

4   What type of compassionate assistance or support would I find beneficial to help heal my old patterns?

5   What changes in destructive patterns would I like to see to make my barn and those I visit more compassionate?

CHAPTER TWENTY-FOUR

Becoming a Global Compassionate Citizen

We acknowledge that by the acceptance and practice of the 25 Principles of Compassionate Equitation, we are on the path to becoming Compassionate Global Citizens and extending the message of The Compassionate Equestrian to the entire world.

Susan Gordon:

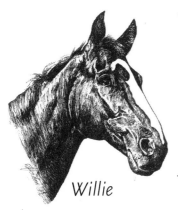

Willie

Willie did not know what nationality he was, nor did he likely care. I was amused when he responded positively when spoken to with a faux German accent, however. On the longe line, when I said "Vil-helm, gall-op!" instead of "Willie, canter!" he would raise his neck and shoulders a little higher, give an audible, "Harrumph!" and elevate into as much collection as he could muster from his old body. There was something very distinguished about him, as there is with many people who come from well-traveled, world-wise backgrounds.

The place I first fell in love with the Hanoverian breed was at Spruce Meadows, the renowned Canadian show jumping facility in Calgary. It was brand new when my beautiful Appaloosa colt was boarded there, and I drooled over the magnificent horses that were flown in from Germany in the 1970s. How I wished I could have gone on an exotic buying-trip to Europe to acquire one of them for myself.

From the people and decorum at Spruce Meadows I learned a lot about the international horse world. I believed then, as I do now, that we can all be cordial and professional when dealing with each other, regardless of nationality or ethnic origin. We, and our horses, can be outstanding global ambassadors who bring collaborative efforts to the forefront in a world that is much in need of peace and compassion.

Willie had an aura of quality and a commanding presence that I respected, and I was always happy to explain his history to people. Horses from around the world can help inspire us to become better global citizens and welcome others with compassion and understanding. We can use our interests in breeds as good reasons to travel, visiting farms, training facilities, and schools, while expanding our own knowledge and bringing the message of The Compassionate Equestrian to all. Willie would say, "Danke!"

One of the most important things I have come to understand about horses is their ability to connect with one another. If a horse on a large piece of property is in trouble, all the others seem to know it. If a horse is cast in his stall, for example, trapped up against the wall, many of his neighbors will be upset, too.

There is usually a lot of whinnying and spinning in stalls when horses "tap into" the distress of another of their species.

I find they seem to tune into an even broader range of energetic connectivity. After the tragic events in the United States on September 11, 2001, we had an unusually high number of colic cases at the Arizona barn where I was boarding Willie. We lost one wonderful mare that we'd only recently acquired. While at the veterinary clinic, we found out they had attended to a record number of colicking horses that week. It really seemed like the horses were experiencing the collective shock and stress of a nation, and a world, stunned by the horrific terror attacks.

If prolific author Rupert Sheldrake's theories of *morphic resonance* and *morphic fields* are correct, they help explain how horses could become aware of shifts in human consciousness.[1] In a 2014 interview with John Horgan in *Scientific American*, Sheldrake explained his theories thusly: "Morphic resonance is the influence of previous structures of activity on subsequent similar structures of activity organized by morphic fields. It enables memories to pass across both space and time from the past. The greater the similarity, the greater the influence of morphic resonance. What this means is that all self-organizing systems, such as molecules, crystals, cells, plants, animals, and animal societies, have a collective memory on which each individual draws and to which it contributes."

We can also begin to understand how the interplay of both compassionate and non-compassionate care and training affect the Global Herd. Imagine the horses in your healthy, joyful, compassionate barn. Now imagine a barn a town or two over that is exactly the opposite. Do you think your "happy horses" know their fellow species are not treated well a hundred miles to the west? I think they do. It is kind of like watching the news every night and feeling upset by seeing one disaster after the other. I feel horses are so sensitive to societal conditions they have their own "inner television" telling them about one stressful event after another. I believe this has contributed to a pervading sense of unwellness in much of the Global Herd—humans and horses included.

> In the November 2010 issue of Noetic Now, *Rupert Sheldrake, PhD, writes: "The easiest way to test for morphic fields directly is to work with societies of organisms. Individual animals can be separated in such a way that they cannot communicate with each other by normal sensory means. If information still travels between them, this would imply the existence of interconnections of the kind provided by morphic fields. The transfer of information through morphic fields could help provide an explanation*

for telepathy, which typically takes places between members of groups who share social or emotional bonds" (http://www.noetic.org/noetic/ issue-four-november-2010/morphic-fields-and-morphic-resonance/).

If one species is sensitive to how humans are interacting with each other and other beings, then it stands to reason that *all* animals are so aware. Therefore, if we turn our local barns into centers of Compassionate Care and Training, they will have a resonating effect on other barns, equestrian-based community developments, private facilities, and backyards, and those who work and ride in them. Because horse people are influential in many segments of society, *their* compassion can move beyond horses and affect other people in their circles of influence. These people may have nothing to do with horses, but the effects of compassion will be seen in their home and work lives. And so, perhaps soon, humanity will be in a different place altogether.

The awareness and practice of compassion in this industry has the potential to expand not only to the Global Herd of equines, but the Global Herd of humanity, as well.

In my late twenties, I was fortunate to have been led to a meditation teacher by my business partner in an advertising agency. Meditation and mindfulness practice produces fascinating and deeply personal revelations over time. The contemplative methods changed my life rather dramatically. With horses, I stayed in the "busy trainer" mindset for quite a long time after beginning meditation practice, partly out of self-defense and partly just because it takes a long time to retrain old habits and rewire imprints. However, as my practice progressed the physiological changes became more noticeable. Most profound was a feeling of *expansiveness*, for lack of a better word. In the quietness and calmness of sitting, watching the breath, comes a connection to a very large field of energy. It would manifest in waves, carrying me further and further outward in space. There was a sense of feeling very grounded and connected to the earth, too, but a much larger awareness was completely palpable.

Expanded awareness can become a part of every minute of your daily activity. It is not limited to meditation time.

As we become Compassionate Global Citizens, we also carry the responsibility of mentoring and developing a Compassionate Youth Equestrian Culture—our emerging Global Herd. Rising costs and limited access have combined with a technology-obsessed society to cause a drop-off in the numbers of young people becoming involved with horses.[2] And yet the lessons they can learn from horses are as invaluable as they always have been.

> *In April, 2014, the* Journal of the American Veterinary Medical Association *reported that "the proportion of horse owners ages 18 to 34 has declined from 24 percent in 2006 to 15 percent in 2009 to 11 percent in 2013....The same goes for the rate of participation in equine competitions, particularly at the local level" (https://www.avma.org/news/javmanews/pages/140415g.aspx?utm_content=javma-news&utm_medium=email&utm_campaign=gen).*

We also need to ensure young horse lovers are supplied with compassionately trained, healthy, well-bred horses so they stay safe, have fun, and can learn the fine skills of riding to one day pass on to another generation. Compassionate leadership means caring not only for ourselves, but also for whoever is "up next."

Dr. Allen Schoen:

The Compassionate Equestrian *approach evolved into a global approach.*

As you have learned throughout these pages, fundamentally, compassion is at the base of every choice we make for our horses. We can expand that to include ourselves, our families, our barns, our communities, society at large, and eventually, the world.

After selling a large part of my veterinary practice, I was going through a period of introspection and retrospection as a veterinarian. What would the next steps on my journey of trying to be of benefit to animals look like? I moved to British Columbia, Canada, to a small retreat island to take time out to reflect on my veterinary journey, but I would still return regularly to Connecticut to see a limited number of my old patients.

It was during this introspective time that I was introduced to the Charter for Compassion (one of our foundational concepts—see p. 7). The founder, religious historian Karen Armstrong, first introduced me to the Charter for Compassion through her award-winning TED talk. Shortly after that I was asked by a local Tibetan Lama, who had been asked by the Dalai Lama, to establish a medicinal plant garden for people and animals at a new monastery in Redding, Connecticut. At that time the monastery had a Tibetan doctor who was developing the medicine garden for people, but they did not have anyone who had training for animals. They found me because of my background and publishing history, as well as my personal journey exploring different spiritual traditions, in particular, Buddhist philosophy.

As part of this project, the Dalai Lama was working with the local university, Western Connecticut State University in Danbury, to establish a Center for Compassion, Creativity, and Innovation. As part of the creation of that center, a conference was organized and I was asked to speak on how I integrated creativity and compassion into my veterinary practice. I realized when addressing the question that this really *was* my entire journey as a veterinarian. My compassion for animals led me to always look for new approaches to help animals that couldn't be helped in any other way. I was never satisfied with the status quo.

At the Compassion, Creativity, and Innovation Conference, I stated that periods of quiet reflection, quieting the mind, and compassionate intention were the keys to interacting with animals on a deeper level. The conference spawned a book entitled *Creativity and Compassion* (Karuna Publications, 2012), to which I contributed a chapter based on my talk: "In the Quiet Space With Animals."

The Compassionate Equestrian *as a book and a movement actually evolved from requests and ideas from the Dalai Lama.*

Yes, there is now a small Tibetan medicine garden for animals at the monastery, but perhaps the greatest seed planted by that garden is this book. And, Karen Armstrong's Charter for Compassion is the root from which the 25 Principles of Compassionate Equitation sprouted. I would encourage all of you to watch her award-winning TED Talk (http://charterforcompassion.org/charter-karen-armstrong).

We have now aligned ourselves with the Charter for Compassion's Sector on the Environment as representatives of the horse world. At this moment this feels like my evolutionary contribution to developing a more expansive, compassionate field of veterinary medicine, based on a deep respect for all beings, and all that is.

"The heart is like a garden: it can grow compassion or fear, resentment or love. What seeds will you plant there?"

Jack Kornfield, Author and Co-founder of the
Insight Meditation Society

The groundwork has been laid for a new awareness and new opportunities for interacting with individual horses, as well as the Global Herd.

The integrative goal of *The Compassionate Equestrian* is to develop a unique approach to our personal heart and mind training in order for us to be more compassionate with our horses, ourselves, and every being that we interact with. We can then expand our love and connection with horses out to all animals, to our local communities, and to the global citizenry, allowing us all to be vessels of loving-kindness, assisting the world to shift to become a more loving, tolerant, humane society.

We have the ability to create this kind of connection based on the latest advances in quantum physics, consciousness studies, and new biology, while using technology to help deliver the information. As you try to understand and integrate the various fields we've referenced, as we strive to create the interdisciplinary field of Compassionate Equitation, you must sometimes go beyond the current limits of conventional study. As a conventionally trained veterinarian, ideally, I may look for the "gold standard" of double-blind, placebo trials to document all studies, and in an ideal world, I would love to see this be the case for all research. But these days, such studies cost a vast fortune to conduct. Only well-funded companies can afford to support them. Much has changed since I was trained at Cornell University in 1978. There has been a drastic cut in independent funding of research that is free of potential conflicts of interest. Universities have to rely more and more on corporate funding and support versus governmental support, which then may create additional conflicts of interest.

More and more research is funded by the companies that have an inherent interest in financial benefits related to the outcome of the study.

I have come to appreciate that there are many things that people cannot comprehend based on the current understandings of physics and biology. Science is a continuing evolution of discovery. The challenge is, sometimes people can fall into the "religion of scientism," feeling that all that exists is only what can be proven by double-blind, placebo-controlled trials. Such is the continued dubious circle of conflict of interest that has evolved. (Although I like to argue that life did exist before double-blind, placebo-controlled studies.) In the textbook that I co-edited, *Complementary and Alternative Veterinary Medicine* (1998), there is an excellent chapter on the foundations of evidence-based medicine, written by a brilliant veterinary epidemiologist, Dr. Brenda Bonnet from the University of Guelph, in Guelph, Ontario, Canada. This reviewed the many levels of evidence-based medicine and the merits and challenges of each. It must be noted that evidence-based medicine also benefits from collections of clinical case studies and individual anecdotal case presentations. Science continues to develop new theories and insights, and evolve beyond current belief systems.

I have come to appreciate the multi-dimensional layers of existence that Albert Einstein, Rupert Sheldrake, Amit Goswami and other scientists have proposed, and how they may be involved in human-animal interactions.

All horsepeople are animal communicators at some level. If when you ride, you talk to you horse, touching him, patting him on his neck, all that is a form of animal communication. There are courses in animal behavior, equine behavior, and nonverbal communication. Any horse trainer or veterinarian routinely communicates with horses at some level, as well.

Still, some individuals go further and sense that they can communicate telepathically with horses and other animals. Skeptics say that this is impossible and a scam. Some of the foundation for the controversial field of animal telepathy or animal communication (also sometimes known for individuals who call themselves "animal psychics") may also be based on quantum physics. Over the years, I have evolved from being quite a skeptic, myself, to being more open-minded due to an

8 HABITS OF TRULY COMPASSIONATE PEOPLE

In June 2014, Lyndsay Holmes published the following list in her article "8 Ways to Tell If You Are a Truly Compassionate Person" on The Huffington Post:

1   You find commonalities with other people

2   You don't put emphasis on money

3   You act on your empathy

4   You're kind to yourself

5   You teach others

6   You're mindful

7   You have high emotional intelligence

8   You express gratitude

accumulation of anecdotal evidence that is difficult to dispute. Individuals identifying themselves as "animal communicators" span a broad spectrum. I have seen a wide range, including well-intentioned, yet naïve individuals who take a weekend course on "animal communication or telepathy" and then advertise themselves as such. I am also aware of less-than-scrupulous individuals looking to charge huge sums of money and take advantage of distraught animal owners. However, I have also witnessed some extremely gifted, unique animal communicators who were able to share significant, validated facts with people about their animals that could only be reasonably explained through quantum physics and the quantum field theory.

I know some animal communicators personally and am quite impressed with their unique abilities. Respected teachers all base their explanations of how they communicate with animals on quantum physics. Yet others seem to defy the logic of linear scientific study. I have observed some results that cannot be explained based on that level of scientific understanding. I acknowledge that because we cannot understand something based on our current scientific knowledge base does not mean it does not exist or work. We can balance our awareness and scientific skepticism between being open-minded, yet looking for scientific validity and scrutiny.

THE ANIMAL COMMUNICATOR

Despite what some skeptical veterinarians might say, I must admit to seeing results from certain animal communicators that really validate the benefits when properly done. One documentary that may really open your mind and ask questions is called *Animal Communicator* (directed by Craig Foster, 2012). You can watch it at the website www.cultureunplugged.com or order the full documentary at www.animalspirit.org.

I feel that as our understanding of this deeper connection unfolds, based on advances in quantum physics, consciousness, and new biology, we are offered fascinating potential for our relationships with all animals and accelerating our creation of a more Compassionate Universe. I recognize that some may believe I am stepping out on a limb here, yet when I discuss the creation of a new animal health paradigm based on integrating quantum physics and neurobiology, I have been pleasantly surprised by the number of veterinary colleagues who have also come to appreciate this concept through their own personal journeys. I believe more veterinarians are recognizing that there is validity to some of these concepts and are open to integrating them into a more expansive animal health-care field, while still using discretion and discernment.

Recently there has been much discussion in veterinary medicine concerning the One Health Approach, which we learned about in chapter 4 (p. 97), combining human medicine, epidemiology, public health, and environmental health.

I was speaking at a major veterinary conference in New Zealand in 2013. The Dean of a US veterinary school lectured on the topic of the One Health approach, and I listened carefully, enthusiastically agreeing with much that was said. Yet, as I listened, there was a distinct overall tone of severe pessimism concerning the state of the world, the environment, anthropogenic climate disruption, and other One Health challenges the world is confronting.

Every proposed solution focused on what needed to happen to the *outside* world and how *outside* situations needed to change, despite the ever-continuing decrease in funding for needed studies and research, as well as the political and business choices that were often the antithesis of what was needed. I pondered this, and the entire concept as it was presented, and felt that perhaps one of the key solutions was not being addressed: our *inner* world, our hearts and minds, our thoughts and emotions, awareness and consciousness, and the impact *that* has on all the *outer* decisions. All the choices being made throughout the world appear to be more and more based on a foundation of transnational corporate greed. But each corporation is still made up of individuals, who at their deepest level may not realize what their cumulative corporate choices mean for the destruction of our environment and the world as we currently know it. Or else some may sadly be in complete denial and just focused on personal short-term financial remuneration with little consideration of rapidly occurring global consequences.

I realized that perhaps the key solution to One Health is to make compassion for all beings *the foundation for all choices made, rather than momentary demands of government and business.*

It is only through a change of consciousness and awareness based on compassionate choices that we can really create the fundamental paradigm shift that is required for a One Health model that incorporates the health of all humans, all animals, and the environment, to work. Most efforts of this ilk seem to be, like the proverbial saying, just "moving furniture around on the Titanic." We feel that expanding on *The Compassionate Equestrian* model to truly become Global Citizens can change the course of things. We cordially invite you to join us and become the change we wish to be.

One of my favorite quotes by one of my favorite human beings, Albert Einstein, summarizes this entire vision beautifully:

> *A human being is part of a whole, called by us the "Universe," a part limited in time and space. He experiences himself, his thoughts and feelings, as something separated from the rest—a kind of optical delusion of his consciousness. This delusion is a kind of prison for us, restricting us to our personal desires and to affection for a few persons nearest us. Our task must be to free ourselves from this prison by widening our circles of compassion to embrace all living creatures and the whole of nature in its beauty.*

Questions to Consider

BASED ON PRINCIPLE 24

1   How do I see myself becoming a Global Citizen based on *The Compassionate Equestrian* model?

2   Do I believe in interspecies communication?

3   How would the One Health Approach be of benefit to me? My family? The world?

4   If there is one choice or action that I could do right now to expand *The Compassionate Equestrian* model to becoming a pathway to Compassionate Global Citizen, what would it be?

CHAPTER TWENTY-FIVE

Forgiveness

We acknowledge that forgiveness is a key to healing emotional and psychological wounds, and pain and suffering within ourselves. We recognize the importance of forgiving ourselves as well as forgiving all others— horses and humans—as a foundation for improving health and happiness. We commit to working on forgiveness within ourselves for the benefit of all beings.

Susan Gordon:

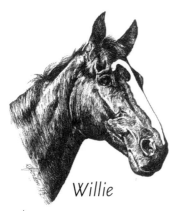

Willie

An important teaching from the Alateen program I was sent to as my mother began alcohol recovery was the lesson of forgiveness. Following the "a day at a time" mantra was invaluable for healing and for learning to forgive others. All too often I observed other family members and friends retain bitterness and unresolved grief, creating circumstances that appeared to eat away at their souls and well-being. Recalling lessons I learned amongst other children of alcoholics, and later, from the Al-Anon Program, for friends and spouses of those with addictions, I have always tried to make forgiveness a priority in my life. Letting go of anger and forgiving others opens the door for an ever-evolving sense of peace and tranquility.

I held no ill will toward the people who had allowed Willie to end up as he did, only gratitude that I could care for him as long as I was able. I was grateful for his adopters when he had to leave my hands as well. As with many other horses that came by my way, I apologized to Willie for the things I could not provide him, and asked his forgiveness for others who had not treated him with the gentleness and tolerance he needed.

Some people might think it is a little silly to talk to horses with such empathic dialogue, but even if they do not understand specifically what we are saying, I believe they can sense the intention behind our words. This is why they may respond less than favorably if the intention behind your words is not authentic. I have had horses alter their behavior simply by offering an apology and asking for forgiveness, either for my own actions or for those of other riders who had worked with the horse previously.

I could make myself crazy thinking about all the times my decisions could have taken a different direction, not only with Willie, but with many other horses. We professional trainers make our living through horses. We know that offering an opinion contrary to a client's, or insisting a horse receive a veterinary workup when he does not appear lame (to the client), or scratching from a class when the horse "isn't quite right," can cost us income-producing business. It all depends on the reasons behind the choices we make. Looking back, although I am very grateful for having apprenticed with other trainers—who were conscientious and highly skilled horsepeople—if I could do it all over again I would adopt a very specific business model based on what we have written within *The Compassionate Equestrian*. These guidelines wouldn't make the choices easier, but they would help ensure the right choices are made for a particular horse in a particular space and time, and encourage a kind, understanding camaraderie amongst everyone at the barn.

"Consider the possibility, and I am only saying consider the possibility, that maybe nothing is unforgivable. Maybe there is a way to find forgiveness even for what we have believed for so long to be unforgivable. Explore this mindfully."

Allan Lokos, "Lighten Your Load,"
Tricycle Magazine (Winter 2010)

EXERCISE IN COMPASSION

Breathe In, Breathe Out

In *Glimpse After Glimpse* (HarperOne,1995), Sogyal Rinpoche offers this simple exercise:

1   Imagine vividly a situation where you have acted badly, one about which you feel guilty, that makes you wince even to think of it.

2   Breathe in. As you do, accept total responsibility for your actions in that particular situation, without in any way trying to justify your behavior. Acknowledge exactly what you have done wrong and wholeheartedly ask for forgiveness.

3   Breathe out. As you do, send out reconciliation, forgiveness, healing, and understanding.

Continue to breathe in blame, and breathe out the undoing of harm; breathe in responsibility, breathe out healing, forgiveness, and reconciliation.

In *Nonviolent Communication* (Puddledancer Press, 2003), Marshall B. Rosenberg, PhD, writes, "Self-judgments, like all judgments, are tragic expressions of unmet needs." In other words, if our self-dialogue is critical, judgmental, and blaming, we are telling ourselves that we are not acting in harmony with *our* own needs. If we apply the critique to others, we are actually saying that *they* are not in harmony with *our* needs. Until we learn to connect with the feelings behind those needs we so want to be satisfied, and empathize with others and ourselves, the prospect of enriching our lives with the ability to forgive remains obscured by a state of self-punishment. A healthier approach is to evaluate ourselves moment by moment in a way that inspires positive change in the direction in which we would like to go, and originates with respect and compassion for ourselves, rather than coming from shame, guilt, or disdain for self. Then we can extend a forgiving hand to all, and find ourselves at "home," in the center of our heart (see p. 346).

The beauty you see around you, including that of your horse, is a direct reflection of the beauty inside you.

Dr. Allen Schoen:

As we worked to complete the 25 Principles of Compassionate Equitation, and as I reviewed them, I realized that *forgiveness* is one of the most important words to emerge. We have only briefly mentioned the subject in the book up to this point, however. Forgiveness is especially key to self-compassion, as we may find it difficult to offer compassion to others if at times our internal dialogue toward ourselves lacks gentleness and tolerance.

The Principles acknowledge that forgiveness is one of the greatest healers, if not the most important. Reflect back on times you would either have liked to ask for forgiveness or perhaps would like to have been moved to forgive another. You are invited now to forgive the horse(s) and human(s), including yourself, that you have not yet found it in your heart to pardon. A forgiving heart is a healing heart.

We probably can all think of moments when we might have done something or said something or acted in some way to someone in a horse barn or to our horses that perhaps we have some remorse about and wish we had done it differently, with more diplomacy and respect. As I reflect back in my life as an equine veterinarian, memories rush through my neural net: horses, trainers, grooms, riders, farriers, veterinarians, employees, family members, and countless others where I would love to just take a moment and apologize. I wish I had been more polite, more positive, made a little more effort, and gone the extra mile. I can also envision situations where I would have liked to offer the option of forgiveness to many of the horsepeople I worked with. I am sure they also had remorse or regrets about the way things may have ended up for various horses; I'm sure they wished they could have made some things turn out differently. No one is perfect. If we are coming from a compassionate, heartfelt, well-meaning place inside, then we are all simply human beings doing the best we can, most of the time.

Self-forgiveness is also a beneficial exercise. I am aware that I am my own worst critic and tend to always be harsher on myself than perhaps I deserve. I chuckle sometimes and have selected a label as a Reluctant Type A Workaholic: passionate about all that I do, yet often pushing myself beyond reasonable limits, and I end up paying for that in countless ways. I can beat myself up and too often ask the questions, "Why can't I work 60-80-100-hour work weeks for decades?" "Why am I so exhausted after weeks on end of 12-hours-or-longer daily work schedules?" "What is wrong with me?" "Why can't I keep on going at that same pace?"

Yes, the voice goes on and on, unless I acknowledge it compassionately and choose to love and care for myself better. One of the latest books that found its way to my hands is *The Joy of Burnout* by Dr. Dina Glouberman (Skyros Books, 2007). It sounds like an oxymoron to me, but it actually has some great thoughts to share on self-compassion. Since my inner self-critic can be one very loud voice, I find that I need to turn it into a more compassionate self-talk. I acknowledge that I really always try to do my best.

I need to forgive myself.

Self-forgiveness is an essential element of compassion for all beings. It is beneficial to forgive all those who are truly doing the best they can within the circumstances they are in.

As we all know, there are some individuals in the horse world who actually may not have all the best intentions for others at certain times, nor the best interests of the horse in mind. They may not be the most scrupulous characters and may be out for themselves rather than anyone else. Their actions may be based on greed or fear. For those individuals, I can actually find it more challenging to forgive. That is part of my journey: learning to forgive those who do not have the best intentions toward horses. It truly saddens my heart when money comes before the welfare of the horse, when greed rules when it does not have to, and at those times I still need to find compassion and forgiveness in my heart.

This is an excellent opportunity for me to use the beautiful method of atonement Ho'oponopono, which we shared on p. 128: "I am sorry, please forgive me, I love you, and I thank you."

Diablo was a nine-year-old-off-the-track Thoroughbred that I was asked to see as a fifth veterinary opinion. He had actually injured one veterinarian, scared away two others, and almost killed the fourth.

The trainer "kind of" warned me of Diablo's behaviors and said he was just a really mean horse, and he did not know what else to do for him before they sent him to the slaughterhouse, as that would have been his likely fate. Someone mentioned that I should have a look and perhaps I could suggest a positive step toward a better outcome.

As soon as I approached Diablo, I could see his ears go back, his eyes squint, and he snorted and moved nervously as his body tightened up. Then he began to lift his right hind leg, aiming to kick me. I did all the nonverbal, loving, compassionate communication I could. I slowly approached him, allowed him to sniff me, and I gently rubbed his neck. He tightened up even more, and I could see him aiming and still swinging that right hind to kick me. I performed the acupuncture point palpation exam as much as I was able. As soon as I reached his right hind over his sacroiliac region, he could no longer restrain himself. Diablo tried to strike me as viciously as possible, missing me by inches, clearly stating, "Don't go there!" I was able to get close enough to perform a bit more thorough examination, and I suggested he go for a bone scan of the right sacroiliac region as I was suspicious of a possible old fracture from the racetrack in the right S-I joint. Few other injuries might cause that much chronic and severe pain in that area. I have seen many off-the-track Thoroughbreds with varying degrees of right sacroiliac injuries from strains, to ligamentous tears, to fractures due to racing too young and always going in the same direction. The trainer and owner refused to heed my advice.

Fortunately, I knew the next rider who ended up with Diablo, and upon my recommendation, she agreed to take the horse to New Bolton Equine Center at the University of Pennsylvania Veterinary School. On the bone scan they did find an old injury to the right sacroiliac joint and through careful sedation, they were able to inject it. The horse's personality instantly changed and he was not nearly as dangerous. Now manageable, Diablo flourished under his new rider's loving, careful attention. The rider was able to rehabilitate the horse and bring him back to being rideable, and even nice most of the time. I rechecked the horse after the sacroiliac injection and was able to do a complete exam without

Forgiveness Exploration

In her book *It's Time, No One's Coming to Save You* (Devarani Publications, 2004), Mary Goldenson, PhD, describes this exercise in forgiveness:

1   Let your body relax, breathe into your heart, and let yourself feel the walls of pressure you are carrying around.

2   Feel the pain that keeps your heart closed that is caused by not forgiving someone or not forgiving yourself.

3   Let yourself feel the ways you have been hurt or how you hurt others, betrayed them, or caused them suffering, knowingly or unknowingly, out of fear, anger, or confusion. Remember and visualize these people and/or horses and feel the sorrow and regret.

4   One by one, picture each memory of hurt that still burdens your heart and say: "I ask for your forgiveness; I ask for your forgiveness."

him trying to kill me. He had been in such pain before that all he could do was defend himself in any way possible. I chuckled and suggested that she change his name to something more fitting for his new, improved personality, and that Diablo was perhaps not appropriate anymore.

I treated the horse with acupuncture and chiropractic care every few months and was able to maintain him pain-free for over a year. After that time, he started to become more defensive around that S-I joint again, so I suggested the owner have her veterinarian or New Bolton Center re-inject the joint. They did so, and he was able to continue work for another year or more. Periodically he would need the S-I joint injected. They eventually moved out of my practice area and I lost touch with them. I hope the former Diablo was able to live a long and happy life, pain-free and with proper maintenance.

I am so grateful to the rider who made the commitment to help Diablo. I am grateful to the veterinarians at New Bolton who were able to evaluate him, diagnose the problem, and treat him appropriately. I forgave Diablo for injuring the other veterinarians and trying to kill me. I found that I also needed to forgive the prior owner and trainer in my heart, for just saying the horse was a mean horse and beating on him instead of truly trying to find and solve the cause of his behavior. In addition, I had to forgive countless others for passing the horse along because he is "mean" without trying to find out what was wrong with him.

I needed to forgive all those involved in the racing industry who do not consider such injuries and try to prevent them. From what I can see in the horses I treat, I believe that right-side sacroiliac injuries are common in off-the-track Thoroughbreds and cause a tremendous amount of pain in many of them. It is not normally part of a differential diagnosis for veterinarians who are not familiar with such injuries in racehorses. I would like to see this condition mentioned more in the veterinary literature in regard to Thoroughbreds that have raced. This is but one example of where I really feel for the horse.

In the horse world, so many people are in such a rush and so preoccupied they often are not able to give a particular horse the attention he needs.

We see this kind of neglect from human caretakers more often than we might like to admit. I try to forgive all of them. Ideally, I would like to see a world where everyone is able to slow down somewhat, be a bit more mindful of each situation and a tad more compassionate with each other. Occasionally and sadly, people are looking for someone else to blame, which can lead to aggressive accusations, as well as litigation. But when there is no conscious malfeasance, and there isn't fear of harm being done to others, discussions, mediation, forgiveness, and understanding might be a more compassionate approach.

Ideally, it might be of great benefit if we each look inside our own hearts and explore whom we might wish to forgive or ask forgiveness from. We may actually be doing our greatest good for ourselves by releasing long-held destructive emotions. Resentment and bitterness may be hurting us more than we know. When it comes to that particular horse—the one we look back on and think that perhaps we could have helped him more—we need to forgive ourselves, learn from the lesson, and hope that what you learned can benefit some other horse or person in the future.

"To not forgive would be unforgivable."

Swami Beyondananda

Questions to Consider
BASED ON PRINCIPLE 25

1   Is there a horse from my past that I wish I could have done something more for? Can I forgive myself, learn from the situation, and strive to help some other horse in the future?

2   Is there a horse I can help more now, based on forgiveness and on this Principle?

3   Is there someone in the barn or who works with my horse who I would like to ask for forgiveness? Do I feel remorse about something I said or did or that I could have done better?

4   Is there someone I would like to forgive in the barn or related to my horses' care?

5   What more can I learn about forgiveness for myself? For others?

Where Will Your Journey Take You?

Practical Steps to Becoming a Compassionate Equestrian

In the process of writing *The Compassionate Equestrian* it became apparent that the long journey to the end is really a journey home to our heart. A radiant heart and mind can expand, as the daily practice of compassion becomes a part of your life. Perhaps these Principles have been the first 25 steps in your personal quest of becoming a Compassionate Equestrian. May each step you choose to take support a transformation of your relationship with your horses and everyone around you.

When the heart glows with compassion, others take notice. They may not be able to see the stream of energy emanating from a compassionate individual, but they may certainly feel it. Your love for others can be based on what is best *for* them, not what you want *from* them. Imagine if all human relationships were based on loving-kindness and not the perception of love that derives from desire and unhealthy attachment. Imagine if you loved your horse and had compassion for him based on what is best *for* him and not what you want *from* him. You might have fallen in love with the way he looks, how he moves, his bloodlines, or the training he has. But as it is with human relationships, that is a likely basis for disappointment. The more we base our love on our own wants and superficial desires, the easier our hearts will be broken when those attributes are not met or our horses do not live up to our idealized images of them.

> "Only a life lived for others is a life worthwhile."
>
> ### Albert Einstein

In some cases, it may turn out to be that the best thing for your horse is to have someone else become his caretaker. Compassion may mean letting go. We learn that, in life, everything is temporary. With compassion, we can let go of our attachments to outcomes, as well.

As you continue to grow on your journey to becoming a more compassionate being, your influence can expand to others who may wish for the same calm, peaceful nature you exude. They may not have begun the journey themselves but will observe the benefits of your mindfulness and caring for others, and then realize they want to be that way too. Be patient with those who are new to a transformative path, as human nature is based on desires, attachments, and personal filters. Some may be envious of your compassionate nature, unaware that they too, can transform and live a more balanced, peaceful life. They, like most, just want to be heard and feel loved. Through it all, you can learn how to manage your own personal boundaries and also have compassion for yourself. This is *your* opportunity to teach, with compassion, that each individual can work toward his or her own path and that everyone has the opportunity to develop an awakened heart and mind.

Bound by the common aspect of an equestrian-based lifestyle, horses present a vehicle for the horseperson to communicate and demonstrate everything that has been taught in this book—from 10 minutes of mindful meditation and breathing (QFI), to the understanding of how horses' behavior problems may be related to pain, compassion truly is a source of energy and strength. The practice can keep us calm and peaceful when others around us may not be. It opens doors and offers an opportunity to expand our hearts and minds by becoming more aware of the suffering of other living beings, and how much we are all alike. It becomes the basis for our actions in the world, and in the world of horses, compassion is needed so very much.

As the Dalai Lama says, "If you want to be happy, practice compassion. If you want others to be happy, practice compassion."

BUILDING COMPASSIONATE
EQUESTRIAN COMMUNITIES

We can see how abiding by the 25 Principles of Compassionate Equitation can be easily enacted in private barns and small-farm scenarios. But how to change the tide in larger facilities, where horses, riders, and trainers come and go on a regular basis?

You can start by posting the Principles in a prominent place: in the lounge, tack room, or on the notice board in the main aisle. Once a barn manager, trainer, or a group of riders at a facility take the Pledge (see p. 408) and commit to following the Principles, they can apply to receive a plaque signifying a Compassionate Barn, and which tells all: "We abide by the Principles of Compassionate Equitation."

Perhaps somewhere in the boarding agreement it could state, "This is a Compassionate Barn, and we do our best to abide by the Principles of Compassionate Equitation." Nobody can do it all the time—it is just that we all need to do the best we can. Such a clause would introduce newcomers to expectations in terms of behavior and communication. It can be an incredibly great tool for barns to create a more Compassionate Equestrian Community.

We presently know indivduals who consciously choose to run their barns in the most compassionate way they are able and only accept boarders who are in compliance. The 25 Principles as we've written them have not been out there for reference and guidance, but some of the barns have learned how to be discerning after years of dealing with difficult, angry clients, and they have said, "No, we only want people who abide by our barn's policies." Part of the purpose of the Principles is to help people acknowledge their ability to be selective about their clientele and begin creating boarding and training contracts that list Compassionate Policies as a fundamental aspect of the industry.

Mapping the Journey

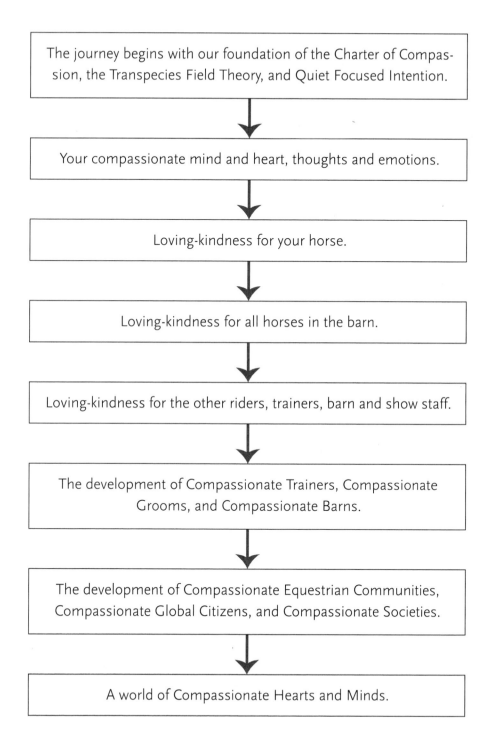

The journey begins with our foundation of the Charter of Compassion, the Transpecies Field Theory, and Quiet Focused Intention.

Your compassionate mind and heart, thoughts and emotions.

Loving-kindness for your horse.

Loving-kindness for all horses in the barn.

Loving-kindness for the other riders, trainers, barn and show staff.

The development of Compassionate Trainers, Compassionate Grooms, and Compassionate Barns.

The development of Compassionate Equestrian Communities, Compassionate Global Citizens, and Compassionate Societies.

A world of Compassionate Hearts and Minds.

One of the first steps on the journey to spreading *The Compassionate Equestrian* approach is to just start being a compassionate horseperson yourself. As Gandhi said, "Be the change that you wish to see in the world." Plant the seeds wherever you go by setting an example. Leave brochures and pamphlets on the 25 Principles of Compassionate Equitation at the barns and shows you attend. Say to others, "This may be something you'll find interesting if you want a better relationship with your horse, a different experience riding, and a more fulfilling barn atmosphere."

In spiritual teachings they say to give 100 percent effort with 0 percent attachment to the outcome.

Plant these seeds without attachments. When you try to demand people change their ways, they will resist—that's what Mother Theresa would say. People asked her how she could work day after day with lepers and people who were dying, and she replied that you do not become attached to the outcome, you just "do it." Following the Principles may be a very difficult thing for some people to do. It may not even be possible for some. I do believe it *is* possible for most, though, and if we do not work, seed by seed, little by little, on creating a new world for horses and their humans, it will never happen.

The Compassionate Equestrian Call to Action: What You Can Do Next

1   Revisit the 10-minute QFI exercise on p. 46 and make it a part of your daily pre-barn ritual.

2   Listen to the Compassionate Equestrian CD meditations regularly (go to www.drschoen.com for more information).

3   Take the Pledge to become a Compassionate Equestrian committed to the Global Herd (see p. 408).

4   Visit *thecompassionateequestrian.com* and apply for an official plaque, declaring your barn "A Compassionate Barn" that abides by the 25 Principles of Compassionate Equitation.

5   Post the 25 Principles of Compassionate Equitation in your barn and invite others to discuss the Principles and what they mean to the facility and to all you do with horses.

6   Write a Compassionate Boarding Clause and a Life-Cycle Management Policy for your barn or facility.

7   Find The Compassionate Equestrian on Facebook and follow The Compassionate Equestrian blog at www.thecompassionateequestrian.net. Weigh in with your own experiences and thoughts and participate in the discussion there regarding the subjects of horses, kindness, tolerance, and forgiveness.

8   Send us short video clips and photos showing how you are being compassionate in your horse life and how this book has influenced your interactions with your horse, your riding friends, and others in the equestrian industry (see our websites for contact information).

9   Ask us about connecting The Compassionate Equestrian to your organization, rescue, or blog.

10   Request to have a ribbon or trophy awarded to the Most Compassionate Equestrian at horse shows and events in which you participate.

11   Participate in or organize retreats or workshops that explore deeper perspectives on the human-animal bond as a vehicle for creating a more harmonious, compassionate world. Dr. Schoen periodically offers retreats or can be scheduled to speak to your group or organization. Contact him or sign up to be on his mailing list at www.drschoen.com.

12   Be the change you want to be.

"We are all connected. When you touch one thing, you are touching everything. Whatever we do has an effect on others. Therefore, we must learn to live mindfully to touch the peace inside each of us. Peace in the world starts with peace in oneself. If everyone lives mindfully, everyone will be healthier, feel more fulfilled in their daily lives and there will be more peace. This collective mindfulness can bring positive change to our families, organizations, communities, nations and future generations."

Thich Nhat Hanh, Poet and Peace Activist

Conclusion

Susan Gordon:

The journey goes by all too quickly. Mine begins with a little girl begging her mom to take her to the park so she can ride a pony, then one day she is saying a final goodbye to her mom, and then eventually a farewell to her last horse.

Spiritual teachings help us understand our connection to life, the impermanence and illusions, and that which makes us suffer. Practicing compassion brings us to a greater awareness of ourselves, and how our interactions with others affect all beings.

The path is about the memories we make, and our relationships with others. It doesn't matter if the memories are happy or sad—they are just simply "there." We can look at them for what they are, without attachment, but with a grateful and loving heart. That is our story, each one an individual, with all of its synchronicities, disappointments, high points, and low. We can embrace ourselves, our horses, and everyone around us, whether physically, or just with a smile and kind words, and understand that in doing so, we can add even a little bit of brightness to somebody else's day, and our own as well.

If you feel as though you might not have understood all the concepts in this book, that's okay. Go back and reread parts, and more thoughts will arise as you add your voice to those seeking a Compassionate World. We felt from the beginning that having two very different voices from the horse world would help broaden the message of compassion across generations and demographics, yet demonstrate common ground in our insights and suggestions, which always seek out the kindest path for our horses.

Willie represents the story of tens-of-thousands of horses worldwide that are in need of caring homes. From burned-out, to backyard, to show barns, to retirement, my life and his interwove in a series of events that can only be described as one, big, transformational adventure. Sometimes we slip, but we learn that when we are tolerant, kind, and empathic toward others, desiring to help where we can, all that loving-kindness is reflected back to us.

In the words of one of my favorite songs by the Moody Blues, "All the love you've been giving, has all been meant for you."

Dr. Allen Schoen:

As we finish this trail ride together—this "safari" as I called it at the beginning of the book—I am grateful that I have been able to follow my heart's desire and ponder the question that has been my life's overriding theme, "What is Ultimate Healing?" My sometimes bumpy ride began with being an idealistic animal lover, getting into the saddle by becoming a holistic, integrative veterinarian, searching for ways to help the hopeless animals, piercing through the bramble that blocked the path sometimes, and exploring trails less traveled by pioneering new approaches. It was a challenging ride, with stormy weather, fog, and blizzards sometimes obscuring the path, allowing only the very next step to be seen and taken in that moment. Sometimes when it seemed like I took a "wrong" turn, blinded by the storms, I later realized that the detours were part of the journey, as well. When I felt I was lost, all I could do was follow the next step, trusting that that was the way home.

For me, at this moment, as I get out of my well-worn saddle, the current answers to my quest for Ultimate Healing are leaving me with a focus on feelings of gratitude, forgiveness, loving-kindness, and compassion for all that is. The horse can be a vehicle for an awakening within us, and one step toward helping the world.

I hope you have enjoyed the ride and found it of some benefit to your own journey. Keep in touch, as it is only the beginning of the ride of your life. As Roy Rogers and Dale Evans—the cowboy and cowgirl of an earlier, slower-paced time—used to sing, "Happy trails to you, until we meet again."

Go forth and do good. May you be of benefit to all that is!

The Pledge of the Compassionate Equestrian

I have read the 25 Principles of Compassionate Equitation and agree to abide by the Principles to the best of my abilities.

As a Compassionate Equestrian, I commit to making compassion the foundation for all decisions regarding my horse, people with whom I interact in the equine community, and all others with whom I interact on a daily basis.

By choosing the most compassionate thoughts and actions, equestrians as a Global Herd can become a movement for creating a kinder, happier, healthier, more compassionate world.

Bibliography

Alberta SPCA. "How Stress Affects a Horse's General Health." 2013. Alberta SPCA CTS Animal Courses. 2014 <http://www.ctsanimals.ca/va3070/resources/toKnow/pdfEquine30_3-1.pdf>.

American Veterinary Medical Association. One Health Initiative. 18 July 2008. *Journal of the American Veterinary Medical Association (JAVMA)*. 2015 <http://www.onehealthinitiative.com/taskForce.php>.

Animal Spirit. "The Animal Communicator." Animalspirit.org. 2014 <www.animalspirit.org>.

Animal Welfare Science Hub. Animal Welfare Hub. February 2015 <http://animalwelfarehub.com/>.

ARIA. American Riding Instructors Association. 2014 <https://www.riding-instructor.com/>.

Armon R, Fisher A, Goldfarb B, Milton C. "Effects of music tempos on blood pressure, heart rate, and skin conductance after physical exertion." 3 November 2012. Ebookbrowse. University of Wisconsin — Madison. 2014 <http://ebookbrowsee.net/effects-of-music-tempos-on-blood-pressure-heart-rate-and-skin-conductance-after-physical-exertion-pdf-d412786566>.

Armstrong, Karen. "Charter for Compassion." 2009. Charter for Compassion. 2014 <http://charterforcompassion.org/>.

Audubon Lifestyles. Equestrian Facilities/Sustainable Equestrian Facility Program. 14 September 2012. The Dodson Group, LLC. 2014 <http://www.audubonlifestyles.org/domains/to%20be%20deleted/test/certification-programs/for-equestrian-facilities >.

Behzadi F, Hamzei M, Nori S, Salehian MH. "The Relationship between Goal Orientation and Competitive Anxiety in Individual and Team Athletes Fields." Annals of Biological Research 2 (6) (2011): 261-268.

Benson-Henry Institute for Mind-Body Medicine. About the Benson-Henry Institute for Mind-Body Medicine. 2015 <http://www.massgeneral.org/bhi/>.

BHS. British Horse Society - Home. February 2015 <http://www.bhs.org.uk/>.

Blue Cross For Pets. Looking after your horse. 2014 <http://www.bluecross.org.uk/2146-2820/safety-around-horses.html>.

British Equestrian Federation. BEF Brochure. 2010. 2014 <http://www.bef.co.uk/repository/downloads/BEF/BEF_Brochure_2010.pdf>.

Canadian Environmental Law Association. Collections/Pollution/Precautionary Principle. 2014 < http://www.cela.ca/collections/pollution/precautionary-principle >.

Canadian Horse Defence Coalition. Canada's $80 Million Horse Slaughter Industry—Statistics and Analysis—What You Can Do. 13 February 2015. 1 March 2015 <https://canadianhorsedefencecoalition.wordpress.com/2015/02/13/canadas-80-million-horse-slaughter-industry-statistics-and-analysis-what-you-can-do/>.

Carman JA, Vlieger HR, Ver Steeg LJ, Sneller VE, Robinson GW, Clinch-Jones CA, Haynes JI & Edwards JW. "A long-term toxicology study on pigs fed a combined genetically modified (GM) soy and GM maize diet." Journal of Organic Systems 8.1 (2013): 38-54.

Carpenter, Siri. "That gut feeling." *Monitor on Psychology* 48.8 (2012): 50.

Center for Investigating Healthy Minds at the Waisman Center. 2013. The Board of Regents of the University of Wisconsin System. 2014 <http://www.investigatinghealthyminds.org/>.

Certified Horsemanship Association. Certified Horsemanship Association - Certified Riding Instructors. 2014 <http://cha-ahse.org/>.

College of Syntonic Optometry. What is Syntonics? February 2015 <http://www.collegeofsyntonicoptometry.com/home.html>.

Compassion Fatigue Awareness Project. Suffering from Compassion Fatigue? Life Stress? 2013. 2014 < http://www.compassionfatigue.org/pages/selftest.html >.

Consumer Lab. Reviews/Ginseng Supplements. 3 March 2014. 2014 <https://www.consumerlab.com/reviews/ginseng_supplements/ginseng/ >.

Corp-Minamiji, Christy. Across the Fence/Under the Blue Tarps. 22 January 2013. Blood-Horse Publications. 2014 <http://cs.thehorse.com/blogs/across-the-fence/archive/2013/01/22/under-the-blue-tarps.aspx >.

Dalla Costa E, Minero M, Lebelt D, Stucke D, Canali E, et al. (2014). "Development of the Horse Grimace Scale (HGS) as a Pain Assessment Tool in Horses Undergoing Routine Castration." PLoS ONE 9.(3) (2014): e92281.

Davidson, Richard. Meng Wu Lecture: Richard Davidson, PhD. 2 October 2012. 2014 <http://ccare.stanford.edu/videos/meng-wu-lecture-richard-davidson-ph-d/>.

Davis, Lloyd W. "Interpersonal Neurobiology." PSYC-8226-3 Biopsychology Debra Wilson, PhD. Prod. Walden University. http://www.pdflibrary.org/pdf/interpersonal-neurobiology-lloyd-w-davis.html, February 2009.

Doheny, Kathleen. "Depression Health Center/Pets for Depression and Health." 2012. WebMD. 2014 <http://www.webmd.com/depression/features/pets-depression >.

Dossey, Larry. A Conversation About the Future of Medicine. 2014 <http://www.dosseydossey.com/larry/QnA.html >.

Dunn, Jancee. "Huffpost Healthy LIving: Everything You Need to Know About Meditation." 1 April 2014. Huffinton Post. <http://www.huffingtonpost.com/2014/04/01/meditation-facts-need-to-know_n_5062845.html>.

Dusek JA, Benson H. "Mind-Body Medicine: A Model of the Comparative Clinical Impact of the Acute Stress and Relaxation Responses." Minn Med. 92.5 (2009): 47-50.

Egenvall, A, et al. "Days-lost to training and competition in relation to workload in 263 elite show-jumping horses in four European countries (Abstract)." Prev Vet Med 112(3-4) (2013): 387-400.

Equine Canada. About Coaching. 2014 <http://www.equinecanada.ca/index.php?option=com_content&view=section&id=126&Itemid=743&lang=en.>.

—. "Equine Life-cycle Management Policy." 2013. EquineCanada.ca. 2014 <http://equinecanada.ca/index.php?option=com_docman&task=doc_view&gid=6457&Itemid=88&lang=en >.

Equine Guelph. Healthy Lands for Healthy Horses. University of Guelph. 2014 <http://www.equineguelph.ca/healthylands.php >.

Equine Performance Institute. FAQs/Stomach Ulcers/Equine Gastric Ulcer Syndrome (EGUS). n.d. 2014 <http://www.equinepi.com/faq/ulcers.html>.

Esch, Tobias and George B. Stefano. "Medical Science Monitor/The Neurobiological Link Between Compassion and Love." 1 March 2011. National Center for Biotechnology Information. 2014 <http://www.ncbi.nlm.nih.gov/pmc/articles/PMC3524717/>.

Esfahani Smith, Emily. Masters of Love. 12 June 2014. June 2014 <http://www.theatlantic.com/health/archive/2014/06/happily—ever—after/372573/ >.

ETH Zurich. "Hereditary trauma: Inheritance of traumas and how they may be mediated." 13 April 2014. ScienceDaily. <http://www.sciencedaily.com/releases/2014/04/140413135953.htm#.UozMllGFOZY.email >.

Fédération Equestre Internationale (FEI). FEI Clean Sport/Welfare. 2010-2012. Lausanne Fédération Equestre Internationale. 2014 <http://www.feicleansport.org/welfare.html >.

FEI. FEI Sustainability Handbook. 2014. 2014 <http://www.fei.org/system/files/FEI_Sustainability_Handbook_for_Event_Organisers.pdf>.

Ferguson CE, Kleinman HG, Browning J. "Effect of Lavender Aromatherapy on Acute-Stressed Horses (Abstract)." Journal of Equine Veterinary Science 33.1 (2013): 67-69.

Ferraro GL, Stover SM, Whitcomb MB. Suspensory Ligament Injuries in Horses. brochure. University of California, Davis. Davis: Center for Equine Health, 1999.

Frazier, Matt. How a Plant-Based Diet Can Make You Fitter, Faster and Happier. 2014 < http://www.nomeatathlete.com/about/ >.

Gangadean, AK. Awakening Global Consciousness: Why it is Vital for Cultural Sustainability. 2004. Awakening Productions. 2014 <http://prelude.awakeningmind.org/pages/agcarticle.php>.

Genetic Roulette: The Gamble of our Lives. Dir. Jeffrey M Smith. Perf. Narrator Lisa Oz. The Institute for Responsible Technology. http://geneticroulettemovie.com/, 2012.

Genetic Science Learning Center. Epigenetics. 2015. Univertsity of Utah. 28 February 2015 <http://learn.genetics.utah.edu/content/epigenetics/ >.

German Equestrian Federation (FN). < http://www.pferd-aktuell.de/biologischevielfalt >.

—. Deutsche Reiterliche Vereinigung. February 2015 <http://www.pferd-aktuell.de/>.

Glouberman, Dina. The Joy of Burnout: How Burning Out Unlocks the Way to a Better, Brighter Future. 3 Rev . Skyros Books, 2007.

Goldenson, Mary. IT'S TIME: No One's Coming to Save You. Devarani Publications, 2004.

Gregoire, Carolyn. "What Neuroscience Can Teach Us About Compassion." 13 May 2014. Huff Post The Third Metric. Huffington Post. 2014 <source: http://www.huffingtonpost.com/2014/05/13/what-neuroscience-can- tea_n_5268853. html?utm_hp_ref=mostpopular >.

Gyatso, Tenzin, Dalai Lama XIV and Howard Cutler. *The Art of Happiness: A Handbook for Living.* Vol. 10th Anniversary Edition. New York: Riverhead Publishing, 2009.

Hanson, Rick. "Relaxed and Contented: Activating the Parasympathetic Wing of Your Nervous System." 2007. Wise-brain.org. 2014 <http://www.wisebrain.org/ParasympatheticNS.pdf >.

—. Sounds True Presents The Compassionate Brain. Sounds True Inc. 2014 <http://live.soundstrue.com/ compassionatebrain/>.

Higgins, Gillian. "Horses Inside Out: Understanding How Your Horse Works Improves Performance." Horses Inside Out. Horses Inside Out Ltd. 2014 <http://www.horsesinsideout.com>.

HIPPOH. Horse Industry Professionals Protecting Our Horses. 2014 <http://www.hippohfoundation.org/>.

Holland, JL. "The Danger of Mycotoxins." 19 May 2014. *TheHorse: Your Guide to Equine Health Care.* 2014 <http://www. thehorse.com/articles/33898/the-danger-of-mycotoxins?utm_source=Newsletter&utm_medium=nutrition&utm_ campaign=05-19-2014 >.

Horse-Canada. Horse-Canada Archives/The Secrets of Equine Body Language. Horse-Canada.com. 2014 <http://www. horse-canada.com/archives/the-secrets-of-equine-body-language/>.

Horses Healing Hearts. Welcome to our site! 2014 <http://www.horseshealingheartsusa.com/ >.

Hoyle, Julie. How to Come Home to Yourself. Lori Deschene. 2014 <http://tinybuddha.com/blog/ how-to-come-home-to-yourself/>.

Humane Society of the United States. The Facts about Horse Slaughter. 17 March 2014. 2014 <http://www.humanesoci-ety.org/issues/horse_slaughter/facts/facts_horse_slaughter.html >.

Indo Asian News Service. Be in horses' company to ease Alzheimer's symptoms. 6 May 2014. June 2014 <https:// in.news.yahoo.com/horses-company-ease-alzheimers-symptoms-090403393.html>.

Institute of HeartMath®. Expanding Heart Connections. 2014 <http://www.heartmath.org/ >.

Institute of HeartMath. Articles of the Heart. 8 October 2012. <http://www.heartmath.org/free-services/articles-of-the-heart/energetic-heart-is-unfolding.html>.

Institute of Noetic Sciences. "IONS Overview." Noetic.org. 2014 <http://noetic.org/about/overview/>.

Integrative Medicine for the Underserved. Mindfulness-Based Patient Handouts. IM4US.org. 2014 <http://im4us.org/ Mindfulness-Based+Patient+Handouts>.

Internatioinal Alliance for Animal Therapy and Healing. Feeding Naturally. 2014 <http://www.iaath.com/feedingnaturally. htm >.

International Association for Veterinary Rehabilitation and Physical Therapy. 2014 <http://www.iavrpt.org>.

Johnson, Sterling C, et al. "Neural Correlates of Self-Reflection." *Brain* 125.8 (2002): 1808-1814.

Journal American Veterinary Medical Association. "Study: Young horse owners dwindling." 2 April 2014. avma.org. 2014 <https://www.avma.org/news/javmanews/pages/140415g. aspx?utm_content=javma-news&utm_medium=email&utm_campaign=gen>.

Just Food. What is CSA? 2014 <www.justfood.org/csa>.

Kane, E. "Vitamin E is essential equine nutrient." 1 May 2004. Veterinary News.DVM 360. *DVM360 Magazine.* 2014 <http://veterinarynews.dvm360.com/vitamin-e-essential-equine-nutrient>.

Kane, Ed. "Filling the nutrition gap: A veterinary order for supplemented stored forages." 31 May 2014. Veterinary News. DVM360. *DVM360 Magazine.* 2014 <http://veterinarynews.dvm360.com/filling-nutrition-gap-veterinary-order-sup-plemented-stored-forages >.

Kentucky Equine Research Staff. "Barn Beat: What Music Style is Best for Horses." 13 May 2013. Equinews: Kentucky Equine Research Nutrition and Health Daily. 2014 <http://www.equinews.com/article/barn-beat-what-music-style-best-horses >.

Ladwig, Jill. "Brain Can Be Trained in Compassion, study shows." 22 May 2013. University of Wisconsin-Madison News. 2014 <http://www.news.wisc.edu/21811>.

LeDoux, Joseph E. "Amygdala." 3 February 2008. Scholarpedia.org. 2014 <http://www.scholarpedia.org/article/ Amygdala>.

Lesimple C, Hausberger M. "How accurate are we at assessing others' well-being? The example of welfare assessment in horses (Abstract)." Frontiers in Psychology 5.21 (2014).

Lesté-Lasserre, Christa. "Study: Post Training Stress Detrimental to Equine Learning." June 20 2013. TheHorse.com. Blood-Horse Publications. 2014 <http://www.thehorse.com/articles/32080/ study-post-training-stress-detrimental-to-equine-learning#ixzz2zv9EidsG>.

Liberman, J. *Light: Medicine of the Future*. Santa Fe: Bear & Company, 1990.

Lipton, Bruce H. *The Biology of Belief*. 13. Hay House, 2011.

Lokos, Allan. "Lighten Your Load." *Tricycle Magazine* 2010.

MacLeod, Clare. Lessons from human sports nutrition. 11 September 2013. 2014 <https://www.pegasushealth.com/blog/lessons-from-human-sports-nutrition/ >.

Mandal, Ananya. What is the Hypothalamus? 28 October 2012. 2014 <http://www.news-medical.net/health/What-is-the-Hypothalamus.aspx >.

Martino, Joe. Mind Over Matter: Princeton & Russian Scientist Reveal the Secrets of Human Aura & Intentions. 10 September 2013. 2014 <http://consciouslifenews.com/mind-matter-princeton-russian-scientist-reveal-secrets-human-aura-intentions/1164859/# >.

McDonough W, Braungart M. *Cradle to Cradle: Remaking the Way We Make Things*. New York: North Point Press, 2002.

McDonough, William. Cradle to Cradle®. LLC MBDC. 1 March 2015 <http://www.mcdonough.com/cradle-to-cradle/#.VPNhMrPF9gA>.

McGreevy, Paul D. "The advent of equitation science." 2007. International Society for Equitation Science. 2015 <http://www.equitationscience.com/documents/Equitation/McGreevy_EquitationScience.pdf>.

McKenzie, E. Exercise Physiology: Are Horses Like Humans & Other Species? June 2013. Blood-Horse Publications. 2014 <http://www.thehorse.com/videos/31915/exercise-physiology-are-horses-like-humans-other-species?utm_source=Newsletter&utm_medium=welfare--industry&utm_campaign=06--27--2013>.

Meadows, C. Taking Charge of Your Health & Wellbeing/Explore Healing Practices/Shiatsu. <http://www.takingcharge.csh.umn.edu/explore-healing-practices/shiatsu >.

Meszoly, Joanne. Pasture Puncture Wounds from *EQUUS* magazine. 8 January 2004. Equine Network. 2014 <http://www.equisearch.com/article/puncture010804>.

Mitchell, Marilyn. "Dr. Herbert Benson's Relaxation Response." 29 March 2013. *Psychology Today*. Psychology Today. 2014 <https://www.psychologytoday.com/blog/heart-and-soul-healing/201303/dr-herbert-benson-s-relaxation-response>.

Morris, Eric. "From Horse Power to Horsepower." Access (Accessmagazine.org) 2007.

Muller-Paisner V, Bradshaw GA. "Freud and the Family Horse: Exploration into Equine Psychotherapy." *Spring: A Journal of Archetype and Culture* Spring.83 (2010): 213-237.

Multi Radiance Medical. Multi Radiance Medical/Veterinary/MR4 Activet. 2014 <- http://www.multiradiance.com/veterinary/mr4activet>.

Murdoch, Wendy. Soft Eyes Get You Where You Want to Go. 3 January 2013. 2014 <http://www.murdochmethod.com/soft-eyes-get-you-where-you-want-to-go/ >.

My Horse Daily. 2015. Cruz Bay Publishing Inc. 2014 <http://myhorse.com/redirects/muscle-pain-form-lameness-limits-movement-horses/>.

National Equine Welfare Council. The Equine Welfare Compendium. 24 October 2011. 2015 <http://www.newc.co.uk/highlights/new-welfare-compedium-launched/>.

National Farm Animal Care Council. Codes of Practice. 2013. 2015 <https://www.nfacc.ca/codes-of-practice/equine>.

National Forage Testing Association. The National Forage Testing Association/Welcome. January 2015 <www.foragetesting.org>.

National Institute for the Clinical Application of Behavioral Medicine. NICABM-Home. 2014 <http://www.nicabm.com/>.

National Institute of Mental Health. How Might New Neurons Buffer Against Stress? 18 July 2014. 2015 <http://www.nimh.nih.gov/news/science-news/2014/how-might-new-neurons-buffer-against-stress.shtml>.

NCMHD Center of Excellence for Nutritional Genomics. Information. 2012. 2014 <http://nutrigenomics.ucdavis.edu/?page=information>.

New Stride Thoroughbred Adoption Society. New Stride - Home. 2014 <http://newstride.com/ >.

Ontario Ministry of Agriculture, Food and Rural Affairs. Nutrient Management Strategies and Horse Barns. Ed. P. Doris - Environmental Specialist/OMAFRA. July 2010. 2014 <http://www.omafra.gov.on.ca/english/engineer/facts/10-057.htm >.

Ortner, Nick. The Tapping Solution. February 2015 <http://www.thetappingsolution.com/>.

Osborn, Liz. How Much Weight Can a Horse Carry? 2008-2015. Current Results Nexus. 2014 <http://www.horsescience-news.com/horseback-riding/how-much-weight-can-a-horse-carry.php>.

P, Torricelli, et al. "Regenerative medicine for the treatment of musculoskeletal overuse injuries in competition horses." *International Orthopaedics* 35.10 (2011): 1569-1576.

Papes F, Logan DW, Stowers L. "The vomeronasal organ mediates interspecies defensive behaviors through detection of protein pheromone homologs." *Cell* 14.4 (2010): 692-703.

Patronek GJ, Loar L, Nathanson, JN. "Animal Hoarding: Structuring interdisciplinary responses to help people, animals and communities at risk." 2006. vet.tufts.edu. <http://vet.tufts.edu/hoarding/pubs/AngellReport.pdf>.

PCUK. The Pony Club - Home. February 2015 <http://www.pcuk.org/>.

Pert, Candace. Where Do You Store Your Emotions? 2014 <http://candacepert.com/where-do-you-store-your-emotions/>.

Podhajsky, Alois. *My Horses, My Teachers.* reprint edition, April 1 1997. Trafalgar Square Books, 1997.

Powell, Debra M, et al. "Evaluation of Indicators of Weight-Carrying Ability of Light Riding Horses." *Journal of Equine Veterinary Science* 28.1 (2008): 28-33.

Psychology Today. Oxytocin. 2014 <http://www.psychologytoday.com/basics/oxytocin >.

Reinisch, Amanda I. "Understanding the Human Aspects of Animal Hoarding." *The Canadian Veterinary Journal* 49.12 (2008): 1211-1214.

Reuter, Coree. "Fix It With Feed Part 4: Prevent Ulcers By Mimicking Nature." 9 February 2011. *The Chronicle of the Horse.* 2014 <http://www.chronofhorse.com/article/fix-it-feed-part-4-prevent-ulcers-mimicking-nature >.

Rinpoche, Sogyal. *Glimpse After Glimpse, Daily Reflections on Living and Dying.* Ed. Patrick D. Gaffney. HarperOne, 1995.

Rosenberg, Marshall B. *Nonviolent Communication: A Language of Life: Life Changing Tools for Healthy Relationships.* Second. Enciinitas: Puddledancer Press, 2003.

Salam, Ranabir and K. Reetu. "Indian Journal of Endocrinology and Metabolism." Jan-Mar 2011. National Center for Biotechnology Information. 2014 <http://www.ncbi.nlm.nih.gov/pmc/articles/PMC3079864/>.

Saving Horses, Inc. PMU/Nurse Mare Foal Rescue. 2014 <http://www.savinghorsesinc.com/PMU_Nurse_Mare_Foal_Rescue.php >.

Schafer KS, Kegley SE. "Persistent toxic chemicals in the US food supply." *Journal of Epidemiology & Community Health* 56.11 (2002): 813-817.

Schoen, A. "In the Quiet Space With Animals." Briggs, J. Creativity and Compassion, How They Come Together. Ed. J Briggs. Wayne: Karuna Publications, 2012. 179-186.

Schoen, Allen M. "Animal Massage: The Touch That Heals." Dr. Schoen . <http://www.drschoen.com/animal-massage-the-touch-that-heals/>.

—. Lyme Disease: Fact from Fiction. 2015 <http://www.drschoen.com/lyme-disease-fact-from-fiction/>.

Schoen, AM. "Fear Response and Generalization Similar Transpecies." 11 May 2011. Dr. Schoen.com. 2014 <http://kindredspiritsproject.com/?p=1066 >.

—. *Veterinary Acupuncture: Ancient Art to Modern Medicine.* St. Louis: Mosby/Elsevier, 2001.

—. What is Integrative Holistic Animal Health Care? 2014 <http://www.drschoen.com/what-is-integrative-holistic-animal-health-care/>.

Schoen, AM, Wynn SG. *Complementary and Alternative Veterinary Medicine: Principles and Practice.* St. Louis: Mosby, 1998.

Sheldrake R, Smart P. "A Dog That Seems To Know When His Owner is Coming Home: Videotaped Experiments and Observations." *Journal of Scientific Exploration* 14 (2000): 233-255.

Sheldrake, Rupert. "Morphic Fields and Morphic Resonance." November 2010. Institute of Noetic Sciences. 2014 <http://www.noetic.org/noetic/issue-four-november-2010/morphic-fields-and-morphic-resonance/ >.

Siegel, Daniel J. "About Interpersonal Neurobiology." 2010. Dr. Dan Siegel. 2014 <http://www.drdansiegel.com/about/interpersonal_neurobiology/>.

—. Mindsight: *The New Science of Personal Transformation.* New York: Bantam, r 2010.

Singer, Michael. *The Untethered Soul; A Journey Beyond Yourself.* Oakland: New Harbiner Publications, 2007.

Skelly, C. "Resources/Did you know? Common Toxins in Equine Feedstuffs." November 2010. My Horse University.

Michigan State University. 2014 <http://www.myhorseuniversity.com/resources/eTips/November_2010/Didyouknow>.

Southlands Farms. Farm Camps and Program. 2014 <http://www.southlandsfarms.com/seasoned-farmers-youth-practicum.html>.

Spector, Lisa and Joshua Leeds. Through a Dog's Ear, Music to Calm Your Canine Companion, Volume 1. 1 March 2008. 2014 <http://www.soundstrue.com/shop/Through-a-Dog's-Ear/581.pd >.

Staff, Mayo Clinic. Healthy Lifestyle Stress Management. 11 July 2013. 2014 <http://www.mayoclinic.org/healthy-living/stress-management/in-depth/stress/art-20046037>.

Stixrud, William and Christopher Clark. Transcendental Meditation/Childhood and Adolescent Disorders. Maharishi

Foundation USA. 2014 <http://www.tm.org/benefits-childhood-and-adolescent-disorders>.

Stone, Kathlyn. Over-the-Counter Medicine/Top selling OTC Drugs by Category, 2012. About.com. 2014 <http://pharma. about.com/od/Over-the-Counter-Medicine/a/Top-selling-Otc-Drugs-By-Category-2012.htm >.

Surya Das, Lama. *The Big Questions: How to Find Your Own Answers to Life's Essential Mysteries.* Rodale Books, 2007.

Thal, Doug. Home - HSVG. 2014. 2014 <http://horsesidevetguide.com/ >.

The Canadian Horse Defence Coalition. Horse Protection Initiatives. 2014 <http://184-69-125-162.cv.gv.shawcable.net/ chdc/ber/horse-protection-initiatives.html>.

The Future of Food. By Deborah Koons Garcia. Dir. Deborah Koons Garcia. Perf. Narrator Sara Maamouri. Prod. Deborah Koons Garcia. http://www.thefutureoffood.com/About.html, 2004.

The Greater Good Science Center. Greater Good/Compassion/What is Compassion? 2015 <http://greatergood.berkeley. edu/topic/compassion/definition>.

Thompson, Jeffrey D. Sound—Medicine for the New Millennium. 2007. 2014 <http://www.neuroacoustic.com/newmil. html >.

Tulku, Tarthang. *Knowledge of Freedom: Time to Change.* Cazadero: Dharma Publishing, 1984.

UMass Medical School Department of Medicine, Division of Preventive and Behavioral Medicine. Center for Mindfulness in Medicine, Health Care, and Society. 2014 <http://www.umassmed.edu/cfm/index.aspx >.

University of Kentucky College of Agriculture, Food, and Environment. "UK Ag News - Pioneering Research: Collaborating With Horses to Develop Emotional Intelligence." 21 June 2013. University of Kentucky. 2014 <http://news.ca.uky. edu/article/pioneering-research-collaborating-horses-develop-emotional-intelligence >.

Unwanted Horse Coalition. "Rehabilitating the Neglected Horse: A Caregivers' Guide." Unwantedhorsecoalition.org. 2014 <http://www.unwantedhorsecoalition.org/resources/rehab_brochure.pdf >.

—. Welcome. 2014 <www.unwantedhorsecoalition.org>.

USDF. United States Dressage Federation. 2014. <http://www.usdf.org/>.

Vitale, Joe and Ihaleakala Hew Len. *Zero Limits: The Secret Hawaiian System for Health, Wealth, Peace and More.* Wiley, 2008.

von Borstel, Uta Ulrike, et al. "Impact of riding in a coercively obtained Rollkur posture on welfare and fear of performance horses." *Applied Animal Behavior* Science 116 (2009): 228-236.

Walmsley, Liz. "Diagnosing and managing muscle tears in horses." Docstoc. 2014 <http://www.docstoc.com/ docs/10575670/Muscle-Tears>.

Weng HY, Fox AS, Shackman AJ, Stodola DE, Caldwell JZK, Olson MC, Rogers GM, Davidson RJ. "Compassion training alters altruism and neural responses to suffering." *Psychological Science* (final edited form) PMC 2013 Oct. 1 (author manuscript) 24.(7) (2013): 1171-1180.

Wikipedia: The Free Encyclopedia. Limbs of the Horse. August 2014. Wikimedia Foundation, Inc. 2014 <http://en.wikipedia.org/wiki/Limbs_of_the_horse>.

—. Physical medicine and rehabilitation. 3 February 2015. 28 February 2015 <http://en.wikipedia.org/wiki/Physical_medicine_and_rehabilitation >.

Wilson, E.O. *Biophilia.* Cambridge: Harvard University Press, 1986.

Winerman, Lea. "The Mind's Mirror." *American Psychological Association Monitor.* 9. Vol. 36. Print. Washington: American Psychological Association, October 2005.

World Anti-Doping Agency. WADA-Home. 2014 <www.wada-ama.org>.

World Commission on the Ethics of Scientific Knowledge and Technology (COMEST). "The Precautionary Principle." 2005.

UNESDOC.UNESCO.org. Scientific and Cultural Organization United Nations Educational. 2014 <http://unesdoc. unesco.org/images/0013/001395/139578e.pdf >.

World Horse Welfare. Home. 2014 <www.worldhorsewelfare.org>.

—. International Work. 2014 <http://www.worldhorsewelfare.org/International-Work >.

Yung-Jong Shiah, Dean Radin. "Metaphysics of the Tea Ceremony: A Randomized Trial Investigating the Roles of Intention and Belief on Mood While Drinking Tea." Explore 9.6 (2013): 355-360.

Zak, Paul. "Dogs (and Cats) Can Love." 22 April 2014. *The Atlantic.* 2014

<http://www.theatlantic.com/health/archive/2014/04/does-your-dog-or-cat-actually-love-you/360784/ >.

Acknowledgments

Susan Gordon:

Thank you to every horse that came my way over the past 45 years. Each one had lessons to teach me. Most have likely passed away by now, and I pray they all had humane completions to their lives.

I am also thankful for all the people who have come into my life, horse-related or otherwise. Especially my first instructor, the late senior show judge and technical delegate, Margaret Ellard and her Warmblood schoolmaster, Grouch, who provided the very best in rider education. In support of this book, I am eternally grateful to my co-author, Dr. Allen Schoen, Tim and Vicki Moore who provided my extraordinary "writer's retreat," Phyllis Wakelyn for her patient listening and counseling, Sara Ratner and her special horse Nick (the white Arabian gelding was responsible for my meeting Dr. Schoen), and the excellent trainers I have known, including the late Michael Patrick (1973 ASPCA Maclay Champion), David Greening, Patricia Ripenburg (née Deptford), Tim Tomkinson, and Bee Gordon (not related)—who gave me the chance to teach and ride as a professional. To Dorie and Ulrich Schmitz for being so accommodating and creating a barn where education and compassion flourishes. Thank you Mrs. Margaret Southern—a bigger influence in my life than she would ever know—and especially all my clients and their horses, without whom many of these stories would not have been possible. Catherin McLellan, and my other spiritual guides, thank you for appearing in the right time and place to introduce me to meditation and energy healing. Thank you to everyone who embarks on this journey for helping us make this a more compassionate world for horses and their people.

To Mom and Dad—thank you for allowing me the freedom to make my own decisions, left turns, right turns, or unusual changes of direction...and no, I never did "grow out" of horses. We'll meet again someday.

To my brother, Ronald Gordon, PhD, thank you for the lessons and patient discussions in neuroscience, sports psychology, and critical thinking.

Dr. Allen Schoen:

I am grateful for all my teachers, two-legged, four-legged, and winged, for all they have taught me through their own journeys. I am grateful to my parents for honoring my need to follow the beat of a different drummer. I am grateful to my sister and all my family who have supported my growth as a holistic veterinarian. I am also grateful to each horse and each and every animal that has taught me so much about animal healing through their own journeys.

I wish to acknowledge all my great teachers throughout college, veterinary school, and my postgraduate training in the various complementary medical modalities that I have studied and incorporated into my approaches to healing.

I am grateful to my various spiritual teachers who have shown me that there is more to life and more to healing than meets the eye. They have opened my windows of perception to the beauty of the interconnectedness of all that is. I am grateful to all these teachers including the Dalai Lama, Amma, Baba Hari Das, Rabbi Shlomo Carlbach, Mother Theresa, and countless others. I am thankful to Garchen Rinpoche, one of my most cherished teachers. I am also grateful to so many Buddhist Rinpoches, Lamas, Taoist guides, and other spiritual guides for sharing their wisdom and insights with the world. It is through their teachings that I have come to realize the importance of a compassionate heart and mind in healing animals, and through them, the world.

I also wish to profusely thank Rebecca Didier, Martha Cook, and Caroline Robbins of Trafalgar Square Books for their foresight, wisdom, clarity, guidance, and bountiful support of our vision to create a more compassionate equestrian community and world. I personally thank Rebecca Didier for her amazing, awesome, wise, clear, compassionate, and insightful guidance as truly one of the best editors I have ever worked with in my career. It has been a true joy creating this book together with her. I feel like I am blessed with a new friend as well as a superb editor!

I wish to acknowledge all of you who have chosen to read this book and join us on this safari ride, trailblazing a new path of healing for all! Thank you!

Index